Serological Cancer Markers

Contemporary Biomedicine

Serological Cancer Markers
Edited by ***Stewart Sell***, 1992
The Red Cell Membrane
Edited by ***B. U. Raess and Godfrey Tunnicliff***, 1990
Handbook of the Hemopoietic Microenvironment
Edited by ***Mehdi Tavassoli,*** 1989
Leukolysins and Cancer
Edited by ***Janet H. Ransom and John R. Ortaldo***, 1988
Methods of Hybridoma Formation
Edited by ***Arie H. Bartal and Yashar Hirshaut***, 1987
Monoclonal Antibodies in Cancer
Edited by ***Stewart Sell and Ralph A. Reisfeld***, 1985
Calcium and Contractility: *Smooth Muscle*
Edited by ***A. K. Grover and E. E. Daniel***, 1984
Carcinogenesis and Mutagenesis Testing
Edited by ***J. F. Douglas***, 1984
The Human Teratomas: *Experimental and Clinical Biology*
Edited by ***Ivan Damjanov, Barbara B. Knowles, and Davor Solter***, 1983
Human Cancer Markers
Edited by ***Stewart Sell and Britta Wahren***, 1982
Cancer Markers: *Diagnostic and Developmental Significance*
Edited by ***Stewart Sell***, 1980

Serological Cancer Markers

Edited by

Stewart Sell

Department of Pathology and Laboratory Medicine,
University of Texas Health Science Center, Houston, TX

Humana Press **Totowa, New Jersey**

999 Riverview Drive
Totowa, New Jersey 07512

Printed in the United States of America

Library of Congress Cataloging in Publication Data

Serological cancer markers / edited by Stewart Sell.
p. cm. -- (Contemporary biomedicine)
Includes index.
ISBN 0-89603-209-4
1. Tumor markers. I. Sell, Stewart, 1935- . II. Series.
[DNLM: 1. Neoplasms--diagnosis. 2. Tumor markers, Biological.
QZ 241 S486]
RC270.3.T84S47 1992
616.99'20756--dc20
DNLM/DLC
for Library of Congress 92-1428
CIP

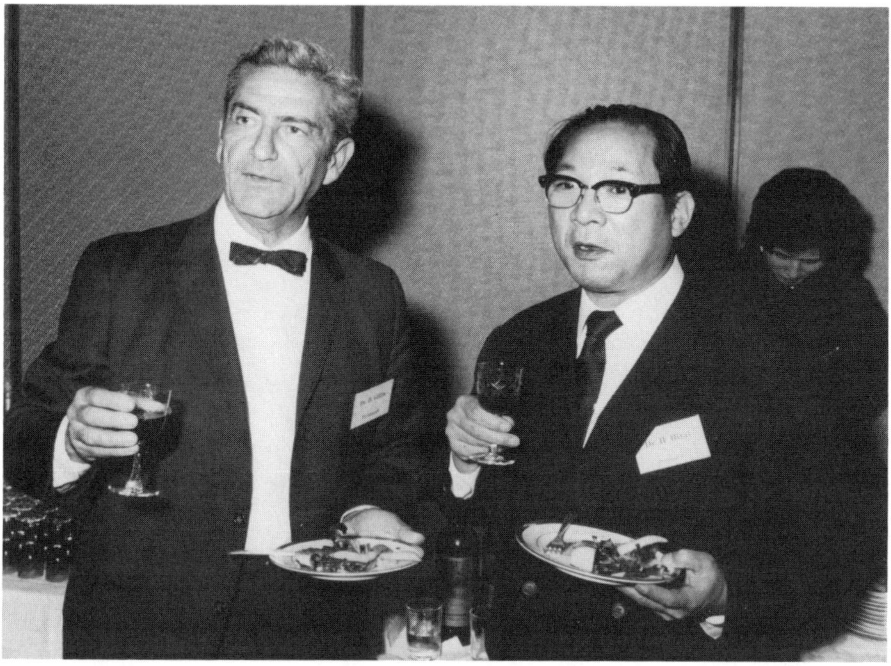

Dedication

To Professor David Gitlin of the USA and Professor Hidematsu Hirai of Japan, seen here at the Third Meeting of the International Society for Oncodevelopmental Biology and Medicine in Tokyo, Japan, 1974. Their early work on alpha-fetoprotein, discovered by Garri I. Abelev of the Soviet Union, set the example for the rest of us.

Preface

The purpose of this book—the fourth volume of a series on Cancer Markers—is intended to provide an updated "status report" on today's use of cancer markers in the diagnosis and monitoring of cancer, with an emphasis on cancer markers detected in the serum. It has been 7 years since the publication of the last volume in this series. The 1980, 1982, and 1985 volumes covered the development of cancer markers, not only in their roles of unraveling the basic biology of cancer, but also as increasingly important players in the management of patients with cancer. During the last 7 years we have seen the application of a number of markers identified by monoclonal antibodies, as well as the beginnings of the use of genetic markers defined by molecular probes. Measurements of oncogenes in tissues or cells promise many applications for the future, but as yet, these genes have not shown to be useful as serum markers of cancer.

The commercial interest in serum markers for cancer, particularly for the diagnosis and monitoring of tumor patients, is indicated in Chapter 24 by Owen, where the total worldwide market for cancer markers is projected to increase from $148 million in 1988 to $232 million in 1993. The degree of research interest in cancer markers is reflected in the fact that in 1988 a separate category for tumor markers was added to *Index Medicus*. The number of publications in this category since 1988 is as follows: 608 in 1988, 858 in 1989, and 803 in 1990.

The major focus of the present book is on the "new" cancer markers detected by monoclonal antibodies. Since our 1985 survey, extensive application of the use of cancer marker assays in the blood for the diagnosis, monitoring of therapy, prediction of recurrence, and determination of prognosis has been carried out. Markers detected in the blood by monoclonal antibody-based tests generally include: carbohydrate epitopes (CA 19-9, CA-50, TAG-72, and CA-242); mucin epitopes (CA 15-3, CA-125, DU-Pan 2, and MCA); and cytoplasmic proteins (SCC and TPA). The data so far indicate that the carbohydrate markers are about equivalent to CEA for colorectal cancer, but somewhat better for pancreatic–biliary cancer. The mucin marker CA

15-3 is slightly better than CEA for detecting metastatic breast cancer, whereas MCA is about the same as CEA. SCC is elevated in patients with metastatic epithelial cancers, and this as well as all markers has its greatest value in monitoring the effect of treatment in patients with elevated levels caused by malignancy. The present status of these markers is described in detail in separate chapters, and the reader is encouraged to refer to the designated article for whichever marker is of interest.

The use of all markers for screening high-risk populations for cancer has been disappointing. The most successful has been alphafetoprotein (AFP), along with myeloma paraprotein, the best serum marker for cancer. In recent studies, particularly in American Eskimos, AFP determinations have been used to detect liver cancer in asymptomatic patients, which has led to marked improvement in survival rates following surgical removal of smaller tumors.

It may be predicted that the use of the reagents developed to measure cancer markers will have an even greater impact on therapy than on the diagnosis of cancer. Monoclonal antibodies are being used to direct drugs or isotopes as "magic bullets," to detect clandestine lesions by specific direction of radioisotopes and immunescintigraphy, or to remove epitope-bearing cancer cells from cell populations, such as bone marrow cells, that can then be used for retransplantation into the patient. Certainly, it may be predicted that the next few years will see even more applications of cancer markers identified by monoclonal antibodies than have been seen in the preceding 7 years.

The author would like to thank the leaders of the two major international organizations for the annual meetings on cancer markers, particularly Professor Hidematsu Hirai of the International Society for Oncodevelopmental Biology and Medicine (ISOBM) and Professor Janis Klavins of the International Academy for Tumor Marker Oncology (IATMO). Their continued enthusiasm has provided outstanding leadership and an invaluable forum for work in this field. I would also like to acknowledge discussions with Dr. J. Hilgers, which provided some stimulating insights and thoughtful ideas for organization.

Stewart Sell

Contents

Contributors

GARRI I. ABELEV • *Laboratory of Immunochemistry, Cancer Research Center of the USSR, Academy of Medical Sciences, Moscow, USSR*

DORIS BALINSKY • *National Cancer Institute, National Institutes of Health, Bethesda, MD*

EMILIO BOMBARDIERI • *Nuclear Medicine Department, National Cancer Institute, Milano, Italy*

DAVID COLCHER • *Laboratory of Tumor Immunology and Biology, National Cancer Institute, National Institutes of Health, Bethesda, MD*

T. MING CHU • *Diagnostic Immunology Research and Biochemistry Department, Roswell Park Memorial Institute, New York State Department of Health, Buffalo, NY*

ABRAHAM FUKS • *Department of Medicine and Oncology, McGill University, Montreal, Canada*

MASSIMO GION • *Centre for Study of Biological Markers of Malignancy, Division of Radiotherapy, General Regional Hospital, Venezia, Italy*

GENNADI V. GLINSKY • *Cancer Research Center, Columbia, MO*

PHIL GOLD • *Professor of Medicine and Physiology, McGill University and The Montreal General Hospital, Montreal, Canada*

JOHN W. GREINER • *Laboratory of Tumor Immunology and Biology, National Cancer Institute, National Institutes of Health, Bethesda, MD*

CAJ HAGLUND • *Fourth Department of Surgery, Helsinki University General Hospital, Helsinki, Finland*

SEN-ITIROH HAKOMORI • *The Biomembrane Institute and University of Washington, Seattle, WA*

PATRICIA HORAN HAND • *Laboratory of Tumor Immunology and Biology, National Cancer Institute, National Institutes of Health, Bethesda, MD*

DANIEL F. HAYES • *Laboratory of Clinical Pharmacology, Dana-Farber Cancer Institute, Harvard Medical School, Boston, MA*

JOHN HILKENS • *Division of Tumor Biology, The Netherlands Cancer Institute, Amsterdam, The Netherlands*

MICHAEL A. HOLLINGSWORTH • *Department of Microbiology and Immunology, Duke University Medical Center, Durham, NC*

HANNU JALANKO • *Department of Bacteriology and Immunology, University of Helsinki, Helsinki, Finland*

ELEONORA R. KARAMOVA • *Laboratory of Immunochemistry, Cancer Research Center of the USSR, Academy of Medical Sciences, Moscow, USSR*

HIROSHI KATO • *Department of Obstetrics and Gynecology, Yamaguchi University School of Medicine, Ube, Japan*

J. V. KLAVINS • *International Academy of Tumor Marker Oncology, Department of Pathology, Catholic Medical Center of Brooklyn and Queens, Inc., Jamaica, NY*

DONALD W. KUFE • *Laboratory of Clinical Pharmacology, Dana-Farber Cancer Institute, Harvard Medical School, Boston, MA*

MASAHIDE KUROKI • *First Department of Biochemistry, Fukuokaniversity, School of Medicine, Fukuoka, Japan*

PENTTI KUUSELA • *Department of Bacteriology and Immunology, University of Helsinki, Helsinki, Finland*

ROLF LAMERZ • *Medical Department, University of Munich, Munchen, Germany*

QIAN LIU • *Landeshauptstadt Stuttgart, Katharinehospital, Institute fur Klinische Chemie and Laboratoriumsmedizin, Stuttgart, Germany*

MANFRED L. LÜTHGENS • *Landeshauptstadt Stuttgart, Katharinehospital, Institute fur Klinische Chemie and Laboratoriumsmedizin, Stuttgart, Germany*

SHAHLA MASOOD • *Department of Pathology, University of Florida Health Science Center, Jacksonville, FL*

RICHARD S. METZGAR • *Department of Microbiology and Immunology, Duke University Medical Center, Durham, NC*

DIANE E. MILENIC • *Laboratory of Tumor Immunology and Biology, National Cancer Institute, National Institutes of Health, Bethesda, MD*

Alfredo Molinolo • *Laboratory of Histopathology, National Academy of Medicine, Buenos Aires, Argentina*

Fredrick J. Montz • *Division of Gynecologic Oncology, UCLA Medical Center, Los Angeles, CA*

Peter Oehr • *Institut fur Klinische und Exp. Nuklearmedizin, University of Bonn, Bonn, Germany*

Noriaki Ohuchi • *Second Department of Surgery, Tohoku University School of Medicine, Sendai, Japan*

N. Coleman Owen • *Fritzsche Pambianchi and Associates, Del Mar, CA*

Adolf L. Pohl • *Institute for Clinical Chemistry and Laboratory Medicine, University of Vienna, Vienna, Austria*

Peter J. Roberts • *Fourth Department of Surgery, Helsinki University General Hospital, Helsinki, Finland*

Norio Sawabu • *Department of Internal Medicine, Cancer Research Institute, University of Kanazawa, Yoneizumi, Kanazawa, Japan*

Jeffrey Schlom • *Laboratory of Tumor Immunology and Biology, National Cancer Institute, National Institutes of Health, Bethesda, MD*

Stewart Sell • *Department of Pathology and Laboratory Medicine, Universy of Texas Health Science Center, Houston, TX*

Hanna M. Sikorska • *Rougier Bio-Tech Ltd., Montreal, Canada*

Torgny Stigbrand • *Department of Medical Biochemistry and Biophysics, University of Umea, Umea, Sweden*

Kazuhisa Taketa • *Health Research Center, Kagawa University, Takamatsu, Japan*

Ann Thor • *Department of Pathology, Harvard Medical School, Boston, MA*

Carlo Tondini • *Laboratory of Clinical Pharmacology, Dana-Farber Cancer Institute, Harvard Medical School, Boston, MA*

Britta Wahren • *Department of Virology, National Bacteriological Laboratory and Karolinska Institute, Stockholm, Sweden*

Chapter 1

Cancer Markers of the 1990s

An Introduction

Stewart Sell

The original goal of the cancer marker program was to be able to measure a marker in serum that could be used to diagnose cancer when it was still small enough to be removed surgically. If this had been possible using a simple serum marker assay, many patients otherwise doomed to die of their cancer, could be cured. Unfortunately, for most cancers, if a malignant tumor cannot be removed surgically, other forms of therapy, though often effective, are usually not curable, and often have serious deleterious side effects. Even a small tumor, the size of a peanut, contains millions of living cancer cells. Chemo-, radio-, or immunotherapy may be able to eliminate 99.99% of the tumor cells. The small fraction of residual viable tumor cell are able to poliferate, develop resistance to further therapy, and eventually kill the patient. Unfortunately, for many cancers, the goal of detecting and localizing cancer, when it is still small enough to be removed surgically, remains the rare exception to the general rule.

The growing interest in different tumor markers is illustrated by the increasing number of published papers in this field (Fig. 1) and the impact of the commercialization of clinical tests for tumor

From: *Serological Cancer Markers* Edited by Stewart Sell ©1992 The Humana Press, Totowa, NJ

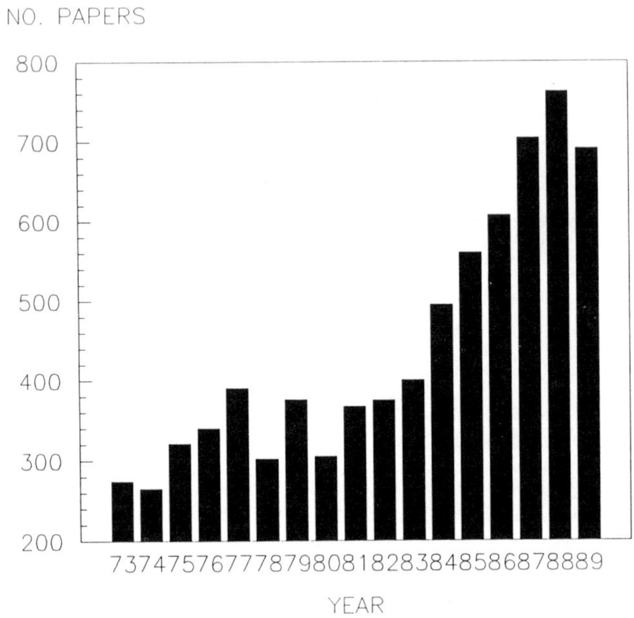

Fig. 1. Publications on cancer markers, 1973–1989. The bars indicate the number of publications listed under "neoplastic antigens" from 1973 to 1989 in *Index Medicus.*

markers (*see* Chapter 24). The "classic" cancer markers are listed in Table 1. Myeloma paraproteins have been useful for making the diagnosis of multiple myeloma for many years since the recognition that "monoclonal pikes" found by electrophoresis of serum were associated with plasma cell tumors. The first cancer marker ever reported was the presence in the urine of the light chain of immunoglobulin, Bence-Jones protein, found in about 75% of myeloma patients (Bence-Jones, 1847). Since its discovery in 1847 by precipitation of a protein in acidified boiled urine, the measurement of Bence-Jones protein has been a diagnostic test for multiple myeloma. Bence-Jones protein was known about for over 100 years before it was identified as immunogloblin light chain. Myeloma paraproteins and/or Bence-Jones protein are found in 99% of patients with plasma cell tumors. However, protein spikes termed "monoclonal gammopathy" may be found in up to 10% of elderly men without other evidence of myeloma. The use of Bence-Jones proteins to monitor therapy of patients with nonplasma-cell B-cell tumors such as chronic lymphocytic leukemia and non-Hodgkin's lymphoma using very sensitive isotachophoresis methodology is discussed by Abelev and Karamova, in their article herein.

The modern era of cancer markers began in the 1960s with the discovery of alphafetoprotein (AFP) and carcinoembryonic antigen (CEA). AFP was first found in the sera of mice with liver cancer and in sera of newborn mice (Abelev et al., 1963) and later in sera of humans with liver cancer (Tatarinov, 1964). Shortly thereafter, CEA was discovered by Gold and Freeman (1965). Prior to the discovery of these markers, myeloma paraproteins and elevated levels of endocrine hormones produced by tumors had been used to diagnose and follow a limited number of cancer patients. For instance, the persistence of human chorionic gonadotropin after termination of pregnancy was used to diagnose choriocarcinomas (Bagshawe et al., 1973). Its presence in men indicated embryonal carcinoma or ectopic hormone production by a tumor (Rosen et al., 1975). In addition the measurement of phosphatases was used to follow the course of tumors, such as acid phophatase for prostate cancer, and alkaline phosphatase when metastases to the bone occurred (Gutman et al., 1936; Pontes, 1983).

AFP and CEA levels in cancer patients were studied extensively in the late 1960s and early 1970s. After a period of high enthusiasm, expectations became more guarded. It soon became clear that elevations of CEA, the most widely applied marker, could not be used alone to make the diagnosis of cancer, since CEA is elevated in a number of noncancerous situations (Go, 1976). However, elevations of CEA were very helpful when used in combination with other diagnostic procedures and could also be used accurately to determine if residual cancer remained after surgical resection of CEA producing tumor. AFP was additionally shown to be useful in the diagnosis and monitoring of patients with liver and yolk sac cancer. In the 1980s screening of high risk populations for liver cancer in China (Xu, 1983) and Alaska (Heyard et al., 1985), dem-

Table 1
Cancer Markers That Have Been Elected

Name	Nature	Normal limit	Type of cancer
Myeloma paraprotein or Bence-Jones protein	Monclonal immunoglobulin or immunoglobulin light chain, ~4% CHO	No protein spike in electrophoresis	Myeloma
Alpha-fetoprotein	70 kDa glycoprotein, 4% CHO	15 μg/mL	Hepatoma, yolk-sac
Carcinoembryonic antigen	200 kDa glycoprotein up to 70% CHO	3–5 μg/mL	GI, pancreas, lung, breast, etc.
Human chorionic gonadotropin	Glycopeptide hormone	3 IU/mL	Choriocarcinoma, embryonal
Prostate-specific antigen	33 kDa glycoprotein	2.5 μg/mL	Prostate
Placental alkaline phosphatase	Heat-inactivated alkaline phosphatase	—	Testicular, ovary
Estrogen receptors	Two 65 kDa membrane units	10,000/cell	Breast, ovary

Modified from Sell, S., Cancer Markers of the 1990's. *Clinics Lab. Med.* **10,** 1–37, 1990.

Table 1 *(continued)*

Use			Sensitivity, %	Specificity, %	Chapter
Diagnosis	Prognosis	Monitoring			
++	+	+++	90	90	22
+++	+	+++	60–90	60–100	3
+	++	+++	42–96	10–90	4
++	+++	+++	60–100	40–90	—
+	++	+++	33–99	82–97	5
+	+	++	35–72	90	6,7
	+++	+	—	—	8

onstrated that AFP could also be used for screening and could detect otherwise clandestine liver cancers in a small but significant number of clinically normal individuals. For instance, in four reported studies from China a total of 3,618,988 healthy individuals were screened by field techniques such as reverse hemagglutination or radiorocket electrophoresis (Xu, 1983). From 11 to 60 positives were found per 100,000 people tested, and 300 individuals with asymptomatic hepatocellular carcinoma were diagnosed. It is estimated that detection of small tumors by this method, followed by surgical treatment, improved the survival rate from 15 to 80% after 1 yr and from 5 to 6% after 3 yr. In the Alaskan study, 3387 AFP determinations were carried out on 1394 individuals. Pregnancies accounted for most of the 129 elevations, however, nine males, with elevations above 300 ng/mL were found to have liver cancer. Six of these were asymptotic and four had small, surgically resectable cancers. The serum AFP levels of these four patients fell to normal after surgery and have remained so for 4–20 mo followup periods, suggesting cure.

Secretion of cancer products into the circulation is a normal process for proteins such as AFP that are rapidly released after synthesis from both normal and cancer cells. However, for other cancer markers, such as CEA, which are normally not secreted into the blood, elevated serum levels are believed to be the result of a change of polarity of the cancer cells that allow release of cancer associated glycoprotein into the circulation or, in the case of epithelial cancer, to the stage of the growth of the cancer when the cancer cells break through surrounding basement membrane. For example, CEA is normally produced by intestinal lining cells and is secreted into the gastrointestinal lumin. There is polarity of the epithelial cells with the CEA being found on the pole of the cell opposite the basement membrane. With malignant transformation, these cells lose their polarity so that CEA secreting cells are no longer "facing" the gastrointestinal lumen. However, the circulating level of the cancer marker most likely does not become significantly increased until the cancer tissue "breaks through" the basement membrane. Tissue invasion permits direct release into the interstitial fluid and subsequent delivery by the lymphatics into the blood.

In the case of epithelial carcinomas, which comprise more than 80% of all cancers in man, the substances shed from cancer cells at first flows with the secretions of the organ, i.e., into the mammary ducts in the case of breast cancer; into alveoli/bronchi in the case of lung cancer; or into the gastrointestinal tract in the case of colon cancer. Only upon breakthrough of the basement membrane of the invading tumor and loss of polarization of the tumor cells do these substances appear in the blood. It follows that early detection of these tumors by elevations of a secreted substance in the blood is theoretically impossible until after invasion of the basement membrane has occurred. In addition, it has not been possible, at least at this date, to detect early *in situ* cancer by interpreting quantitative or qualitative differences in tumor marker levels in the secretions of the various organs where adenocarcinomas develop.

Although great activity directed to finding other serum cancer markers followed the discovery of AFP and CEA, the results were generally disappointing. These approaches followed the plan originally used for CEA. Animals (rabbits) would be immunized with human cancer tissue, the antisera obtained after immunization absorbed with normal tissue of the same organ at the origin of the cancer, and the reactivity of the antisera to the cancer tissue extract determined. Although this approach was applied to many different human cancers, only one other marker, prostate specific antigen (PSA, *see* Chapter 5), has stood the test of time. PSA was shown to be better than acid phosphatase for detection of prostate cancer and it proved to be very useful for detection of residal tumor after surgical resection. For diagnosis rectal examination by an experienced physician remains a very effective technique. However, the results of this technique are quite dependent on the experience of the examining physician and up to 50% of small prostatic tumor may be missed. Some of the "cancer markers" that were identified and studied but not found to be particularly useful are listed in Table 2.

Table 2
Some Cancer Marker Candidates that Were Not Elected[a]

			Reactivity	
Name	Immunogen	Antisera	Tumor tissue	Fatal tissue
Beta-oncofetal antigen	Colon CA metastases	Rabbit	Many	Epithelial
Carcinofetal ferritin	Fetal liver	Rabbit	Many	Liver
Fetal gut antigen	Fetal gut	Rabbit	GI	GI
Fetal sulfoprotein	Gastric CA	Rabbit	GI	GI
Gamma-fetoprotein	—	CA patient	Many	Serum
Pregnancy-specific protein-I	Placental	Rabbit	Germ cell	Pregnancy sera

[a]Modified from Sell, S., *Clinics Lab. Med.* **10,** 1–37, 1990.

In the final chapter in this section, Glinsky presents his interesting results on glycoamines in cancer patients, including a wide ranging hypothesis on the role of glycoamines in tumor biology and immunology. With the development of hybridoma technology and application of hybridomas to the production of monoclonal antibodies to detect putative tumor antigens, a new era in cancer markers arrived.

The availability of monoclonal antibodies that detect a large number of different epitopes associated with molecules produced in cancer tissue has led to marked increase in the number of items on the cancer marker menu. The most important of these are presented in different chapters in this book. Hakomori (Chapter 10) writes that many of these detect carbohydrate structures that are altered because of changes in the level of glycosylating enzymes; secondary consequences to the processing of carbohydrates including mainly aberrant fucosylation or sialylation; or to abnormalities of cancer cell metabolism resulting in changes in density of molecules on the cell surface and exposure of molecules usually covered by other cell surface molecules. These "antigens" have often been identified by labeling of tissue sections fixed in a manner that preserves carbohydrate structures.

A partial listing of the "nouvelle cuisine" of cancer makers is presented in Table 3. This table includes the author and page number of the chapter in this text devoted to this marker. This table includes carbohydate markers, as well as mucin marker and cellular proteins, including squamous cell carcinoma antigen (SCC). In addition, tissue polypeptide antigen (TPA), one of the first markers to be discovered, has been reincarnated as a useful marker for monitoring *(see below).*

The first test of carbohydrate antigens to be appled clinically is now referred to as CA 19.9, developed in the early 1980s by Steplewski's group at the Wistar Institute (*see* Magnani et al., 1982). It is now one among several tests measuring antigens in the blood of the Lewis and other blood group series of carbohydrates. These may not only measure such antigens in "free" form, but also in a form attached to proteins from tumors of the gastrointestinal tract. In addition to CA 19.9, other carbohydrate markers include CA-50, TAG-72, and CA 242.

Very prominent among the new cancer markers are the mucins: glycoproteins with a high level of *O*-glycosidic and a low level of *M*-glycosidic bound carbohydrates. The prototypes of these tests, such as MAM-6, were developed in the early 1980s by a number of laboratories (*see* the Hilkens chapter). The commercially available CA 15.3 assay has become widely accepted in this context and has been confirmed by a variety of other tests (MCA, BCM, CA 549, CAM 26, CAM 29, TAG 12) that detect epitopes on simi-

Table 3
Cancer Markers Now Running For Office

Name	Nature	Normal limit	Type of cancer
I. Carbohydrates			
CA-19-9	Sialyated Lewis X^A	37 U/mL	GI pancreas, ovary
CA-50	Sialyated Lewis X-1, afucosyl form	14 U/mL	GI, pancreas lung
TAG-72	Sialyl Tn	4–7 U/mL	Breast, ovary GI
CA-242	Sialyated carbohydrate co-expressed with CA-50	200 U/mL	GI, pancreas
II. Mucins			
CA 15-3	Transmembrane molecule-episialin 200 kDa, up to 50% CHO	30 U/mL	Breast, ovary lung (adeno)
CA-125	High mol wt glycoprotein	35 U/mL	Ovary (epidermal) endometrial
DU-PAN-2	1000 kDa Mucin (peptide epitope)	400 U/mL	Pancreas, ovary GI, lung
MCA	350 kDa glycoprotein	11 U/mL	Breast, ovary GI
III. Cytoplasmic Proteins			
SCC	48-kDa glycoprotein	1.5 ng/mL	Cervix, lung head and neck (squamous)
TPA	Cytokeratins: 8, 18, and 19	85 U/L	Multiple, squamous

Modified from Sell, S., *Clinics Lab. Med.* **10,** 1–37, 1990.

Table 3 *(continued)*

Use			Performance		
Diagnosis	Prognosis	Monitoring	Sensitivity, %	Specificity, %	Chapter
+	++	+++	33–89	89–97	13
					14
+	++	+++	40–78	80–98	20
++	++		9–72	97	18
+	++	++	44–83	75	17
+	++	+++	88–97	30–90	12
+	++	+++	40–86	86–99	19
+	+	+++	34	86	16
+	++	+++	20–80	84–90	15
	+	+++	33–86	92–98	21
	+	+++	67–80	75	9

lar molecules, and it has been applied to a wide variety of cancers, in particular carcinoma of the breast. Other examples of mucin markers are presented in more detail in chapters by Montz (Chapter 19), by Metzgar (Chapter 16), and by Bombardieri (Chapter 15).

Some abundant cellular proteins, present inside the cells rather than on the cell membrane and normally thought to be shed into the circulation in very low amounts, namely SCC *(see* Chapter 21) and TPA (*see* Chapter 9), appear to be released into the circulation in relatively high amounts by many types of carcinomas, notably epithelial cells of squamous type. These tumor types do not often show elevations of mucin and/or carbohydrate antigens and are among the most difficult cancers to monitor. Therefore, the markers may become very useul for monitoring squamous cell carcinomas.

TPA was originally discovered in 1957 by Bjorklund and Bjorklund (1957) as an insoluble heat-labile tumor antigen detected by immunofluorescence in malignant cells, but not normal tissue. Thus the discovery of TPA predated that of AFP and CEA. However, until recently the use of TPA as cancer markers was controversial. It has now been found to be useful for monitoring cancer patients. TPA is identified by antibodies that react with cytokeratins 8, 18, and 19 (Weber et al., 1984). Since these are produced by both normal and malignant cells, elevations in the serum are not restricted to cancer patients, but are found in a variety of noncancerous conditions, e.g., inflammation or pregnancy; processes associated with a high rate of cell turnover. However, in patients who are known to have cancer and an elevation of TPA, the TPA level has now achieved its place as a useful marker for monitoring the TPA secreting tumor tissue.

Most of the "new" cancer markers detected by monoclonal antibodies have been found to be useful for monitoring the effects of therapy of a patient with a cancer that produces an elevated serum concentration of the marker. Falling levels indicate successful therapy and reelevations indicate regrowth or development of metastases. High serum levels at the time of diagnosis of the tumor generally indicate a poor prognosis, whereas low or normal levels indicate a good prognosis. However, elevations of these markers are frequently found with nonmalignant conditions, so that they may only be used as an adjunct to other diagnostic techniques. Some, such as CA 15.3 and SCC, may be very useful to indicate the presence of metastases if levels continue to be high after removal of a primary tumor.

The combined use of more than one cancer marker may greatly increase sensitivity, but may also greatly decrease the specificity of detection of cancer (*see* Chapter 23). For instance, in the studies of Bhargava et al. (1988), using placental alkaline phosphatase and CA-125 as markers for ovarian cancer, the sensitivity was 59% for CA-125 and 31% for PL-ALP, but by using both CA-125 and PL-ALP the sensitivity was increased to 67%. On the other hand the specificity with PL-ALP was 94% and with CA-125 was 87%, whereas using both, the specificity dropped to 82%. The application of multiple makers is fraught with many difficulties in interpretation. For instance, as pointed out by Pohl, setting the specificity of each cancer marker the 95th pecentile and using multiple marker increases the likelihood of a false positive diagnosis of cancer. A normal person who has 13 separate cancer marker tests has, by chance alone, a probability of 50% for being diagnosed as having cancer. It is, in fact, the potential for the overdiagnosis of cancer that has contributed largely to the limited approval for cancer marker tests by the United States Food and Drug Administration panel.

The choice of marker to be measured and the criteria to be used in evaluation is now under active consideration by a "Working Group on Tumor Marker Criteria" (Bonfer, 1990). This committee has addressed criteria (1) for establishing reference values (use of age-matched healthy controls and international tumor staging classifications), (2) for accurate diagnosis by histologic examination of the tumor, and (3) for interpretation of changing levels for evaluation of recurrence or to follow the effects of therapy (monitoring). Standardization of the application of the use of cancer marker tests is essential to provide a basis for establishing clinical correlations and acceptable standards of interpretation.

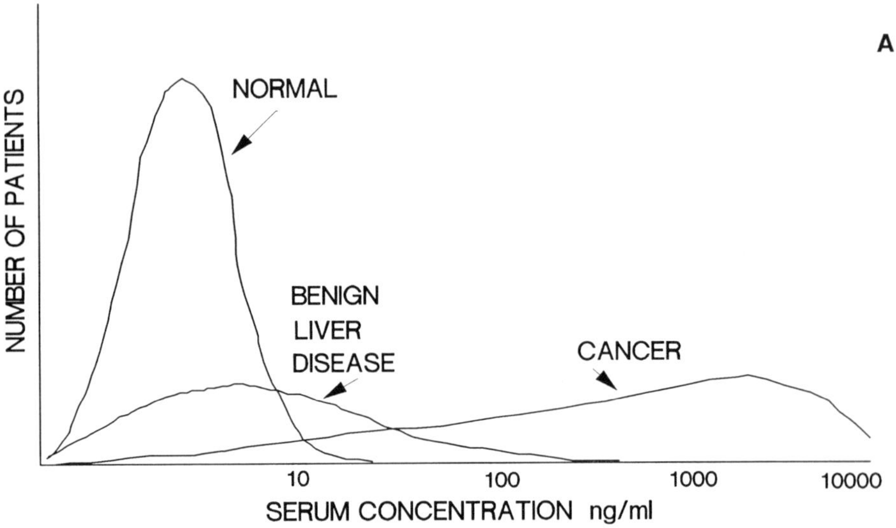

Fig. 2. (**A**) Distribution of the serum concentrtion of AFP in groups of normal patients (NP), patients with benign liver disease (BLD), and patients with hepatocellular carcinoma (HCC) based on data in the literature.

At this point the author would like to make a plea for the use of receiver-operator curve analysis of laboratory tests for cancer markers. A hypothetical example based on data in the literature for AFP is given in Fig. 2. Separation of controls into normal and benign liver disease groups clearly illustrates the importance of the appropriate selection of controls in using a test to diagnose cancer. For example, if a group of normal healthy controls is used as the reference population with a cutoff value of 25 ng/mL, many patients with benign liver disease would be included, thus producing many false positive results. However, when patients with HCC are compared to patients with benign liver disease a cutoff value above 400 ng/mL will eliminate more than 99% of patients with benign liver disease while maintaining a sensitivity of approx 70% for patients with HCC. Of all the cancer markers, AFP may be the only one for which claim can be made that elevations above a selected limit (for example, 500 ng/mL) are diagnostic of cancer.

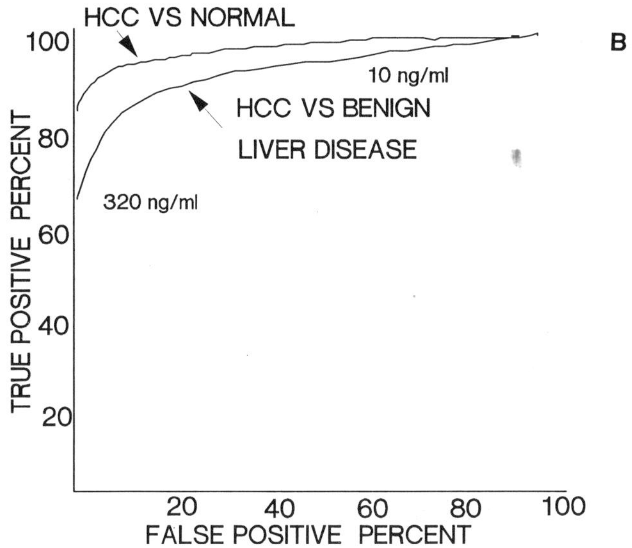

Fig. 2 (**B**) Receiver-operator curve for data in A. The upper limit of normal for AFP is 10 ng/mL. Although this is based on 95% confidence limits for normals, the serum levels of approx 40% of patients with benign liver disease (cirrhosis, hepatitis, and HBsAg carriers) ranges between 110 and 320 ng/mL, so that the cutoff value for the diagnosis of HCC should be 320 ng/mL. The receiver-operator curve will be different depending on whether the normal or benign disease group is used for comparison to the HCC group. Thus a cutoff value of 25 g/mL is indicated for separation of normal and HCC (curve A), but because patients with benign liver disease will have levels between 25 and 320 ng/mL, a higher cutoff value is more appropriate when comparing this group with HCC patients. Approximately 70% of patients with HCC will have serum AFP levels above 320 ng/mL. Approximately 3% of patients with benign liver disease will have levels above 320 ng/mL and less than 1% levels greater than 400 ng/mL. (Based on data from Chen and Sung, 1977.)

Patients with serum levels above 500 ng/mL who prove with further examination and testing not to have hepatocellular cancer are rare enough to be written up as case reports. The receiver-operator curve clearly describes the usefulness, as well as the limitations, of a laboratory test.

The therapeutic application of monoclonal antibodies to deliver toxins, drugs, or radioisotopes to tumor is being attempted in a number of clinical trials. This topic is not covered in detail in this text. However, a number of clinical trials have revealed difficulties in the application of this exciting approach. Some of the difficulties and ways to deal with them by genetically engineering the monoclonal antibodies are now under active investigation. For instance, host immune response to the mouse immunoglobulin may be largely eliminated by construction of hybrid monoclonal antibodies that retain the mouse variable regions (paratope) to bind to the antigen, while replacing the constant regions of the antibody with human-derived segments. Substitution of Fc region with desirable functions (ADCC, complement fixation) has also been described, as well as the construction of expression systems that permit the generation of large amounts of genetically engineered antibodies with desired properties.

The commercial impact of cancer markers is discussed in Chapter 24. In the future, marker analysis profiles individually selected for a given patient may be expected to provide information for initial diagnosis, estimation of prognosis and evaluation of therapy that will direct treatment in ways much more effective than now realized. This approach is reflected in the estimate that the world market for cancer markers will increase more than threefold in the next 5 yr. The oncodevelopmental or oncofetal nature of cancer markers and their application in the future is addressed by Klavins in the final chapter of this text.

The articles in this book were selected to provide a detailed overview of the current status of serological markers of cancer. In addition to the serological markers there are many cytological markers of cancer, including cell surface markers, cytoplasmic proteins, and nuclear markers. The study of these has contributed not only to the understanding of the nature and origin of cancer, but have also led to major advances in diagnosis by the pathologist. The cytological markers of cancer will be presented in a separate volume of this series.

References

Abelev, G. I., S. D. Perova, N. I. Khramkova, Z. A. Postnikova, and I. S. Irlin (1963), *Transplantation* **1,** 174–180.

Bagshawe, K. D., H. Wilson, P. Dublon, A. Smith, M. Baldwin, and A. Kardana (1973), *J. Ob. Gyn.* **80,** 461.

Bence-Jones, H. (1867), *Lancet* **2,** 269.

Bjorklund, B. and V. Bjorklund (1957), *Arch. Allergy* **10,** 153.

Bonfer, J. M. G. (1990), *Tumor Biol.* **11,** 287.

Chen, D. S. and J. L. Sung (1977), *Cancer* **40,** 779.

Go, V. (1976), *Cancer* **7,** 562–566. 197.

Gold, P. and S. O. Freeman (1965), *J. Exp. Med.* **121,** 439.

Gutman, E. B., E. E. Sproul, and A. B. Gutman (1936), *Am. J. Cancer* **28,** 485.

Heyward, W. L., A. P. Lanier, B. J. McMahon, M. A. Fitzgerald, S. Kilkenny, and T. R. Paprocki (1985), *J. Am. Med. Assoc.* **254,** 3092.

Leong, A. S.-Y. and J. Wright (1987), *Histopathology* **11,** 1295.

Magnani, J. L., B. Nilsson, M. Brockhaus, D. Zopf, Z. Steplewski, H. Koprowski, and V. Ginsburg (1982), *J. Biol. Chem.* **257,** 14365.

Pontes, J. E. (1983), *J. Urology* **130,** 1037–1047.

Rosen, S. W., B. D. Weintraub, J. L. Vaitukaitis, H. H. Sussman, J. M. Hershman, and F. M. Muggia (1975), *Ann. Inter. Med.* **82,** 71–83.

Tatarinov, Y. (1984), *Vopr. Med. Khim.* **10,** 90, 91.

Weber, K., M. Osborn, R. Moll, B. Wiklund, and B. Lüning (1984), *EMBO J.* **3,** 2707.

Xu, K. L. (1983), in *Oncodevelopmental Markers* (Fishman, W., ed.), Academic, San Diego, pp. 395–408.

Chapter 2

Clinical Cancer Markers

Diagnosis, Prognosis, and Monitoring

Manfred L. Lüthgens and Peter Oehr

1. Introduction

Owing to their relatively small concentrations, exact quantitative analyses of cancer markers are performed by highly sensitive immunological methods. Despite the development of various types of nonisotopic immunoassays, isotopic immunoassays are still considered the methods of first choice in marker analysis, by some investigators.

Improvements of the assays in recent years have been effective with respect to quality and handling. The production of monoclonal antibodies against separate antigen epitopes was an essential contribution to this with two goals: the improvement of specificity, and homogeneity of the product. The first euphoria of obtaining high tumor site specificities by using monoclonal instead of polyclonal antibodies has been replaced in the meantime by a more reasonable consideration. On the contrary, it has been proven to be advantageous to combine two or more monoclonal antibodies against different epitopes to give results similar in their reactivity to polyclonal assays.

From: *Serological Cancer Markers* Edited by Stewart Sell ©1992 The Humana Press, Totowa, NJ

Results of tumor marker tests can be evaluated by reliable, well-established methods in general diagnostics (Remein and Wilkerson, 1961). They are fundamental in the determination of the range limits of each assay, such as low detection limit, upper limit of the normal range, specificity, sensitivity, or positivity, respectively. Difficulties arise, however, in the assessment of the patient's clinical status; even with sophisticated diagnostic and invasive methods, sufficient staging is often not obtainable. Also in patient surveillance, it is necessary to follow-up the patient's tumor activity grade.

Although marker analysis can be helpful in preoperative diagnosis (staging), its main aims are considered by Lüthgens and Schlegel (1987) to be:

1. Documentation of the therapeutic success by values returning to, or distinctly tending toward, the normal range.
2. Early detection of tumor reactivation in order to begin a curative therapy.
3. Rapid detection of a therapy failure in order to change the treatment.

2. Analytical Assays

Most assays for the determination of cancer markers were first developed as radioimmunoassays (RIA) or, more recently, as immunoradiometric assays (IRMA). Actually, the development of suitable RIAs for CEA by Thomson et al. (1969) and Hansen et al. (1971) prepared the way for the extensive use of this first cancer marker in clinical routine. The handling of the assays has been definitely simplified by changing from RIA to IRMA. This latter technique, especially in combination with monoclonal antibodies, has also considerably increased the quality of results.

For several years, nonisotopic techniques have been available for the analysis of some cancer markers. In these assays, enzymes, instead of the radioactive nuclide ^{125}I are used as tracers, allowing measurements in photometers and automation. In addition, fluorescence and luminescence tracers have been developed in order to compensate for various disadvantages of the enzymatic techniques in comparison to IRMA.

3. Populations

3.1. Normal Controls

The group of normal controls used for reference range determinations should exclusively be comprised of clinically healthy individuals, i.e., without any symptoms of disease or pathologic clinical findings (Sunderman, 1975). Additionally, in the case of some markers, for instance in CEA, one has to consider exogeneous disturbances, such as alcohol or nicotine abuse as well as extreme physical stress. Among the endogeneous factors, a slight age dependency may be important, whereas sex, race, or biorhythms are negligible. The use of healthy blood donors, regularly checked by blood donation institutions, is the most reliable way to obtain normal controls. It is recommended to balance this population with respect to sex and age distribution.

3.2. Patients With Benign Diseases

It is well documented that elevated marker levels occur in benign diseases. In inflammatory diseases these elevations may exceed by tenfold the value of the upper limit of the normal range; they are, however, almost exclusively of a temporary nature. Thus, a discrimination between elevations caused by malignancy or by inflammation may be resolved by follow-up, if not clarified by other diagnostic means. In untreated malignancies, the marker values tend to increase or remain at a higher level, whereas decreasing values indicate a benign process.

3.3. Cancer Patients

Whereas the primary therapy of tumor patients is based on a pathogram consisting of histology with grading, staging by TNM, and receptor analysis, if applicable, for therapy monitoring, an ex-

Table 1
Tumor Activity Grades[a]

Tumor Activity Grade	International Term	Abbreviation
A0	No evidence of disease Complete remission	NED CR
A1	Questionable tumor activity	QA
A2	Partial remission Stable disease	PR SD
A3	Progressive disease	PD

[a]Internationally used terms according to Schlegel et al. (1981).

act classification of the tumor activity status is of great importance. In cancer marker analysis, a grouping of the patients in accordance with Table 1 has been successfully proved.

It is possible to classify tumor patients into three main grades, those with A0, A2, and A3. It allows, with regard to duration and extent of remission, to distinguigh between partial and complete remission. For patient surveillance, especially in therapy monitoring, a discrimination of a marker at least between A0 and A3 is required. It is thus necessary to register the current tumor activity grade at each clinical check-up.

4. Assessment of Marker Results

4.1. Specificity and Sensitivity

The evaluation of marker results follows approaches proved in other diagnostic methods using specificity and sensitivity as terms clearly defined by Remein and Wilkerson (1961). Herein sensitivity is, e.g., the percentage recognized by the test of true positives in a group of tumor patients based on the specificity, which is the percentage recognized by the test as true negatives within the group of healthy persons. People comprising this group but suffering from any kind of disease should be omitted. In cancer marker analysis, this is especially true for patients with benign tumors or malignancies. In order to avoid any imponderables, even with healthy controls, it has become common practice to calculate sensitivities on the basis of 95% specificities (Lüthgens and Schlegel, 1987).

The term "specificity" has been interpreted in different ways. Some oncologists may be led by the misconception that cancer markers should recognize cancer patients exclusively, and therefore, elevated values in other diseases are regarded as "false" positives. The use of this interpretation will cause a shift in the basis depending on the composition of each selected population. The situation becomes even more complicated if a marker is expected to recognize "specifically" just one primary tumor site or histological type of cells. Obviously, this demand is too great for the presently available markers, since it would approach their use as a tool for screening whole populations.

For calculating sensitivity, only patients with active tumors (activity grade A3, Table 1) ought to be included, since in groups with other activity grades A2, A1, and A0, the percentage of patients with active tumors decreases. Despite the fact that, by definition, in grade A0, no active tumor should occur, one has to assume a certain number of subclinical unidentified reactivations.

4.2. Negativity and Positivity

Using patient populations of any kind as a basis for comparison with a group of patients having active tumors, it would be incorrect to call the rate of positives "sensitivity." As shown above, sensitivity is based on the specificity of healthy controls (Remein and Wilkerson, 1961). If a group of patients is used with benign diseases or with the tumor activity grade A0 for comparison, one should rather utilize the term "positivity" instead. Consequently, the rate of true negatives of these groups is the negativity. Positivity should be calculated on the basis of the 90% negativity. The

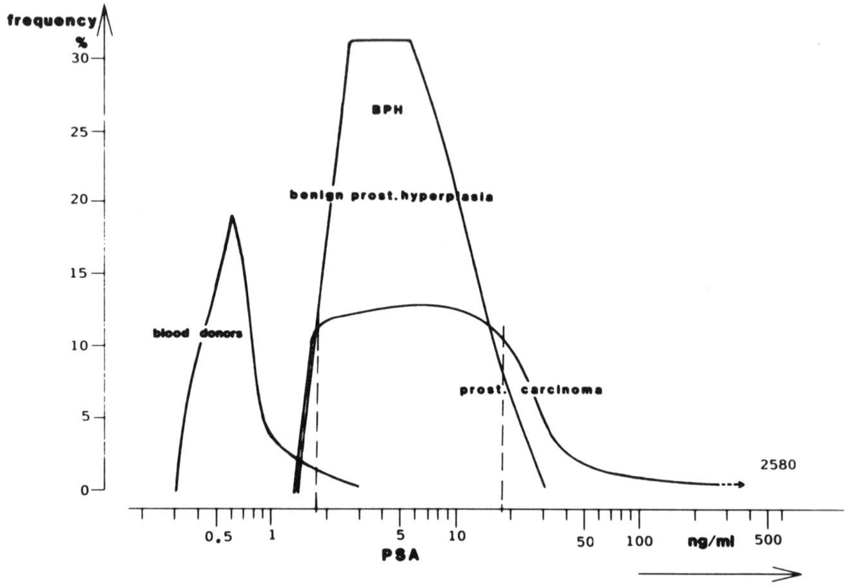

Fig. 1. Distribution of PSA values in blood donors and patients having either benign prostate hyperplasia (BPH) or untreated prostate carcinoma.

utilization of the 90th percentile instead of the 95th percentile is substantiated by a larger gray zone of subclinical unidentified marker elevations in the groups with either benign diseases or activity grade A0.

An example of how the three groups (healthy controls, patients with benign tumors, and patients having active tumors [A3]) overlap is shown in Fig. 1 in case of the distribution of prostate specific antigen (PSA) serum levels. Whereas the 95th percentile (95% specificity) of healthy controls at 1.8 ng/mL hardly overlaps the group of patients having untreated carcinoma (A3), leaving a sensitivity of 98.6%, the 90th percentile of the patient group having benign prostate hyperplasia (BPH) is 18 ng/mL overlapping the A3-group almost completely. Consequently, the positivity is only 36.8%. This example well demonstrates why benign diseases cannot be utilized for calculating sensitivities and cutoff values; important information in the assessment of cancer markers would be lost.

4.3. Distribution Function, ROC-Diagram, and Youden-Index

The relation between specificity and sensitivity or negativity and positivity, respectively, is expressed by distribution functions as well as Receiver Operating Characteristic (ROC) diagrams, according to Oehr et al. (1980). For calculation of distribution functions, first, the marker values are listed in ascending order followed by a percental classification depending on their frequency within a total population. Then the cumulative frequency is plotted vs the marker concentration for each group. In particular, as demonstrated in Fig. 2, the upper limit of a group of blood donors may be 90 U/L at 95% (5% in the graph). The sensitivity can be easily determined following the dotted vertical line to the point where it crosses the distribution curve of the A3-patient group. In our example it corresponds to 76%. This result may be compared with a positivity of only 72% when using the 90th percentile (negativity) of an A0-group as basis.

A more direct relation between specificity and sensitivity or negativity and positivity is accomplished by ROC-diagrams. They allow a comparison of different markers as well as patient groups. Figure 3 gives an example of such a comparison of three different markers. In addition to relations between normal and A3-patients, their positivities on the basis of the negativities of A0-patients are shown, yielding flatter curves than the sensitivities. Comparisons of different methods of marker analysis as well as calculations of optimal limits to differentiate between various patient groups can be achieved by the Youden-Index (Youden, 1950; Ebert et al., 1990).

4.4. Surveillance

In patient surveillance, the actual goal of cancer markers, especially in therapy monitoring, it becomes necessary to plot the marker courses for each individual patient. This can be performed

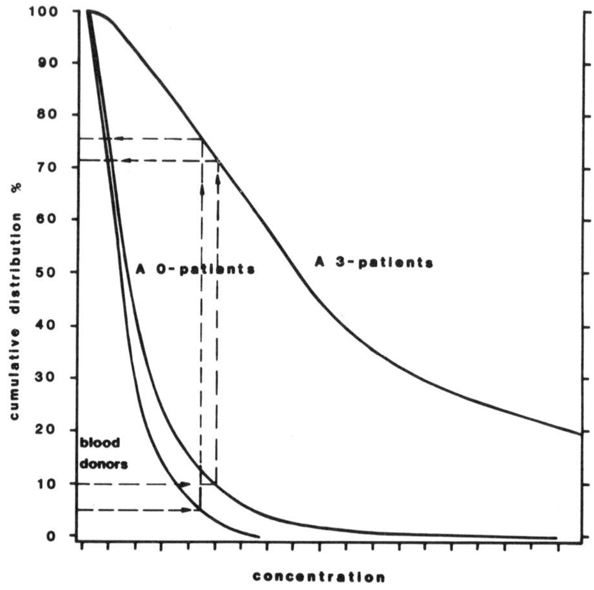

Fig. 2. Cumulative distribution of cancer marker concentrations in blood donor and patient groups. The dotted lines indicate the connections between specificity of blood donors (5% in the graph) and sensitivity (76%) or negativity of A0-patients (10%) and positivity of A3-patients (72%), respectively.

either by a computer plotter with an appropriate software program or graphically. The information should contain remarks regarding tumor activity grade, remission, and therapy regimen. Cancer marker time-courses can vary individually as well as between each other. In general, there are five patterns as described by Falkson et al. (1982) in the follow-up of breast cancer patients with CEA (Fig. 4).

4.5. Prognosis

The determination of cancer marker concentrations can also be of prognostic value. As in cancer therapy assessment, survival diagrams of Kaplan and Meier (1958) provide a valuable aid in the discrimination of pretherapeutic marker levels with respect to sur-

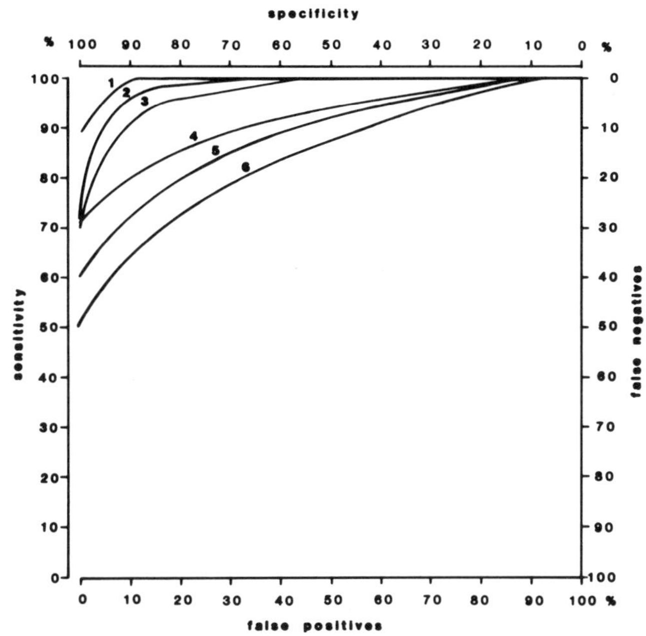

Fig. 3. ROC-diagrams for comparisons of different markers (1, 2, 3) and sensitivities vs positivities (1, 2, 3 vs 4, 5, 6).

vival. Detailed results will be presented in conjunction with the particular markers.

4.6. Significance

For a discriminance analysis of marker results, various statistical models and suitable programs are available. As with other biochemical parameters, marker levels are not normally distributed. Thus, significances should be calculated either free of distribution, for instance, by Kruskal (1952) and by Mann and Whitney (1974) or after logarithmic transformation they are accessible to the Student's *t*-test. Accordingly, probabilities are significant with $p < 0.05$ and highly significant with $p < 0.001$, and so on. Very high significances ($p < 0.0001$) have been obtained with several markers in a wide field of applications, which is indicated by both high

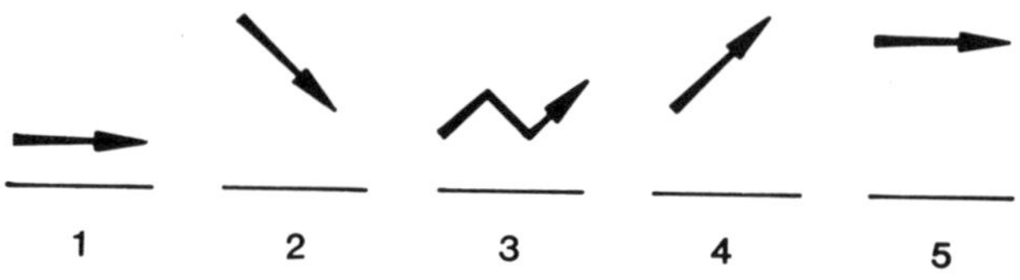

Fig. 4. Patterns of marker courses as outlined by Falkson et al. (1982) with respect to CEA: 1 = in normal range, 2 = decreasing toward normal range, 3 = fluctuation at or above the normal range, 4 = increasing above the normal range, 5 = persisting high level.

sensitivities and high specificities. In case of low sensitivities, the analyst often tends to calculate significances only, in order to probe at least a slight discriminance between the populations or markers.

The discriminance analysis between the various tumor activity grades is a different subject. Here again, very high sensitivities are a prerequisite for significant differences between the A0- and A3-, especially between the A0- and A2-, or A2- and A3-patient groups, respectively. For therapy monitoring with markers, a distinct discrimination between the A0- and A3- patient groups is necessary. In prognosis, the probability *p* of two survival diagrams to be equal or different may be calculated by the logrank-test (Peto et al., 1977) in connection with a chi-square table.

References

Ebert, W., G. Hug, A. Stabrey, and H. Bülzebruck (1990), *Tumor Diagn. Ther.* **11,** 60–67.

Falkson, H. C., G. Falkson, M. Portugal, J. Vander Watt, and H. S. Schoeman (1982), *Cancer* **49,** 1859–1865.

Hansen, H. J., K. E. Lance, and J. Krupey (1971), *Clin. Res.* **19,** 143–147.

Kaplan, E. L. and P. Meirer (1958), *Am. Stat. Ass. J.* **53,** 457–481.

Kruskal, W. H. (1952), *Ann. Math. Stat.* **23,** 525–540.

Lüthgens, M. and G. Schlegel (1987), in *Tumormarkersystem CEA-TPA,* Tumor-Diagnostik, Leonberg, FRG 13–21.

Mann, H. B. and P. R. Whitney (1974), *Ann. Math. Stat.* **18,** 50–60.

Oehr, P., G. Derigs, and R. Bormann (1981), *Tumor Diagn.* **2,** 283–290.

Peto, R., M. C. Pike, P. Armitage, N. E. Breglow, D. R. Cox, S. V. Howard, N. Mantel, R. McPherson, J. Peto, and P. G. Smith (1977), *Br. J. Cancer* **35,** 1–39.

Remein, Q. R. and H. L. C. Wilkerson (1961), *J. Chron. Dis.* **13,** 6–21.

Schlegel, G., M. Lüthgens, G. Eklund, and B. Björklund (1981), *Tumor Diagn.* **2,** 6–11.

Sunderman, F. W. (1975), *Clin. Chem.* **21,** 1873–1877.

Thomson, D. M. P., J. Krupey, S. O. Freedman, and P. Gold (1969), *Proc. Natl. Acad. Sci. USA* **64,** 161–167.

Youden, W. J. (1950), *Cancer* **3,** 32.

Chapter 3

Alpha-Fetoprotein in the 1990s

Kazuhisa Taketa

1. Introduction

Alpha-fetoprotein (AFP) is a well-established marker of hepatocellular carcinoma, yolk sac tumor, and other AFP-producing tumors mostly of gastrointestinal origin. The high sensitivity as well as the high specificity of AFP among other cancer markers was established by Abelev et al. (1963) and Tatarinov (1963, 1964), using an immunodiffusion technique by their evolutional discovery of an oncofetal nature of AFP. Following the development of sensitive radioimmunoassay (Ruoslahti and Seppälä, 1971; Nishi and Hirai, 1973), the specificity of AFP as a marker of hepatocellular carcinoma was somewhat reduced, since low but frequently increased serum levels of AFP were demonstrated in patients with hepatitis and liver cirrhosis, a known underlying condition of hepatocellular carcinoma. Furthermore, the diagnostic sensitivity of AFP became lower as a result of instituting an ultrasonographic screening system for early detection of hepatocellular carcinomas, although AFP measurement itself is included in this system (Okuda, 1986; Liaw et al., 1986; Regan, 1989). Thus, this is not to deny the

From: *Serological Cancer Markers* Edited by Stewart Sell ©1992 The Humana Press, Totowa, NJ

value of AFP as a marker of hepatocellular carcinoma. On the other hand, it is now possible to restore or even increase the specificity of AFP by analysis of its sugar chain heterogeneity with lectins (Breborowicz et al., 1981; Miyazaki et al., 1981).

In this article, the current status of AFP measurement as a diagnostic and monitoring marker of hepatocellular carcinoma and other cancers is described by focusing the review on the lectin-dependent microheterogeneity forms of AFP.

2. Induction Mechanisms

The production of AFP was initially considered to be tightly geared with the DNA synthesis or cell division (Abelev, 1971; Hirai, 1979). However, Taketa and his group were able to dissociate AFP production from DNA synthesis in experiments with rats (Watanabe et al., 1976a,b). In fact, the serum AFP level does not rise after partial hepatectomy in man (Alpert and Feller, 1978), whereas it increases up to several thousand nanograms per milliliter in hepatitis and liver cirrhosis (Sugimoto et al., 1987). The AFP elevation in benign liver diseases is considered to be the result of hepatic injury *per se* (Watanabe et al., 1976a,b), or owing to a restitutive mechanism (Sell et al., 1974, 1976).

The mechanisms of AFP induction at the cellular level have been elucidated in a series of studies made by Abelev and his group (Gleiberman and Abelev, 1985; Abelev, 1989; Gleiberman et al., 1989a,b). They showed that the cell-to-cell and cell-to-matrix contacts inhibit AFP synthesis, whereas the isolation of cells acts as a trigger of AFP production, indicating the importance of junctional communication in the regulation of AFP production. However, this theory alone does not fully explain the more or less random activation of AFP gene in neoplastic cells. The heterogeneous expression of phenotypes in individual tumors is considered an important facet of cancer markers (Taketa et al., 1988, 1990b).

Tamaoki and his coworkers (Sawadaishi et al., 1988) have substantiated the presence of a hepatoma-specific nuclear factor, which is present in AFP-producing, but not in AFP-nonproducing, hepatocellular carcinoma cells, and regulates the promotor and enhancer activities. This fits in their proposed model of transcriptional regulation of AFP gene involving the *cis*- and *trans*-acting elements and their interplay (Tamaoki, 1989). Incidentally, a sequence with an AT-rich core in the pre-S1 promotor region of hepatitis B virus DNA is shown to interact with the hepatoma nuclear factor (Nakao et al., 1989).

3. Circulating and Tissue Levels

3.1. Diagnostic Significance

The normal adult range of serum AFP determined by radioimmunoassay (Masseyeff et al., 1974) is between 0.1 and 5.8 ng/mL (mean ± SD, 2.6 ±1.6 ng/mL). Highly sensitive nonradioisotope methods of AFP analysis, such as immunoenzymatic or immunochemiluminometric assays (Weeks et al., 1983), are currently available. However, none of the commercially available kits cover the lower normal range, which is essential for the early detection of tumors with AFP levels below 10 or 20 ng/mL. A normal range with the 95% prediction band for early infancy is given by Tsuchida et al. (1978) to assist the diagnosis of neonatal hepatitis, biliary atresia, and AFP-producing tumors. A recently reevaluated familial disease, hereditary persistence of AFP (Ferguson-Smith et al., 1983; Greenberg et al.,1990), and similar benign elevation of AFP (Okimoto et al., 1989) should be thought of before considering pathologic conditions, not only for children, but also for adults.

Significant but small AFP rises up to 1000 ng/mL are frequently seen in adult patients with hepatitis and liver cirrhosis. The AFP elevations in the type-B chronic hepatitis are considered to be associated with the seroconversion from hepatitis B e antigenemia to e antibody (Liaw et al., 1986), accompanied by a bridging necrosis of the liver. Thus, the elevation of AFP should not necessarily be considered a beneficial sign or a favorable course. The normal hepatocyte regeneration as may be seen after partial hepatectomy does not lead to an increased serum level of AFP in humans, as mentioned earlier (Alpert and Feller, 1978), and the suggested favorable prognostic sign of raised serum AFP in fulminant hepatitis (Karvountzis and Redecker, 1974) is not supported by a subsequent study by Bloomer et al. (1974). The rising levels of AFP on serial determination in hepatitic and cirrhotic patients cannot be differentiated from those caused by hepatocellular carcinoma simply by comparing their time-courses, because an unexplained decline in serum AFP level is seen in hepatocellular carcinomas (Chen et al., 1984). However, steadily increasing serum levels of AFP above 1000 ng/mL are generally accepted as indicating the presence of AFP-producing tumors (Sell, 1990). Other benign conditions associated with increased serum levels of AFP and predisposed to neoplastic diseases are hemochromatosis, hereditary tyrosinemia, ataxia telangiectasia, and cystic fibrosis.

One of the factors that determine the serum levels of AFP in patients with hepatocellular carcinoma is how early the tumors are detected. According to the recent reports of the Liver Cancer Study Group of Japan (1987, 1988), 34.0–45.5% of hepatocellular carcinomas have AFP levels above 1000 ng/mL. In small hepatocellular carcinomas with diameters less than 3 cm, 25–46% (Okuda, 1986; Chen, 1988; Sonoda et al., 1989) of the cases have circulating AFP levels below 20 ng/mL. Well-differentiated hepatocellular carcinomas smaller than 2 cm in diameter are mostly negative for serum AFP (Kondo et al., 1989) and for AFP staining at the tissue level (Brumm et al., 1989). Among the AFP-positive tumors other than hepatocellular carcinoma, yolk sac tumor, hepatoblastoma, and mixed cholangiocellular/hepatocellular carcinoma, gastric carcinoma or pancreas carcinoma has the highest incidence, followed by cholangiocellular carcinoma and other tumors of entodermal origins, most of them being gastrointestinal tumors. Nonentodermally derived tumors, such as those in the kidney (cf Taketa et al., 1989a) and the breast (Sarcione and Biddle, 1987) also produce AFP. Low levels of AFP in leukemia patients appear in literature (Mihalev et al., 1978) without proving the production of AFP by malignant cells. Several lines of evidence are now available to suggest the production of AFP by transformed lymphocytes (Lafarge-Frayssinet et al., 1989).

3.2 Prognostic Significance

Patients with chronic hepatitis and liver cirrhosis having increased serum levels of AFP show a high risk of developing hepatocellular carcinoma (Hirai, 1987). Hepatocellular carcinoma patients having increased AFP levels at the time of diagnosis have poor prognosis in tumor size-matched cases (Nomura et al., 1989) compared to AFP-negative cases. Thus, AFP serves as a prognostic marker. Serum levels of AFP decline after tumor resection with a half-life of approx 4 d. Patients with longer half-lives show poor survival rates (Sell, 1981; Urabe et al., 1990). Recurrence could be readily predicted by a reelevation of AFP, although a negative response is reported in patients having residual tumors (Curtin et al., 1989). Similar time-courses of serum AFP in orthotopic liver transplantation for malignant disease are reported (Tuchman et al., 1985; Andorno et al., 1989). Rises in AFP level after the transplantation may be explained either by recurrent hepatic cancer or by liver cell damage associated with viral replication in the transplanted liver. No increased AFP levels have been observed during the phases of rejection.

3.3. Radionuclide Imaging

The radionuclide imaging of AFP-producing tumors and their targeting is the ultimate goal of cancer marker studies. Hirai and his groups (Koji et al., 1980; Ishii et al., 1984) first localized AFP-producing hepatocellular carcinomas with radiolabeled antibodies to AFP; however, the results accumulated to date are not promising, generally with low sensitivities of one-third to one-half in hepatomas (Duclos et al., 1989; Springolo et al., 1989) and in germ cell tumors (Hitchins et al., 1989), and with less marked specificity when liver cirrhosis is present. The specific staining of AFP-producing cells may be limited to the cases with membrane-bound AFP (Hosokawa et al., 1989). The use of radioiodinated AFP to localize the AFP receptor, which is widely expressed in cancer cells (Moro et al., 1984), has also been attempted.

4. Molecular Heterogeneity

4.1. Sugar Chain Heterogeneity

AFP exhibits several forms of microheterogeneity as revealed by electrophoretic, isoelectric focusing, and chromatographic techniques. Part of the charge heterogeneities can be explained by the difference in fatty acid content (Parmelee et al., 1978) and in the number of sialic acids attached to the carbohydrate residues. AFP has one asparagine-linked biantennary complex-type oligosaccharide per molecule as a fundamental structure with additional major and minor sugar chain heterogeneities, as reported by Yoshima et al. (1980) on hepatocellular carcinoma AFP and by Yamashita et al. (1983) on yolk sac tumor AFP.

4.2. Reactivities to Lectins

The structural diversity of the carbohydrate moiety of AFP can be detected by analysis of the whole AFP molecule with lectins having different oligosaccharide specificities. Lectin-dependent fractionation of AFP was first demonstrated by Smith and Kelleher (1973), using an affinity chromatographic technique with a concanavalin A (Con A)-bound agarose column. Bøg-Hansen et al. (1975) developed a system of crossed affinity immunoelectrophoresis with free Con A in agarose gels to separate differently glylcosylated glycoproteins. Several microheterogeneous forms of AFP have been demonstrated by this method (Kerckaert et al., 1979), although the sensitivity is too low to be applied to clinical studies, requiring samples with AFP concentrations above 1000 ng/mL (Aoyagi et al., 1984) or 910 ng/mL (Tsuchida et al., 1989). The low sensitivity for detection of separated AFP bands has been circumvented by using the sensitive detection system of antibody-affinity blotting (Taketa et al., 1985). By this method, AFP bands separated with samples having an AFP concentration as low as 50 ng/mL could be quantitatively detected (Taketa and Hirai, 1989). Furthermore, a parallel assay of a larger number of samples in a shorter period of time is possible. Modified crossed immunoaffinoelectrophoresis of Albanese et al. (1986) still requires larger amounts of serum relative to the concentrations of lectins used and are not essentially improved, compared to the originally described method of enzymatic amplification of immunoprecipitates (Taketa, 1983).

AFP bands separated by affinity electrophoresis with different lectins, detected by the antibody-affinity blotting, are shown in Fig. 1, including Con A, *Lens culinaris* agglutinin A (LCA-A), erythroagglutinating phytohemagglutinin of *Phaseolus vularis* (E-PHA), *Allomyrina dichotoma* agglutinin (allo A), *Ricinus communis* agglutinin-120 (RCA-120), and *Datura stramonium* agglutinin (DSA). Separated AFP bands may be readily identified by the nomenclature of Taketa et al. (1990b), as explained in the figure. Correspondence of the AFP bands defined by the present system of nomenclature to the peaks or fractions separated by other methods may be readily understood; e.g., AFP-C1 and -C2 correspond to AFP-N-C and -R-C, or Con A-unbound and -bound AFPs, respectively; and AFP-L1, -L2, and -L3 to AFP-N-L, -W-L, and -S-L, or LCA-unbound, -weakly bound and -strongly bound AFPs, respectively (Breborowicz et al., 1981). Each band does not necessarily represent a single molecular species of AFP with respect to its sugar chain structure. Some of the bands can be further subdivided by prolonged electrophoresis with the same lectins or by two-dimensional affinity electrophoresis with other lectins (Taketa et al., 1989b). AFP-P3 bands of gastrointestinal tumors and yolk sac tumors move faster than those of chronic liver diseases and hepatocellular carcinoma, although no further attempts to distinguish them have been made. Postulated oligosaccharide structures for these AFP bands have been reported elsewhere (Taketa et al., 1989b, 1990a).

4.3. Diagnostic Significance

Breborowicz et al. (1981) and Miyazaki et al. (1981) demonstrated increased proportions of Con A-nonreactive AFP and LCA-weakly reactive AFP in patients with yolk sac tumors and metastatic liver tumors, and of LCA-strongly reactive AFP in hepatocellular

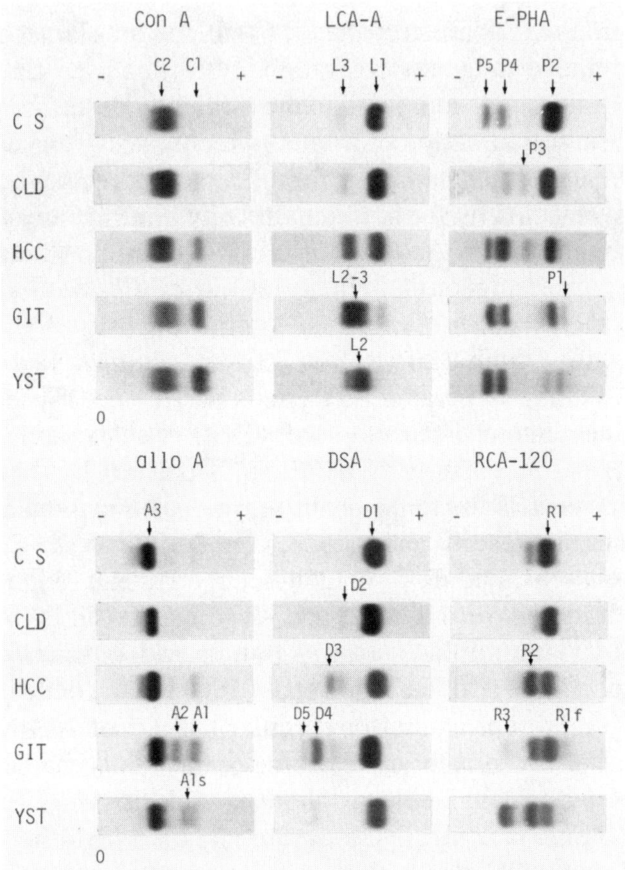

Fig. 1. Representative AFP bands for different pathophysiologic conditions. AFP bands were separated by affinity electrophoresis with different lectins under conditions described by Taketa et al. (1990a) for DSA; by Taketa et al. (1986) for RCA-120, which was used in place of RCA-I with identical results; and for the rest of the lectins used by Taketa (1987). CS, cord serum at full-term delivery; CLD, sera from patients with chronic liver disease; HCC, hepatocellular carcinoma; GIT, gastrointestinal tumors; and YST, yolk sac tumor. Major AFP bands are numbered consecutively from the anode, giving the lowest Arabic number, 1, to the most anodal band, and the numbers are suffixed to capitalized initial letters of the lectins used. Minor or infrequently appearing bands are identified by adding "s" for slow-migrating and "f" for fast-migrating bands relative to the major bands. Fused bands are expressed by hyphenating two bands.

carcinomas. The clinical significance of these observations has been confirmed by several other workers (Ishiguro et al., 1986b; Aoyagi et al., 1988; Tsuchida et al., 1989). The results of quantitative analysis of AFP bands separated by affinity electrophoresis with several lectins having different oligosaccharide specificities are summarized in Fig. 2 for benign and malignant diseases of clinical importance. Only major AFP bands that show significantly increased proportions on malignant transformation are included. The lectin-reactive patterns of AFP may be classified into the following four types, instead of the three proposed by Tsuchida et al. (1989): cord serum or liver type with predominant AFP-C2, -L1, -P2, -A3, -D1, and -R1, hepatocellular carcinoma type with predominant AFP-C2, -A3, and -D1 with variably increased AFP-L3, -P4, and -R2, gastrointestinal tumor type with increased AFP-C1, -L3, -P4 and -P5, together with the appearance of AFP-L2, -A1, -A2, -D4, -R1f, and -R3, and yolk sac tumor type with major AFP-C1, -L2, -L3, -P4, -P5, -A1s, and -R3, with a frequent appearance of AFP-P1 and -R1f. It is apparent that AFP-A1 and -A2 characterize gastrointestinal tumors and AFP-A1s is relatively specific to the yolk sac tumor AFP. Hepatoblastoma appears to produce hepatocellular carcinoma-type AFP in lectin reactivity (Tsuchida et al., 1989). Unclassified patterns of AFP in lung cancer (Moriwaki et al., 1987), renal cell carcinoma (Taketa et al., 1989a), and Sertoli-Leydig cell tumor (Motoyama et al., 1989) may, in part, represent the tumor heterogeneity in the expression of sugar chains (Taketa et al., 1990b). The hepatocellular carcinoma-type pattern of AFP bands present in fulminant hepatitis (Fig. 2) could be interpreted as indicating an undifferentiated phenotypic expression by hepatic injuries, as is also known for other cancer markers (Asaka et al., 1983; Taketa et al., 1988), including the increased total level of AFP in fulminant hepatitis. Increased levels of AFP in ataxia telangiectasia showed a liver-type pattern of lectin reactivity (Ishiguro et al., 1986a). On the other hand, LCA-reactive AFP is reported to increase in hereditary tyrosinemia (Smith and Kelleher, 1989), the pattern being compatible with a severe hepatic damage or premalignant liver.

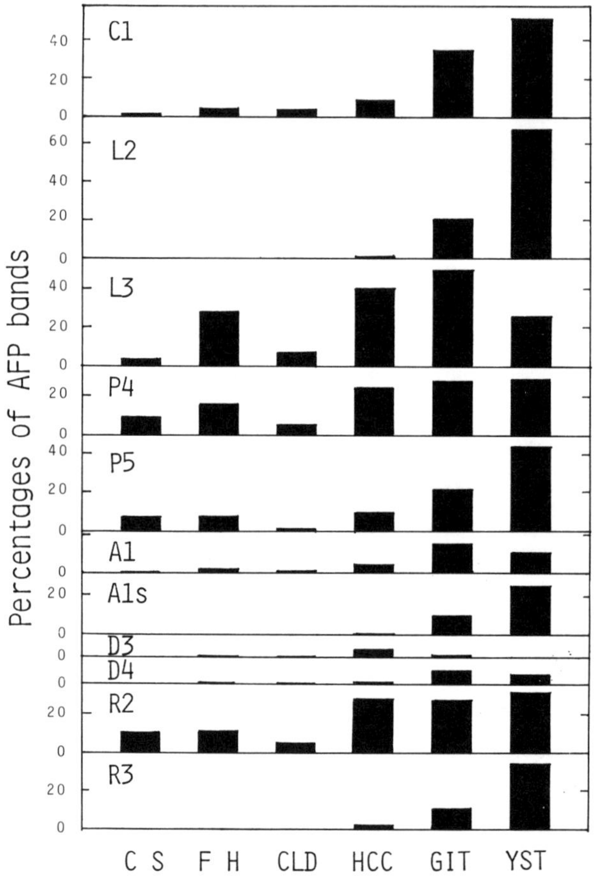

Fig. 2. Mean percentages of AFP bands separated by affinity electrophoresis with different lectins for varying pathophysiologic conditions. Only AFP bands that show increased proportions on malignant transformation and that have a diagnostic importance are shown. Scales are the same for all the AFP bands presented. Data are taken from the following sources: Taketa et al. (1990a) for AFP-D3 and -D4, Taketa et al. (1990b) for AFP-C1, -L2, -L3, -P4, -P5, -A1, and -A1s, and unpublished observation of Taketa et al. for AFP-R2 and -R3, which were analyzed on comparable populations.

When cutoff levels of the AFP bands were set to give a high specificity of 99.9% for a diagnostic purpose of differentiating patients with chronic hepatitis and liver cirrhosis from those with hepatocellular carcinomas, AFP-P4 had a sensitivity of 88% and AFP-L3 78% for cases with increased AFP levels above 200 ng/mL, and AFP-L3 and AFP-P4 in combination (positive when either alone or both exceeded the cutoff levels) had an increased sensitivity of 97% without significant reduction of the specificity (99.7%) (Taketa et al., 1990b). For cases of hepatocellular carcinoma with AFP levels below 200 ng/mL, the positive rates of AFP-L3 and AFP-P4 decreased to 68 and 63%, respectively, and to 88% in combined evaluation. The decreased sensitivities with lower levels of AFP may be accounted for by the masking effect of low levels of AFP produced by the host cirrhotic livers. Increased sensitivities in the combined evaluation of AFP-L3 and AFP-P4 is based on their independent expression, which reflects the tumor heterogeneity with respect to the AFP sugar chain (Taketa et al., 1990b).

Monoclonal antibodies directed to the epitopes of these altered sugar chains have been reported, although the specificities are too low to be applied to clinical studies (Kitagawa et al., 1986; Sittenfeld and Moreno, 1988; Suzuki et al., 1990). AFP antibody-lectin enzyme immunoassay of AFP sugar chain (Kinoshita et al., 1989) would have clinical application if the reproducibility were improved.

4.4. Prognostic Significance

In follow-up studies of patients with liver cirrhosis having increased serum levels of AFP, patients with increased proportions of AFP-L3 and/or AFP-P4 without demonstrable localized lesions of tumor were shown to develop hepatocellular carcinomas in a limited period of time (Taga et al., 1988; Taketa, 1990).

In patients with hepatocellular carcinoma having increased proportions of AFP-L3 and/or AFP-P4, the recurrence of tumors after surgical intervention could be readily predicted by the reappearance of unchanged lectin-reactive patterns of AFP, together with increasing serum levels of AFP.

5. Conclusion

Evidence is given to show that a considerable number of hepatocellular carcinomas and other AFP-producing tumors have been detected by the determination of total serum levels of AFP. The lectin-dependent fractionation of AFP would further provide a specific tool for differential diagnosis of hepatocellular carcinoma and its precursor lesions. Thus, AFP is still the "gold standard" of cancer markers, not only for screening and monitoring, but also for making diagnosis of hepatocellular carcinomas and other AFP-positive tumors.

It is hoped that this review article will assist the government in the understanding of AFP as a useful cancer marker and in improving the current status of its limited clinical use, not only in the United States (Sell, 1981), but also in Japan and other countries with a potential demand.

References

Abelev, G. I., S. D. Perova, N. I. Khramkova, Z. A. Postnikova, and I. S. Irlin (1963), *Transplant. Bull.* **1,** 174–180.

Abelev, G. I. (1971), *Adv. Cancer Res.* **14,** 295–357.

Abelev, G. I. (1989), *Tumor Biol.* **10,** 63–74.

Albanese, E. A., B. L. Bachl, and G. M. Mulcahy (1986), *Anal. Biochem.* **158,** 302–306.

Alpert, E. and E. R. Feller (1978), *Gastroenterology* **74,** 856–858.

Andorno, E., M. Salizzoni, R. Schieroni, and B. De Hemptinne (1989), *J. Nucl. Med. Allied Sci.* **33 (Suppl. to No. 3),** 132–134.

Aoyagi, Y., Y. Suzuki, M. Isemura, K. Soga, T. Ozaki, T. Ichida, K. Inoue, H. Sasaki, and F. Ichida (1984), *Gann* **75,** 809–815.

Aoyagi, Y., Y. Suzuki, M. Isemura, M. Nomoto, C. Sekine, K. Igarashi, and F. Ichida (1988), *Cancer* **61,** 769–774.

Asaka, M., K. Nagase, T. Miyazaki, and E. Alpert (1983), *Gastroenterology* **84,** 155–160.

Bloomer, J. R., T. A. Waldmann, K. R. McIntire, and G. Klatskin (1974), *Clin. Res.* **22,** 354A (Abstr.).

Bøg-Hansen, T.C., O. J. Bjerrum, and J. Ramlau (1975), *Scand. J. Immunol.* **4 (Suppl. 2),** 141–147.

Breborowicz, J., A. Mackiewicz, and D. Breborowicz (1981), *Scand. J. Immunol.* **14,** 15–20.

Brumm, C., C. Schulze, K. Charels, T. Morohoshi, and G. Klöppel (1989), *Histopathology* **14,** 503–513.

Chen, D. S. (1988), *Ital. J. Gastroenterol.* **20,** 287–290.

Chen, D. S., J. L. Sung, J. C. Sheu, M. Y. Lai, S. W. How, H. C. Hsu, C. S. Lee, and F. C. Wei (1984), *Gastroenterology* **86,** 1404–1409.

Curtin, J. P., S. C. Rubin, W. J. Hoskins, T. B. Hakes, and J. L. Lewis, Jr. (1989), *Obstet. Gynecol.* **73,** 893–895.

Duclos, B., J. L. Demangeat, L. Manil, P. Chamouard, R. Baumann, C. Demangeat, B. Bruno, D. Jaeck, A. Constantinesco, and J. P. Weill (1989), *Gastroenterol. Clin. Biol.* **13,** 910–915 .

Ferguson-Smith, M. A., H. M. May, E. O'Hare, and D. A. Aitken (1983), *J. Med. Genet.* **20,** 458 (Abstr.).

Gleiberman, A. S. and G. I. Abelev (1985), *Int. Rev. Cytol.* **95,** 229–266.

Gleiberman, A. S., Y. Y. Sharovskaya, and L. M. Chailakhjan (1989a), *Expt. Cell Res.* **184,** 228–234.

Gleiberman, A. S., E. I. Kudrjavtseva, Y. Y. Sharovskaya, and G. I. Abelev (1989b), *Mol. Biol. Med.* **6,** 95–107.

Greenberg, F., E. Rose, and E. Alpert (1990), *Gastroenterology* **98,** 1083–1085.

Hirai, H. (1979), *Methods Cancer Res.* **18,** 39–97.

Hirai, H. (1989), *Tumor Biol.* **8,** 86–93.

Hitchins, R. N., R. H. Begent, A. J. Green, F. Searl, V. van Heynigen, and K. D. Bagshawe (1989), *Nuklearmedizin* **28,** 29–33.

Hosokawa, S., M. Muramatsu, and K. Nagaike (1989), *Cancer Res.* **49,** 361–366.

Ishiguro, T., K. Taketa, and R. A. Gatti (1986a), *Dis. Markers* **4,** 293–297.

Ishiguro, T., H. Sakaguchi, M. Fukui, and I. Sugitachi (1986b), *Jpn. J. Surg.* **16,** 16–21.

Ishii, N., K. Nakata, T. Muro, R. Furukawa, K. Kondo, Y. Kusumoto, T. Koji, S. Nagataki, S. Nishi, Y. Tsukada, and H. Hirai (1984), *Ann. NY Acad. Sci.* **417,** 270–276.

Karvountzis, G. and A. Redecker (1974), *Ann. Intern. Med.* **80,** 156–160.

Kerckaert, J.-P., B. Bayard, and G. Biserte (1979), *Biochim. Biophys. Acta* **576,** 99–108.

Kinoshita, N., S. Suzuki, Y. Matsuda, and N. Taniguchi (1989), *Clin. Chim. Acta* **179,** 143. Published erratum appears in *Clin. Chim. Acta* 1989, **182,** 239.

Kitagawa, H., E. Ohkouchi, J. Hata, Y. Tsuchida, A. Kitagawa, and T. Tada (1986), *Gann* **77,** 1012–1017.

Koji, T., N. Ishii, T. Munehisa, Y. Kusumoto, S. Nakamura, A. Tamenishi, K. Kobayashi, A. Hara, Y. Tsukada, S. Nishi, and H. Hirai (1980), *Oncodev. Biol. Med.* **1,** 359–368.

Kondo, F., K. Wada, Y. Nagato, T. Nakajima, Y. Kondo, N. Hirooka, M. Ebara, M. Ohto, and K. Okuda (1989), *Hepatology* **9,** 751–755.

Lafarge-Frayssinet, C. H., J. M. Torres, M. Laborda, M. Frain, and J. Uriel (1989), *Biochem. Biophys. Res. Commun.* **159,** 112–118.
Liaw, Y. F., D. I. Tai, C. M. Chu, D. Y. Lin, I. S. Sheen, T. J. Chen, and C. C. Pao (1986), *Gastroenterology* **90,** 263–267.
The Liver Study Group of Japan (1987), *Cancer* **60,** 1400–1411.
The Liver Study Group of Japan (1988), *Acta Hepatol. Jpn.* **29,** 1619–1626.
Masseyeff, R., C. Bonet, J. Dronet, P. Sudaka, and C. Lalanne (1974), *Digestion* **10,** 17–28.
Mihalev, A., D. Tzingilev, and L. M. Sirakov (1978), *Neoplasma* **23,** 103–107.
Miyazaki, J., Y. Endo, and T. Oda (1981), *Acta Hepatol. Jpn.* **22,** 1559–1568.
Moriwaki, Y., K. Higashino, K. Taketa, T. Hada, S. Tamura, and K. Yamaguchi (1987), *Am. J. Gastroenterol.* **82,** 1207–1211.
Moro, R., C. Heuguerot, J. Vercelli-Retta, W. Fielitz, J. J. Lopez, and R. Roca (1984), *Nucl. Med. Commun.* **5,** 5–12.
Motoyama, I., H. Watanabe, A. Gotoh, S. Takeuchi, N. Tanebe, I. Nashimoto (1989), *Cancer* **63,** 2047–2053.
Nakao, K., Y. Miyao, Y. Ohe, and T. Tamaoki (1989), *Nucleic Acids Res.* **17,** 9833–9842.
Nishi, S., and H. Hirai (1973), *Gann Monogr. Cancer Res.* **14,** 79–87.
Nomura F., K. Ohnishi, and Y. Tanabe, (1989), *Cancer* **64,** 1700–1707.
Okimoto, Y., T. Fujihara, M. Tsuda, M. Kinoshita, M. Takaoka, Y. Uchida, Y. Fukuda, and H. Imura (1989), *Jpn. J. Gastroenterol.* **86,** 2812–2815.
Okuda, K. (1986), *Hepatology* **6,** 729–738.
Parmelee, D. C., M. A. Evenson, and H. F. Deutsch (1978), *J. Biol. Chem.* **253,** 2114–2119.
Regan, L. S. (1989), *Arch. Intern. Med.* **149,** 1741–1744.
Ruoslahti, E. and M. Seppälä (1971), *Int. J. Cancer* **8,** 374–383.
Sarcione, E. J. and W. Biddle (1987), *Dis. Markers* **5,** 75–79.
Sawadaishi, K., T. Morinaga, and T. Tamaoki (1988), *Mol. Cell. Biol.* **8,** 5179–5187.
Sell, S., R. D. Reynolds, and W. Reutter (1974), *J. Natl. Cancer Inst.* **53,** 289–291.
Sell, S., D. Stillman, and N. Gochman (1976), *Am. J. Clin. Pathol.* **66,** 847–853.
Sell, S. (1981), *Hum. Pathol.* **12,** 959–963.
Sell, S. (1990), *Clin. Lab. Med.* **10,** 1–37.
Sittenfeld, A. and E. Moreno (1988), *J. Immunol. Methods* **106,** 19–26.
Smith, C. J., and P. C. Kelleher (1973), *Biochim. Biophys. Acta* **317,** 231–235.
Smith, C. J. P., and P. C. Kelleher (1989), in *Biological Activities of Alpha$_1$-Fetoprotein,* vol. 2 (Mizejewski, G. J., and H. I. Jacobson, eds.), CRC, Boca Raton, FL, pp. 35–43.
Sonoda, T., K. Shirabe, K. Takenaka, T. Kanematsu, K. Yasumori, and K. Sugimachi (1989), *Hepatology* **10,** 1003–1007.

Springolo, E., M. C. Kew, J. Esser, M. Beyers, J. D. Conradie, and J. Levin (1989), *Hepatology* **9,** 116–120.

Sugimoto, M., T. Itsukaichi, K. Ishii, Y. Sumino, S. Sugano, T. Abei, and Y. Imanura (1987), *Am. J. Gastroenterol.* **82,** 69–71.

Suzuki, Y., Y. Aoyagi, M. Muramatsu, K. Igarashi, A. Saito, M. Oguro, M. Isemura, and H. Asakura (1990), *Ann. Clin. Biochem.* **27,** 121–128.

Taga, H., H. Hirai, H. Ishizuka, and H. Kaneda (1988), *Tumor Biol.* **9,** 110–115.

Taketa, K. (1983), *Electrophoresis* **4,** 371–373.

Taketa, K. (1987), *Electrophoresis* **8,** 409–414.

Taketa, K. (1991), *Affinity Electropohoresis: Principles and Clinical Application* (Breborowicz, J. and A. Mackiewicz, eds.), CRC, Boca Raton, FL, in press.

Taketa, K. and H. Hirai (1989), *Electrophoresis* **10,** 562–567.

Taketa, K., E. Ichikawa, H. Taga, and H. Hirai (1985), *Electrophoresis* **6,** 492–497.

Taketa, K., E. Ichikawa, K. Umetsu, and T. Suzuki (1986), *Cancer Lett.* **31,** 325–331.

Taketa, K., J. Shimamura, M. Ueda, Y. Shimada, and K. Kosaka (1988), *Cancer Res.* **48,** 467–474.

Taketa, K., E. Ichikawa, H. Sakuda, T. Iwamasa, M. Hayakawa, H. Taga, and H. Hirai (1989a), *Tumor Biol.* **10,** 275–280.

Taketa, K., E. Ichikawa, J. Sato, H. Taga, and H. Hirai (1989b), *Electrophoresis* **10,** 825–829.

Taketa, K., E. Ichikawa, T. Yamamoto, H. Kato, S. Matsura, H. Taga, and H. Hirai (1990a), *Tumor Biol.*, **11,** 220–228.

Taketa, K., C. Sekiya, M. Namiki, K. Akamatsu, Y. Ohta, Y. Endo, and K. Kosaka (1990b), *Gastroenterology*, **99,** 508–518.

Tamaoki, T. (1989), *J. Tumor Marker Oncol.* **4,** 161 (Abstr.).

Tatarinov, Yu. S. (1963), 1st Int. Biochem. Congress of the USSR, *Abstr. Acad. of Sci. USSR,* Moscow-Leningrad **2,** 274 (Abstract).

Tatarinov, Yu. S. (1964), *Vopr. Med. Khimii* **10,** 90–91.

Tsuchida, Y., Y. Endo, S. Saito, M. Kaneko, K. Shiraki, and K. Ohmi (1978), *J. Pediatr. Surg.* **13,** 155–156.

Tsuchida, Y., M. Kaneko, M. Fukui, H. Sakaguchi, and T. Ishiguro (1989), *J. Pediatr. Surg.* **24,** 350–355.

Tuchman, M., D. K. Freese, H. L. Sharp, C. B. Whitley, M. L. Ramnaraine, R. A. Ulstrom, J. S. Najarian, N. Ascher, N. R. M. Buist, and A. B. Terry (1985), *J. Inher. Metab. Dis.* **8,** 21–24.

Urabe, T., S. Hayashi, S. Terasaki, M. Terada, E. Matsushita, S. Kaneko, Y. Inagaki, M. Yoneshima, M. Unoura, K. Kobayashi, and N. Hattori (1990), *Jpn. J. Gastroenterol.* **87,** 100–108.

Watanabe, A., M. Miyazaki, and K. Taketa (1976a), *Cancer Res.* **36,** 2171–2175.

Watanabe, A., M. Miyazaki, and K. Taketa (1976b), *Experientia* **32,** 470–471.
Weeks, I., A. K. Campbell, and J. S. Woodhead (1983), *Clin. Chem.* **29,** 1480–1483.
Yamashita, K., A. Hitoi, Y. Tsuchida, S. Nishi, and A. Kobata (1983), *Cancer Res.* **43,** 4691–4695.
Yoshima, H., T. Mizuochi, M. Ishii, and A. Kobata (1980), *Cancer Res.* **40,** 4276–4281.

Chapter 4

Carcinoembryonic Antigen

Hanna M. Sikorska,
Abraham Fuks, and Phil Gold

1. Introduction

Carcinoembryonic antigen (CEA), a glycoprotein with a mol mass of 180 kDa was first described in 1965 by Gold and Freedman (1965). The protein core consists of a single polypeptide chain, containing a 107 amino acid NH-terminal domain and three highly homologous domains of 178 amino acids each (Beauchemin et al., 1987; Oikawa et al., 1987a). The C-terminal domain consists of 26 amino acids and is strongly hydrophobic, providing a potential attachment site for CEA to the plasma membrane through a phosphatidylinositolglycan anchor (Hefta et al., 1988). Carbohydrate side chains constitute more than half of the mol mass and 28 potential N-linked glycosylation sites on CEA have been identified (Beauchemin et al., 1987; Oikawa et al., 1987a). CEA, an oncodevelopmental human tumor marker, is associated with carcinomas, especially those from the gastrointestinal tract (Shively and Beatty, 1985; Sikorska et al., 1988).

From: *Serological Cancer Markers* Edited by Stewart Sell ©1992 The Humana Press, Totowa, NJ

Immunobiochemical studies revealed a number of closely related molecules and suggested the existence of a gene family. Among these molecules are the nonspecific crossreacting antigen (NCA), biliary glycoprotein (BGPI-II), meconium antigen (MA), pregnancy-specific β-glycoproteins (PSβG), and tumor-extracted antigen (TEX) (Thompson and Zimmermann, 1988). The exact size of this family and relationship between it and other known glycoproteins has been difficult to ascertain, probably owing to mol wt variation dependent on glycosylation, degradation, or aggregation, and variations in immunospecificity of antibody probes (Engvall et al., 1978; Kessler et al., 1978).

Cloning the genes for CEA and related antigens proved to be difficult, caused largely by the high level of glycosylation of these proteins, which made protein sequencing a major task (Shively and Beatty, 1985). Once that obstacle had been overcome (Paxton et al., 1987), the screening of cDNA libraries using either synthetic oligonucleotides based on known protein sequence (Beauchemin et al., 1987; Zimmermann et al., 1987a), or anti-CEA antibodies for identification of protein expressed in suitable vectors (Oikawa et al., 1987a; Kamarck et al., 1987), led to the isolation of cDNA clones for CEA and related family members. The CEA family consists of at least 10 genes that are localized to two clusters on chromosome 19 (Kamarck et al., 1987; Thompson et al., 1987; Zimmermann et al., 1988). Thus far, sequence data for at least six of these genes have been obtained and the complete primary structures deduced for: CEA (Beauchemin et al., 1987; Oikawa et al., 1987a; Zimmermann et al., 1987a), NCA (Tawaragi et al., 1988; Neumaier et al., 1988), PSβG (Streydio et al., 1988; Watanabe and Chou, 1988a,b; Khan and Hammarström, 1990), PSβ/FL-NCA (Khan and Hammarström, 1989; Khan et al., 1989), and BGP (Hinoda et al., 1988).

The high degree of sequence conservation between these proteins suggests a common ancestry (Thompson and Zimmermann, 1988). Predicted protein and DNA sequence comparisons have revealed that the CEA gene family is a subset of the immunoglobulin supergene family (Beauchemin et al., 1987; Oikawa et al., 1987b; Paxton et al., 1987; Williams, 1987).

The expression of the CEA gene family has been studied in a number of tumors and normal tissues (Cournoyer et al., 1988; Zimmermann et al., 1988). Several mRNA species belonging to the CEA family have been reported to be expressed in chronic myeloid leukemia granulocytes, choriocarcinoma, fetal liver, colon, pancreas, gall bladder, colonic adenocarcinomas (CEA and NCA), squamous lung carcinoma (NCA only), normal colon (CEA and NCA), breast carcinoma (NCA only), and first trimester human placenta (PSβG) (Barnett et al., 1987; Cournoyer et al., 1988; Sato et al., 1988; Zimmermann et al., 1988; Khan and Hammarström, 1989; McLenachan and Mansfield, 1989).

The biological function of the CEA protein family is still unclear, although discovery of CEA-like genes in mice and rats and the opportunity of CEA expression in transfected Chinese hamster ovary cells, mouse fibroblasts, and transgenic mice will be important in the identification of its biological function (Beauchemin et al., 1989; Kodelja et al., 1989; Hefta et al., 1990). Cell–cell recognition, adhesion, cell differentiation, enhancement of metastasis, or bacterial recognition have been recently suggested as possible biological functional roles of CEA (Shuster et al., 1980; Streydio et al., 1988; Benchimol et al., 1989; Khan and Hammarström, 1989; Hostetter et al., 1990; Leusch et al., 1990).

The relationship, if any, between CEA and growth factors, protooncogenes and "tumor suppressor genes" (Chakrabaity et al., 1988; Marx, 1989) in carcinogenesis, are not clear. The recent molecular identification in the NIH 3T3 mouse cell line of a CEA-like gene whose expression is strongly induced by *ras* and *mos* oncogenes (Klemenz et al., 1989), hints at the involvement of oncogenes in triggering the expression of CEA and PSβG in gastrointestinal cancer cells.

2. The Role of Serum CEA Measurements in Cancer Diagnosis and Prognosis

Colon cancer is the second most common fatal malignancy in North America. This is in part owing to the late stage at which it is often diagnosed (Mayer, 1988). In the search for tumor markers to aid in the early diagnosis of cancer, several oncodevelopmental entities have been described, most of which have limited clinical utility (Garrett and Kurtz, 1986). Currently, the most clinically useful of these oncofetal markers is CEA.

Since its discovery 25 years ago, a large body of literature has been published (Gold and Freedman, 1965; Ladenson and McDonald, 1980; Beatty and Terz, 1982; Cooper and O'Quigley, 1982; Fletcher, 1986; Sikorska et al., 1988) describing the value of serum CEA measurements in the care of cancer patients. Information concerning the clinical usefulness of CEA has also been reviewed in two major consensus conferences held in 1977 and 1980 (Proceedings of the First International Conference on the Clinical Use of Carcinoembryonic Antigen, 1978; Neville, 1981; Goodyear et al., 1984).

The history of CEA, like that of many other novel clinical techniques, is checkered. The initial high expectations were tempered by the finding of elevated plasma CEA levels in several benign diseases (Table 1) (LoGerfo et al., 1972; Deleriche et al., 1973; Pusztaszeri and Mach, 1973; Lowenstein and Zamcheck, 1978; Chu et al., 1979; Endo et al., 1979; Wittekind et al., 1981; Stockley et al., 1986). Today, with refinements in assay technique and the accumulation of data, we understand that the differences in CEA levels between normal and tumor-bearing individuals are quantitative rather than qualitative in nature. The circulating CEA level in a given patient is the end result of various factors, including the level of gene expression, rate of synthesis of CEA, its subsequent release by the tumor, the half-life of CEA in the circulation, the degree of necrosis and vascularization of the tumor, as well as the rate of CEA catabolism by the liver.

Despite the complexity of the system, the CEA assay has taken its place in the management of patients with cancer. Although guidelines for the appropriate use of CEA assays have been reported, Fletcher (1986) argues that physicians in practice apparently have greater confidence in the practical value of CEA measurements than do "experts" in the field. In one study in 1979, over 50% of physicians believed that a CEA assay was worthwhile for initial detec-

Table 1
Some Nonmalignant Conditions Associated[a] with Elevated Plasma Levels of Carcinoembryonic Antigen

Liver diseases
Alcoholic hepatitis
Chronic active hepatitis
Primary biliary cirrhosis
Cryptogenic cirrhosis
Obstructive jaundice
Bowel diseases
Peptic ulcer
Pancreatitis
Diverticulitis
Inflammatory bowel disease
Breast diseases
Fibrocystic breast disease
Lung diseases
Bronchitis
Other
Smoking
Renal failure

[a]In general, the CEA levels in the above conditions are stable when measured serially.

tion of colonic cancer and that elevated serum levels of CEA in a nonsmoking person without symptoms should prompt an aggressive search for colonic cancer. Both premises were questioned by investigators in the CEA field at that time (Vest and Roche, 1982), and this skepticism continues to the present.

2.1. "Normal" CEA Values

Levels of 2.5–5.0 ng/mL (depending on the assay used) are commonly used as cutoff points for distinguishing normal from abnormal levels. In two large surveys of apparently normal persons, 85–87% had antigen levels of less than 2.5 ng/mL, 95–98%

had levels of less than 5 ng/mL, and virtually no one had a level greater than 10 ng/mL (Herbeth and Bagrel, 1980; Tabor et al., 1981). CEA concentrations are, in general, more often elevated in smokers than in nonsmokers (Stevens and Mackay, 1973; Stevens et al., 1975; Clarke et al., 1980; Merril et al., 1981; Stockley et al., 1986), and in men than in women (Beaudonnet et al., 1981). The same is true for older subjects (Berardi et al., 1977; Touitou et al., 1984). Racial differences in the frequency of serum elevations of CEA have been suggested (Haines et al., 1979), but not established.

2.2. Screening for Cancer with CEA

Screening in medical practice is the procedure of searching for a disease in asymptomatic individuals in order to detect a particular disease process at an early stage. Early detection can often lead to more effective treatment than is possible if the disease is detected after it has become symptomatic.

Currently available CEA assays cannot be used as screening tests for colorectal cancer insofar as false-negative tests can be obtained. The earlier the stage of colorectal cancer (Duke's Stages A and B), the less likely it is that the CEA level is elevated. Assays for CEA more readily detect advanced colorectal cancer of Duke's Stages C and D (Williams et al., 1977; Wanebo et al., 1978a; Herbeth and Bagrel, 1980; Goldenberg et al., 1981; Fletcher, 1986).

CEA assays perform no better in screening for other cancers commonly associated with elevated CEA levels, again because of the lack of sensitivity of existing tests. Elevated plasma levels of CEA, or CEA-reactive material, have been described in advanced breast cancer (De Jong-Bakker et al., 1981; Falkson et al., 1982; Laurence et al., 1972; Steward et al., 1974; Tormey et al., 1975, 1977), pancreatic cancer (Laurence et al., 1972; Zamcheck et al., 1972; Deleriche et al., 1973; Ona et al., 1973; Fitzgerald et al., 1978; Kalser et al., 1978; Medical Research Council Tumour Products Committee, 1980; Podolsky et al., 1981; Begent, 1984; Tsutsumi et al., 1984; Fabris et al., 1985; Del Favero et al., 1986b), lung cancer (Laurence et al., 1972; Lokich, 1982), and other noncolonic adenocarcinomas (Gold et al., 1979; Persijn, 1980; Te Velde et al., 1982), but they do not, for the most part, detect early stages of these diseases (Table 2 [Klavins et al., 1985]). This relatively low sensitivity of CEA assays, in the context of their specificity profiles, together with the low prevalence of cancer in asymptomatic populations, lead to too many false-positive and false-negative results to be a useful screening test for detecting early cancers. This is supported by data from the large, population-based cohort, Framingham study, in which serum samples from patients with newly detected cancers were examined for CEA levels (Williams et al., 1977). The conclusion is also in agreement with the recommendations of the National Institutes of Health Consensus Development Conference of 1981 (Goldenberg et al., 1981).

2.3. Tumor Diagnosis with CEA Assays

A diagnostic test for cancer is one that confirms or rules out the presence of cancer in patients who are suspected of having the disease.

2.3.1. Colonic Adenocarcinoma and Polyps

Although 70–80% of patients with colonic adenocarcinoma have circulating CEA, as described originally by Gold and Freedman (1965), the CEA assay should not be used as the sole diagnostic test for suspected cancer. Positive CEA in symptomatic patients cannot be interpreted as indicating the presence of malignant growth as various benign conditions are associated with elevated CEA levels (Table 1). Foremost among these is liver disease (Lowenstein and Zamcheck, 1977); over 90% of patients with chronic liver disease and 50% of those with acute liver disease have raised plasma levels of CEA, or CEA-like substances (Bullen et al., 1977). In addition to the conditions listed in Table 1, there are numerous single case reports of elevations of CEA, or CEA-like substances in a variety of conditions. However, benign conditions are rarely a cause of substantial elevations (>10 ng/mL) and such conditions do not give rise to the progressive increases in CEA levels seen in cancerous conditions. CEA levels are likely to be higher in symptomatic,

Table 2
Incidence of Elevated Serum CEA in Malignant Neoplasms[a]

Neoplasms	%	Neoplasms	%
Colon carcinomas	100	Primary uveal melanomas	36
Choriocarcinomas[b]	100	Neuroblastomas	35
Medullary thyroid Ca.	85	Seminomas	33
Osteosarcomas	81	Basal cell Ca.	33
Retinoblastomas	80	Gastric carcinomas	32
Ovarian cystadenoca.	77	Laryngeal Ca.	31
Mycosis fungoides	75	Endometrial Ca.	30
Hepatomas	70	Uterine cervix	
Esophageal carcinomas	67	intraepithelial Ca.	29
Adenoca. of cervix	68	Ca. of buccal mucosa	27
Lung carcinomas	67	Craniopharyngiomas	25
Ca. of small intestine	67	Embryonal	
Urinary bladder Ca.	60	rhabdomyosarcomas	24
Renal Ca.	36	Carcinomas of oropharynx	23
Neural crest tumors	43	Brain tumors	22
Breast carcinomas	42	Testicular teratomas	9
Prostatic Ca.[c]			

[a]The table is reproduced after Klavins et al., 1985.
[b]Human chorionic gonadotropin is more specific for this tumor.
[c]Prostatic acid phosphatase is more specific for this tumor.

rather than asymptomatic, colorectal cancer patients, but such patients are more likely to have advanced disease (Sculier et al., 1987).

Both the frequency of positive CEA assays and the absolute CEA levels found in the plasma of patients rise with increasing tumor burden. Thus, the incidence of positive CEA assays may range from 20% in patients with Duke's Stage A to 90% in Duke's Stage D colon cancer. Holyoke et al. (1975) demonstrated significant CEA elevations of 18, 53, 62, 65, and 79% in patients with colon cancer of Duke's Stages A, B_1, B_2, C_1, and C_2, respectively. Similar results have been reported by Booth et al. (1974) and recently by Goldberg et al. (1989). Increased CEA has also been observed in fecal samples from 50% of colorectal carcinoma patients; the antigen appears as a membrane-bound form, reflecting the abrasive destruction of epithelial cells (Sugamo et al., 1989).

Adenomatous colonic polyps are the precursors of invasive cancer. Colonic polyps are usually not associated with elevated serum CEA levels, and serum CEA levels are not presently useful for distinguishing locally invasive polyps from benign lesions (Fuks et al., 1980; Goldberg et al., 1989). Similar comments apply to the CEA assay in distinguishing benign from early malignant lesions of the stomach and pancreas (Holyoke et al., 1979; Zamcheck and Martin, 1981b; Castelli et al., 1986; Del Favero et al., 1986a).

2.3.2. Other Malignancies

Sensitive radio- and enzyme immunoassays have shown that serum CEA may be elevated in neoplastic diseases of the lung, breast, prostate, bladder, and stomach, as well as in various gynecologic malignancies (Cooper et al., 1979).

As in the case of colorectal cancer, CEA measurements are not sufficient as the sole parameter for diagnosis of early *breast cancer* (Concannon et al., 1973; Meeker et al., 1973; Livingstone et al., 1974; Borthwick et al., 1977; Baylin et al., 1978; Haagensen et al., 1978a; Varnavides et al., 1978; Rimstein et al., 1979; Breslin and Healy, 1981; Doyle et al., 1981; Waalkes et al., 1984). Approximately 30% of patients with breast carcinoma do not produce CEA, whereas an elevated CEA was observed in some women with benign breast diseases (4–18%) (Concannon et al., 1973; Meeker et al., 1973; Wang et al., 1975; Borthwick et al., 1977; Haagensen et al., 1978a; Varnavides et al., 1978; Rimstein et al., 1979; Breslin and Healy, 1981).

It is apparent from published data that the plasma CEA level is strongly related to the stage of breast cancer (Steward et al., 1974; Baylin et al., 1978; Myers et al., 1978; Wahren et al., 1978; Coombes et al., 1981; Silva et al., 1982; Gray, 1984; Fletcher, 1986; Loprinzi and Ahmann, 1986; Bates and Longo, 1987). The more advanced the clinical stage, the higher the CEA level at the time of diagnosis.

The prevalence of elevated CEA in stage I patients with breast cancer is 9% (range 0–15%), in stage II, 23% (range 0–43%), and in stage III highly metastatic patients, the prevalence is 45% (31–64%). The highest frequency of raised CEA occurs in disease stage IV. Overall, 58% of patients (29–100% range) with metastases have positive CEA tests. The correlation between CEA level and occurrence of metastases varies with the site of metastases (Baylin et al., 1978). Patients with bone or visceral involvement have more frequent elevations (48–100%) and higher levels than patients with soft tissue involvement (9–52%).

In lung cancer, CEA can also be a useful biomarker. It is elevated in about two-thirds of patients with nonsmall-cell lung cancer and one-third of those with small-cell lung cancer when compared to those with benign lung diseases (Waalkes et al., 1980; Goslin et al., 1983; Sculier et al., 1987). Determination of CEA concentration can be used as a diagnostic tool of malignancy in pleural effusions, as 40–70% first punctures show positive CEA (Sculier et al., 1987).

Although investigated much less, the determination of CEA levels in cerebrospinal fluid seems useful in diagnosing meningeal carcinomatosis (Yap et al., 1980), whereas analysis of gastric juice CEA is useful in identifying high-risk patients for gastric cancer (Tatsuta et al., 1988). Serum CEA has not proved satisfactory as an indicator of early gastric cancer (Ellis et al., 1978), but elevated CEA levels were detected in the majority of patients with advanced carcinoma of the stomach (Dittrich et al., 1985; Goldberg et al., 1989).

3. Prognostic Value of Serum CEA

3.1. Colorectal Cancer

Although serum CEA assays have not been as useful as had been envisaged initially in the screening and diagnosis of colonic carcinoma, they have a definite role in the clinical management of patients with colorectal adenocarcinomas (Zamcheck, 1981a). Preoperative serum CEA levels in diagnosed colorectal cancer are elevated in 40–70% of patients (Mach et al., 1974a; Martin et al., 1976; Tomoda and Furusawa, 1981; Lunde and Havig, 1982). Preoperative serum CEA concentrations correlate inversely with tumor grade and directly with pathological stage (LoGerfo and Hester, 1975; Zamcheck et al., 1975; Jubert et al., 1978; Wanebo et al., 1978a; Zamcheck, 1978; Beatty et al., 1979; Arnaud et al., 1980; Goslin et al., 1980; Wolmark et al., 1981; Midiri et al., 1983; Lewi et al., 1984; Onetto et al., 1985; Aabo et al. 1986; Lazorthes et al., 1986). Thus, CEA is raised in 95% of patients with well-differentiated tumors, whereas the level is raised in as few as 30% of those with poorly differentiated adenocarcinomas (Goslin et al., 1980; Armitage et al., 1984a).

The higher the preoperative CEA level, the more likely is a postoperative tumor recurrence. A significant negative correlation between preoperative elevated plasma CEA levels and patient survival has been observed (LoGerfo and Hester, 1975; Herrera et al., 1977; Evans et al., 1978; Jubert et al., 1978; Beatty et al., 1979; Goslin et al., 1980; Kohler et al., 1980; Stabb et al., 1981; Onetto et al., 1985; Nap et al., 1985). Despite disagreement among various groups that have explored the relationship between preoperative CEA and prognosis, most studies report that a high preoperative CEA level is indicative of a poor prognosis. This association is often as discriminating as pathological staging and grading (Herrera et al., 1976; Wanebo et al., 1978a; Goslin et al., 1980; Kohler et al., 1980; Lavin et al., 1981; Wolmark et al., 1981; Steele et al., 1982; Northover, 1986; Barone et al., 1990; Stamatiadis et al., 1990). On the basis of these observations, the National Institutes of Health suggested in their 1981 Consensus Statement that CEA determination should be used as an adjunct to clinicopathological staging (Summary of an NIH Consensus Statement, 1981). However, it is still uncertain what absolute preoperative CEA value reliably discriminates high-risk from low-risk cases for postoperative recurrences (LoGerfo and Hester, 1975; Herrera et al., 1977; Jubert et al., 1978; Evans et al., 1979; Beatty et al., 1979; Goslin et al., 1980; Stabb et al., 1981; Aabo et al., 1986).

3.2.1. Other Cancers

CEA is also an important marker of prognosis for mammary cancer. Preoperative CEA levels have been studied as prognostic factors in early breast cancer by many investigators. The results are variable and controversial (Laurence et al., 1972; Chu and Nemoto, 1973; Wang et al., 1975; Tormey et al., 1977; Falkson et al., 1978; Haagensen et al., 1978a,b; Myers et al., 1978, 1979a; Pompecki et al., 1978; Tormey and Waalkes, 1978; Waalkes et al., 1978; Beatty et al., 1979; Rimstein et al., 1979; Shousha et al., 1979; Cantwell et al., 1980; Koch et al., 1980; Bezwoda et al., 1981; Chatal et al., 1981; Cillari et al., 1981; De Jong-Bakker et al., 1981; Doyle et al., 1981; Mansour et al., 1983; Mughal et al., 1983; Lang et al., 1984; Palazzo et al., 1984, Palazzo, 1986; Wang et al., 1984; Fletcher, 1986; Zimmerman et al., 1987b), but generally there seems to be sufficient evidence to consider the CEA level a marker of prognosis for breast cancer (Wang et al., 1975; Haagensen et al., 1978b; Myers et al., 1978, 1979a; Coombes et al., 1981; Tormey et al., 1982; Mansour et al., 1983; Fletcher, 1986; Palazzo, 1986).

In most cases, preoperatively raised CEA levels have been found to be associated with a poorer prognosis. The higher the level the more likely the tumor is to recur, or relapse will occur sooner. Serial postoperative plasma CEA level measurements in clinically disease-free patients appears to be an accurate indicator of the development of metastatic disease (Haagensen et al., 1978a; Neville et al., 1978; Loprinzi and Ahmann, 1986). In the majority of cases rising CEA levels indicate development of metastases and a poor prognosis.

An elevated or rising CEA level preceded clinical recurrence by 1–31 mo in some patients (Baylin et al., 1978; Neville et al., 1978; Coombes et al., 1980).

Reported clinical evidence also indicates that both pre- and posttherapy CEA levels could serve as prognostic markers in stomach (Shek, 1984) and lung (Concannon et al., 1978; Stokes et al., 1980) cancers, although the evidence is not as compelling and well documented as for colon and breast.

4. CEA in Monitoring the Course of Cancer Treatment

A rise in the blood CEA concentration in a patient after apparently successful surgical treatment for cancer has repeatedly been shown to signal a recurrence of the tumor. Although the best evidence for this phenomenon is found in colorectal cancer, similar data have been obtained in other CEA-expressing tumors.

Following a complete surgical resection of colorectal cancer, the blood CEA concentration, if elevated before surgery, falls to the normal range in nearly all patients (Arnaud et al., 1980). The fall usually occurs within 1 mo, but sometimes takes up to 4 mo (Mach et al., 1978). If levels do not fall to the normal range, it is likely that an incomplete resection has taken place or the disease has already metastasized. After the initial fall, it is not uncommon for transient, small elevations in CEA levels to occur in the absence of recurrent tumor. However, a sustained and progressive rise is strong evidence for recurrence. Serial CEA monitoring is currently advocated as the best noninvasive technique for detecting recurrent colorectal cancer (Herrera et al., 1977; Shani et al., 1978; Sugarbaker et al., 1978; Wanebo et al., 1978b; National Institute of Health Consensus Development Conference, 1981; Szymendera et al., 1982).

The literature suggests various parameters for predicting tumor recurrence based on postoperative CEA monitoring for colorectal carcinomas (Mach et al., 1978; Moertel et al., 1978; Beatty et al., 1979; Wood et al., 1980; Beart et al., 1981, 1983; Steele et al., 1982; Szymendera et al., 1982; Boey et al., 1984). These include:

1. CEA levels exceeding a predetermined cutoff value; and
2. Progressively rising CEA levels exceeding a specific rate of change.

Different cutoff values ranging from 4 to 20 ng/mL have been suggested depending on assay sensitivity and the patient population studied. Studies based on such "decision rules" have yielded a variety of sensitivity/specificity ratios. Moreover, the multiplicity of rules, each one tested in different patient cohorts, has led to difficulties in data interpretation and, clearly, standardization is required.

More recently, it has been suggested that when CEA increases faster than an average of 12.6% per mo, recurrence should be suspected (Denstman et al., 1986). Serial CEA determinations may, therefore, allow initiation of antitumor chemotherapy, radiotherapy, or "second-look" surgery at an earlier stage of progression of recurrent colorectal cancer and offer the possibility of remission to some patients. Because the overall prognosis for patients with recurrent disease after surgical resection is dismal, serum CEA determination may offer the only chance of a cure for a select group of individuals.

There is a general agreement that the regular and sequential assay of plasma CEA provides valuable information in the post-operative surveillance of patients receiving drug therapy, and as a pretreatment predictor of recurrence in patients with other non-gastrointestinal cancers, such as those of the breast (Lokich et al., 1978; Ahlemann et al., 1980; Coombes et al., 1980; Chatal et al., 1981; Falkson et al., 1982; Mughal et al., 1983; Lang et al., 1984; Andrew et al., 1986; Burgess, 1986) and lung (Gropp et al., 1978; Waalkes et al., 1980; Aroney et al., 1984; Krischke et al., 1988; Sculier et al., 1987), and in meningeal carcinomatosis (Yap et al., 1980). CEA levels also correlate well with regression or progression of cancer growth during chemotherapy and radiotherapy of cancers of the gastrointestinal tract, lung, and breast, and the test may be useful in monitoring the effectiveness of such treatments (Vider et al., 1974; Sugarbaker et al., 1976; Mayer et al., 1978; Shinkai et al., 1986; Barone et al., 1990).

Thus, the available data indicate that the assay for CEA is useful, both preoperatively and postoperatively, in the management of patients in whom the diagnosis of cancer has already been established. Major advances in treatment of recurrent disease will further increase the clinical utility of the CEA assay.

5. Immunohistochemical Diagnosis of Neoplastic Tissue with CEA-Specific Antibodies

Immunoperoxidase staining of neoplastic tissues is a simple, sensitive method widely used in today's clinical pathology laboratory. The value of tissue CEA staining in cancer diagnosis depends greatly on the immunoreactivity of the antibodies used for detection. A wealth of monoclonal antibodies to CEA has been generated. They exhibit various degrees of crossreactivity to other members of CEA family, but nevertheless, several monospecific, excellent pathological reagents are available commercially.

Immunohistochemically, CEA has been identified in cancer of colorectum (Primus et al., 1981; DeLellis and Lee, 1984; Pavelic et al., 1990), breast (Robertson et al., 1989), lung (Beplev et al., 1989), uterine cervix (Duk et al., 1990), gall bladder (Dowling and Kelly, 1986), stomach (Mori et al., 1988), pancreas (Shimizu et al., 1990), neuroendocrine carcinomas of larynx, lung, thyroid (Smets et al., 1990), liver (Wong and Yazdi, 1990), prostate, urinary bladder, and uterus (Nap, 1986; Nap et al., 1988). There have been numerous attempts to compare the incidence of immunohistochemical CEA staining with plasma CEA levels, tumor differentiation, disease stage, histologic tumor type, CEA intensity, distribution, cellular localization, and clinical prognosis for various carcinomas (Denk et al., 1972; Sorokin et al., 1974; Shousha and Lyssiotis, 1978; Shousha et al., 1979; Wagener et al., 1981; Ahneen et al., 1982; Kojima et al., 1983; Mansour et al., 1983; Hamada et al., 1985; Castelli et al., 1986; Mori et al., 1988; Beplev et al., 1989; Robertson et al., 1989; Duk et al., 1990).

A positive correlation between serum CEA and the intensity of tissue CEA staining has been reported for cancer of the colorectum (Cunningham et al., 1986; Pagé et al., 1986), breast (Martinez and Azzopardi, 1979; Böcker et al., 1985), pancreas (Denk et al., 1972), as well as for gestational and nongestational choriocarcinomas (Lind and Haghighi, 1986). No correlation was observed for gastric cancer (Castelli et al., 1986).

Overall, the incidence of positive colorectal cancer tissue staining is similar to the frequency of elevated serum CEA levels (75 vs 73%), but occasionally higher sensitivity of tissue staining than serum CEA levels (90 vs 42%) has been reported.

Conflicting results have been published regarding the relationship between tissue CEA staining and tumor differentiation in colorectal carcinomas. Cunningham et al. (1986), Bordes et al. (1973), and Rognum et al. (1982) showed no correlation, whereas the work of Denk et al. (1972), Zamcheck (1981a), and Goslin et al. (1981) demonstrated a relationship between tumor staining for CEA and the degree of differentiation of the tumor. Obviously, study design, different reagents (antibodies), and method of interpretation result in differing observations.

There is good reason to regard colonic inflammatory diseases, and adenomas, as premalignant lesions (Böcker et al., 1985). Immunoperoxidase staining for CEA supports the concept of a polyp–adenoma–cancer sequence (Jetha et al., 1986). Studies of the localization of CEA in benign colonic polyps showed either weak or moderately strong staining for CEA, whereas 100% of polyps that were graded as being severely dysplastic were strongly positive for CEA. These findings thus indicate that immunoperoxidase staining of apparently benign polyps for CEA may be of value in indicating a need for further monitoring of patients with recurrent colorectal polyps.

Both chronic inflammatory bowel disease and colorectal adenomas show higher tissue CEA concentrations than normal colonic mucosa, suggesting that these situations can be regarded as precancerous conditions (Davidson et al., 1989; Fischbach et al., 1990). Strong CEA positivity was also observed in chronic pancreatitis (Shimizu et al., 1990), cystic fibrosis (Scheele et al., 1989), gall bladder hyperplasia, and chronic cholecystitis (Dowling and Kelly, 1986).

Anti-CEA antibodies stain normal colon mucosa (Gold and Freedman, 1965; Khoo et al., 1973; Fritsche and Mach, 1977;

Quetmeler et al., 1987; Savoie and Sikorska, 1990); that is not surprising in view of the findings that normal colon mucosa cells produce CEA in culture (Breborowicz et al., 1975; Kuroki et al., 1988), and that CEA mRNA is actively expressed in the normal mucosa (Oikawa et al., 1987a; Zimmermann et al., 1987a, 1988; Cournoyer et al., 1988; Sato et al., 1988). CEA has also been demonstrated histochemically in normal epithelial cells of the respiratory system (Matsuoka et al., 1990).

CEA has been demonstrated immunohistochemically in 77% of pancreatic tumors but the technique has no value in discriminating between chronic pancreatitis and carcinoma, since a significant proportion of inflamed tissues stain for CEA (Allum et al., 1986b; Shimizu et al., 1990).

Immunohistochemical demonstration of CEA in breast tumors has been attempted by several groups and it is evident from these studies that CEA is positive in mammary carcinomas in the majority of cases, whereas benign lesions are virtually all negative.

Results on correlation between the positivity of CEA immunohistochemistry and histologic grade, lymph node stage, locoregional recurrence, disease-free interval, or patient survival are very controversial. Data of Böcker (1985), Shousha (1978, 1979), and Wahren (1978) indicate that a significant relationship exists between CEA-positivity of mammary carcinomas and the presence of lymph node metastases, 5-year survival rates, and histological type.

A nearly 90% correlation between grade III breast cancer with lymph node metastases and CEA positivity, as opposed to 40–45% CEA positivity in grades I and II breast cancers, has been shown (Böcker et al.,1985). Invasive ductal carcinoma usually showed more intense tissue CEA staining, compared to tubular, cribriform, and invasive lobular carcinoma. CEA staining was associated with a worse prognosis.

However, the studies of Walker (1980), Van der Linden et al. (1985), Von Kleist et al. (1982), Gilchrist et al. (1985), Persijn and Korsten (1977), and recently, Robertson et al. (1989) clearly indicate the contrary. No correlation could be found between tissue CEA and estrogen receptor status (Persijn and Korsten, 1977). Thus, it appears that the role of immunohistochemistry in diagnosis of breast tumor and prognosis of recurrent lesions is limited. There is not enough convincing evidence that pathologists can reliably interpret the CEA content and relate it to the biological course of the cancer. Results do not indicate that tissue CEA could identify high-risk patients.

CEA staining is strongly positive in gastric tumors (Castelli et al., 1986; Mori et al., 1988; Nap et al., 1988; Nasierowska-Guttmejer and Szawlowski, 1989; Savoie and Sikorska, 1990) and its distribution apparently correlates with histologic type, degree of differentiation, and tumor prognosis.

Staining for CEA has been reported to differentiate between primary hepatocellular carcinoma and metastatic carcinoma to the liver in fine needle aspiration biopsy specimens (Wong and Yazdi, 1990). Most of the CEA stained hepatocellular carcinomas (90%) showed a predominantly bile canalicular pattern, whereas metastatic carcinoma cases demonstrated a diffuse cytoplasmic pattern.

A few reports have described CEA immunostaining in small-cell lung carcinoma (Sehested et al., 1981; Goslin et al., 1983; Beplev et al., 1989), but no correlation between the degree of immunostaining and clinical parameters was reported. The majority of cervical adenocarcinomas show positive staining for CEA but no relation to clinical and histopathological tumor characteristics was demonstrated (Nanbu et al., 1988; Duk et al., 1990).

According to Nap (1986), the consistent lack of CEA positivity in tumors of the kidney, the prostate, and the liver, and the restriction of CEA positivity to medullary carcinoma of the thyroid and the mucinous and endometrioid tumors of the ovary, may allow CEA immunohistochemistry to be used in differentiating primary from metastatic tumors of various organs. According to these findings, a CEA positive epithelial tumor in the liver, kidney, or prostate would be considered metastatic until proven otherwise. Nap suggests that, in the ovary, not only is the presence or absence of CEA in epithelial tumors important, but that the distribution of the antigen within the tumor can provide useful information. Primary ovarian tumors that produce CEA are the mucinous and endometrioid types, and the characteristic staining pattern is that of a focal distribution (Charpin et al., 1982; Fleuren and Nap, 1983). Since the majority of metastatic tumors to the ovary originate from the digestive tract (Scully, 1978), where CEA staining of the tumor is much more diffuse, the distribution of CEA is an important factor to consider in differentiating between primary and metastatic adenocarcinomas of the ovary.

CEA positivity in medullary thyroid, breast, lungs, gall bladder, pancreas, or urinary bladder tumors might be regarded as an ectopic production of CEA, resulting from altered DNA expression in malignant cells developed from tissues that normally do not show CEA positivity during normal development (Nap et al., 1984, 1985, 1988; Nap, 1986). Undoubtedly, new evidence arising from the molecular cloning of CEA gene family will clarify these clinical observations.

As the impact of CEA immunohistochemistry becomes increasingly important, it must also be underlined that CEA can easily be demonstrated retrospectively in routinely fixed, paraffin-embedded sections.

6. Radioimmunolocalization of Cancers with Anti-CEA Antibodies

6.1. Introduction

Radioimmunolocalization (RIL) procedures using "tumor specific" antibody have the potential to differentiate between malignant and benign tissues in vivo. RIL of tumors was pioneered by Pressman and Korngold in 1953, using osteosarcomas as the target. In 1974, Reif et al. (1974) attempted to detect metastatic cancer in a patient with advanced colon carcinoma using radiolabeled antibody to CEA. The radiolabel did not localize to the cancer tissue. The first successful reports demonstrating specific localization of anti-CEA antibodies in xenografts of human tumors in animals were published by Goldenberg and Primus (Primus et al., 1973; Goldenberg et al., 1974) and Mach et al. (1974b). Subsequently, extensive studies demonstrated the RIL of antibodies against human tumor markers in both animal models and patients. Owing to crossreactivity of polyclonal anti-CEA antibodies with NCA-like antigens, only affinity-purified anti-CEA polyclonal antibodies and/or monoclonal antibodies with minimal or no crossreactivity with normal tissue epitopes or plasma components are likely to be effec-tive as targeting agents, in order to avoid the pitfalls encountered by Dillman et al. (1984).

6.2. Animal Models of Radioimmunolocalization with Anti-CEA Antibodies

Preclinical Studies

A human tumor xenograft in the nude mouse has been widely employed as a model to resolve some of the central problems of RIL, namely, how to maximize the specific localization of anti-CEA antibody at the tumor site while minimizing nonspecific accumulation of label in normal organs. Despite its limitations, the model enables several pharmacokinetic factors, such as absorption, distribution, and clearance, to be examined under different in vivo conditions. It also permits the study of how the parameters of time, antibody dose, antibody specificity, type of label, tumor size, vascularization, patterns of blood flow, extent of necrosis, tumor CEA content, and distribution of antibody uptake pertain to the quality of imaging.

The choice of the particular human tumor xenograft may influence the outcome of studies and may cause difficulties in interpretation when results from different laboratories are compared, since the kinetics of CEA synthesis, expression, distribution, and secretion can vary substantially between different tumor cell lines (Shi et al., 1983). Thus, caution must be exercised in direct extrapolation of xenograft findings to the human situation, and it must be recognized that this is an unavoidable initial compromise. The review by Rogers (1986) describes limitations and achievements associated with the use of labeled antibodies against CEA in the xenograft model.

The efficiency of RIL with anti-CEA antibody appears to be related to several factors, including:

1. The degree of expression of CEA in and on the cancer cells;
2. The size of the tumor being localized;
3. The type of antibody being used for the CEA epitope(s) under consideration;
4. The circulating blood pool of CEA;
5. The vascularity of the tumor; and
6. Radiolabeling.

6.2.1. The Effect of Tumor CEA Content on the Tumor Radiolabel Uptake

There is evidence that increased CEA content of xenografted tumor influences the uptake of a radiolabeled MAb anti-CEA (Hedin et al., 1982; Philben et al., 1986). The larger the CEA content, the higher the tumor uptake. Nevertheless, CEA content cannot entirely predict scintiscan and biodistribution results. Thus, CEA is constantly being manufactured in tumor cells and secreted into the interstitial fluid. The production, secretion, and clearance rates may vary from one tumor to another, and may not be reflected directly by tumor CEA content. Tumor heterogeneity must also play a role.

6.2.2. The Effect of Tumor Size on the Tumor Radiolabel Uptake

Conflicting findings emerged when attempts were made to cor-relate tumor size with quality of imaging. Hedin et al. (1982) found no association between tumor size and imaging. Mann et al. (1984) found that tumor uptake was directly related to tumor size, with larger tumors producing better images. Philben et al. (1986), on the other hand, reported that when tumor size was plotted against tumor uptake, there was an exponential curve with a negative correlation, but when scanning tumors of various sizes, the scintiscan quality was similar and independent of the size of the tumor.

When Duewell et al. (1986) and Hagan et al. (1985, 1986) studied the dependence of anti-CEA MAb uptake on xenograft size, they found a relative negative correlation between tumor uptake and tumor size.

The reasons for the varying results from one laboratory to another are not completely clear, but a multitude of parameters can potentially affect the relationship between tumor size and antibody uptake. These include changes in blood flow, degree of tumor necrosis, and the relative levels of intratumoral and interstitital CEA as tumor size increases (Pimm and Baldwin, 1986). In addition, the presence of circulating CEA can influence tumor deposition and the half-life of the radiolabeled antibody (Hagan et al., 1985).

6.2.3. The Effect of Circulating CEA on Tumor Imaging

The effect of circulating CEA was studied in the nude mouse carrying a human tumor xenograft. The formation of circulating CEA complexes resulted in decreased tumor uptake of the labeled antibody (Martin and Halpern, 1984; Hagan et al., 1985). In animals in which high levels of serum CEA immune complexes occurred, the radiolabeled complexes were cleared by the liver and/or spleen with an attendant increased radiation dose to those organs, and a parallel decrease in tumor concentration of the radiolabel.

However, the amount of circulating CEA in patients' sera did not significantly influence immunoscintigraphic visualization of CEA-expressing tumors (Bosslet et al., 1988) in those patients. Analysis of patients' sera revealed conformational changes in serum CEA, causing a decreased affinity of serum CEA to anti-CEA antibody.

6.2.4. Comparative Imaging with Intact Antibodies and Their Derivatives

It has been suggested that $F(ab')_2$ and Fab fragments might give greater tumor discrimination than intact antibodies because of the potentially more favorable biodistribution of antibody lacking the Fc fragment (Mach et al., 1981; Buchegger et al., 1983). Studies with $F(ab')_2$ antibody fragments (Mach et al., 1980a, 1983a; Buchegger et al., 1983; Larson et al., 1983a,b; Wahl et al., 1983; Carrasquillo et al., 1984; Chatal et al., 1984; Beaumier et al., 1985) have demonstrated faster blood clearance, reduced uptake in nontarget organs, such as liver, lung, and spleen, that greatly improves tumor penetration and tumor/normal organ localization ratios.

A major drawback to using fragments for localization is an appreciably lower absolute concentration in the tumor (Buchegger et al., 1983; Wahl et al., 1983; Harwood et al., 1985a). The residence time of the fragment in the tumor is much shorter (24 h) than that of intact antibody (more than 3 d). Unless the residence of fragments in the tumor can be extended or compensated for by increased or repeatedly injected doses, whole immunoglobulin may be more favorable for future experimental and clinical investigations aimed at using high doses of radiolabel in antitumor therapy.

6.2.5. The Choice of Radiolabel

^{131}I, ^{125}I, and, more recently, ^{111}In and Tc-99m have become the most commonly used isotopes for tumor imaging studies. The use of radioiodine as the tracer adds to the complexity of interpretation of in vivo data. This is particularly true if the antigen, as in the case of CEA, appears in the circulation (Bradwell et al., 1985; Hagan et al., 1985; Beatty et al., 1986a). First, in vivo dehalogenation frequently occurs and is probably variable in magnitude depending on the type of antibody employed, its metabolic breakdown, and the method of iodination used (Krohn et al., 1972; Stern et al., 1982; Sullivan et al., 1982; Halpern et al., 1983a; Paxton et al., 1985). On the other hand, ^{111}In appears to be a more reliable agent for tumor imaging (Halpern et al., 1981, 1983b; Bernhard et al., 1983; Rainsbury, 1984; Beatty et al., 1986a; Hagan et al., 1985; Duda et al., 1986) as it is associated with greater stability of the antibody–radionuclide complex, and is probably less likely than iodine to dissociate once metabolism of the monoclonal antibody has occurred (Krejcarek and Tucker, 1977). The major problems with ^{111}In include the long biological half-life of the conjugate resulting in a higher total absorbed radiation dose and the strong uptake of the conjugate by the normal liver.

Technetium-99m (Tc-99m) is the radioisotope of choice for routine nuclear medicine imaging studies because of its short half-life, its near ideal gamma ray energy spectrum, its lack of particulate radiation, and its low cost (generator produced). Early attempts to label antibodies with Tc-99m met with considerable frustration as bonding of the reduced technetium to the protein was unstable and quickly dissociated in vivo. These initial difficulties have been overcome recently and several instant, easy radiolabeling kits for anti-CEA antibodies are available (Rhodes et al., 1986; Schwarz and Steinsträsser, 1987; Goldenberg et al., 1990). It has to be emphasized, however, that neither in vitro characteristics of anti-CEA antibodies nor radiolabeling, biodistribution, and imaging studies in mice with human tumor xenografts are able to fully predict the behavior of antibodies in patients.

6.3. Clinical Studies

The pioneering work of Goldenberg et al. (1978a, b, 1980a) and Mach et al. (1980a), using affinity purified, iodine-labeled polyclonal antibodies to localize advanced neoplastic disease in humans, led to a number of clinical studies of RIL over the past decade. The availability of sophisticated nuclear imaging technology and the development of high affinity MAbs has subsequently improved imaging quality.

In humans, many of the early reported results of tumor imaging with labeled anti-CEA antibodies were inconsistent and rather dicouraging (Reif et al., 1974; Mach et al., 1980a, 1983a; Sullivan et al., 1982; Dillman et al., 1984; Bradwell et al., 1985). The reasons for this included the distribution of the conjugate and free isotope between normal and tumor tissues, and blood pooling in tissues. Any residual anti-CEA antibody crossreactivity (MAbs or polyclonal antisera) with antigens on normal cells, might have also contributed to the problem. However, the majority of results to date indicate that, despite the technical and biologic problems outlined, primary and secondary cancers can be successfully imaged (Goldenberg et al., 1978a,b, 1980a, 1990; Dykes et al., 1980; Berche et al., 1982; Fairweather et al., 1983; Allum et al., 1986a; Armitage et al., 1986; Beatty et al., 1986a; Duda et al., 1986; Holzheimer et al., 1986; Paganelli et al., 1986; Vanderick et al., 1986; Abdel-Nabi et al., 1987, 1988; Henze et al., 1987; Edington et al., 1988; Gasparini et al., 1988; Patt et al., 1988; Riva et al., 1988; Siccardi et al., 1989; Doerr et al., 1990; Kairemo, 1990; Sharkey et al., 1990) (Table 3).

Studies of gastrointestinal cancers with antibodies to CEA have demonstrated appropriate RIL in 70 to over 90% of patients. Hepatic metastases, on the other hand, appear to be much more difficult to image because of the high background uptake of radioactivity by normal liver tissue, particularly with ^{111}In, and relatively low uptake in the metastatic lesions. The reported sensitivities for detection of liver metastases have ranged from 0–94% in different studies. To improve the uptake of antibody-bound radiolabel by hepatic metastatic lesions, intraperitoneal (Paganelli et al., 1986) and intraaortic (Holzheimer et al., 1986), rather than intravenous injections, have been attempted with some success.

In an attempt to "block" the high normal liver uptake, unlabeled MAb was injected simultaneously with the labeled antibody. The resulting improved scintigrams of metastatic lesions suggest that the "blocking" effect of unlabeled MAb influences the nonspecific distribution of labeled MAb primarily through reduction of liver uptake of isotope-labeled antibody, thus increasing the sensitivity of detecting metastases (Lamki et al., 1986; Patt et al., 1988). The use of nuclear scintiscans to detect potentially operable recurrences showed variable success rates (Table 3) depending on tumor localization and immunoconjugate used. In one case, the immunolymphoscintigraphy of breast tumor metastases was exceptionally high, with sensitivity of 90% and specificity of 88%.

The most complete clinical study reported so far was conducted in Italy (Gasparini et al., 1988; Riva et al., 1988; Siccardi et al., 1989). $F(ab')_2$ fragments of CEA monoclonal antibody F023C5, determined to be more suitable than intact IgG or Fab fragments for immunoscintigraphy, were labeled with ^{131}I or conjugated to DTPA for ^{111}In-labeling. The reagents were administered intravenously (2–3 mCi/0.5 mg) to 509 patients in 11 nuclear medicine departments: 284 patients had gastrointestinal adenocarcinomas, 204 had nongastrointestinal adenocarcinomas, and 21 were controls. Serum CEA was elevated in 169 patients, normal in 115, and not

Table 3
Summary of Radioimmunolocalization Studies in Cancer Patients Using Anti-CEA Antibodies

Reference	AB-type[a]	Tumor type/site	No. of patients scanned	Positive scan % sensitivity	Authors' rating[b]
Goldenberg, 1978a,b	^{131}I-AP goat IgG	Primary/colorectal, ovary, cervix, breast, lung endometrium, chotedochus	18	94	1
Mach et al., 1980b	^{131}I-AP goat IgG	Primary/colorectal	27	40.7	2
Goldenberg et al., 1980	^{131}I-AP goat IgG	Primary/colorectal	142	85	1
		Ovary		88	
		Cervix		90	
		Lung		71	
Dykes et al., 1980	^{131}I-AP sheep IgG	Primary/colorectal	13	80	1
		Liver metastases		72.7	
Berche et al., 1982	^{131}I-McAb	Liver metastases	17	94	1
Sullivan, 1982	^{131}I-AP goat or baboon IgG	Primary/colorectal	33	50	2
		Breast		15	
		Thyroid		0	

Fairweather et al., 1983	^{111}In or ^{131}I sheep IgG	Mixed	11	90	1
Mach, 1983a	^{131}I-McAb	Primary/colorectal pancreas	28	50	2
Dillman et al., 1984	^{111}In-McAb	Metastases/liver		0	2
Riva et al., 1986	^{111}In and ^{131}I-McAb $F(ab)'_2$	Primary/lung Metastases/pulmonary	45	87 83	1
Moscatelli et al., 1986	^{111}In-McAb $F(ab')_2$	Thyroid medullary	1	100	1
Vanderick et al., 1986	^{111}In and $^{131}1$-McAb IgG and $F(ab')_2$	Primary/colorectal	10	37	1
Paganelli et al., 1986	^{131}I-McAb $F(ab')_2$	Primary/colorectal Metastases/liver	60	80 59 iv vs 82ip	1
Holzheimer et al., 1986	^{131}I-McAb IgG	Metastases/liver	13	69	1
Allum et al., 1986	^{131}I-McAb IgG	Primary/gastric, esophageal colorectal	50	85	1
		Recurrent gastric and colorectal		61	2

(continued)

Table 3 *(continued)*

Reference	AB-type[a]	Tumor type/site	No. of patients scanned	Positive scan % sensitivity	Authors' rating[b]
Beatty et al., 1986a	^{111}In-McAb IgG_1	Primary/colorectal	40	69	1
		Metastases/liver		42	2
		Recurrent extraheptic		0	2
Duda et al., 1986	^{111}In-McAb IgG_1	Primary/colorectal	21	71	1
		Metastases/liver		0	2
Armitage et al., 1986	^{111}In-McAb IgG_1	Primary/colorectal	7	100	1
		Metastases (and recurrence/s) various	9	72	1
Henze et al., 1987	^{131}I-McAb $F(ab')_2$ (Behringwerke AG, TuMAK BW431/31)	Metastases (and recurrence/s) liver, lung	9	55	2
	^{131}I-McAb IgG_1	Metastases (and recurrences)/ liver, lungs	5	0	2
Abdel-Nabi et al., 1987	^{111}In-McAb IgG_1 (Hybritech Inc. ZCE-025)	Primary/colorectal residual	15	90	1
		Metastases liver, lung, lymph node			

Edington et al., 1988	^{111}In-McAb IgG_1 (Hybritech Inc. ZCE-025)	Thyroid medullary carcinoma (metastatic)	1	100	1
Abdel-Nabi et al., 1988	^{111}In-McAb IgG_1 (Hybritech Inc. ZcE-025)	Primary/colorectal	16	56	1
		Metastases/liver	3	100	1
		Lymph node	4	25	
Gasparini et al., 1988	^{131}I-McAb $F(ab')_2$	Primary/colorectal	25	68	1
		Metastases/liver	16	25	2
	^{111}In-McAb $F(ab')_2$ (F023C5)	Recurrences local	23	87	1
Riva et al., 1988	^{131}I-McAb $F(ab')_2$	Primary/colorectal	25	76	1
	^{111}In-McAb $F(ab')_2$ (F023C5)	Metastases/lymph node	9	89	1
		Liver	9	33	2
		Abdomen	1	100	1
		Lung	5	100	1
		Bone	2	100	1
		Recurrences	194	70	1
		Primary/lung	51	96	1

(continued)

Table 3 *(continued)*

Reference	AB-type[a]	Tumor type/site	No. of patients scanned	Positive scan % sensitivity	Authors' rating[b]
		Metastases/various	37	78	
		Recurrences	31	87	1
		Primary/breast	–	–	–
		Metastases/various	103	75	1
		Other tumors	77	83	1
		GI metastases ip administration	95	83	1
Siccardi et al., 1989	^{131}I-McAb $F(ab')_2$	GI adenocarinomas	284	66	1
	^{111}In-McAb $F(ab')_2$ (F023C5)	Non-GI adenocarcinomas	204	69	1
Yehuda, 1988	^{111}In-McAb IgG_1 (Hybritech)	Metastases/nonliver	34	36	1
		Metastases/ liver	34	36	1
Doerr et al., 1990	^{111}In-McAb IgG_1 (Hybritech)	Recurrences on metastases	13	85	1

Kairemo, 1990	^{99m}Tc-McAb IgG_1 (Behringwerke BW431/26)	Breast cancer metastases to lymph nodes	20	90	1
Goldenberg et al., 1990	^{99m}Tc-McAb $F(ab')_2$ (Immuno-medics NP-4)	Various primaries and metastases	23	95	1
	^{123}I-McAb $F(ab')_2$ (Immunomedics NP-4)	Various primaries and metastases	38	96	1

[a]AB Antibody. AP, Afffinity purified.
[b]1, Encouraging. 2, Disappointing.

determined in 225. The following results were obtained: (a) no adverse reactions; (b) total tumor images with both isotopes in 324 patients (in particular, in 81.5% CEA-seropositive and in 69.0% CEA-seronegative patients); (c) no significant difference in sensitivity among the results of the 11 departments; (d) no significant difference in overall sensitivity between ^{131}I- and ^{111}In-labeled immunoradiopharmaceuticals; (e) the fraction of documented lesions imaged by other methods (true positives) was 73.3% in CEA-seropositive and 53.7% in CEA-seronegative patients; (f) the detection of liver metastases was hampered by nonspecific radioactivity uptake, particularly when using the ^{111}In-labeled reagent; (g) the major cause of negative immunoscintigraphy was a lack of CEA in tumor lesions, as documented by immunohistochemistry; (h) lesion size is also important since the sensitivity was 64% for lesions up to 2 cm in diameter and 84% for larger lesions; (i) many "unexpected" radiolocalizations were recorded. Many (35.8% with ^{111}In-reagent vs 27% with ^{131}I- reagent) were identified as occult tumor lesions. In 35 patients, this finding contributed to the early clinical detection of tumor recurrences.

The variation in results reported by various groups reflects a gamut of potential variables, such as radiolabel, route of administration, tumor size and location, vascularity, patient population studied, imaging technology, subjective interpretation of scans, and antibody preparations used. Direct comparisons are difficult, because different techniques for imaging tumors have been employed. Several studies have utilized a subtractive technique using Tc-99m-labeled serum albumin and pertechnetate to help delineate the tumors (Goldenberg et al., 1978a, b, 1980a; Dykes et al., 1980; Mach et al., 1980b; Sullivan et al., 1982). It should be noted, once again, that early studies that used polyclonal antisera may have been limited by crossreactivity with certain epitopes present in normal tissues. Even when MAbs are utilized, they are of diverse specificities with regard to CEA epitopes, of variable affinities and degrees of cross-reactivity with both known and yet undefined tissue epitopes. Moreover, initial studies made use of radioiodine as a label, while more recent imaging work has used ^{111}In.

Although many of the nuclear scintiscan studies have utilized correlative data from other imaging modalities (X-rays, CT scan, nuclear scan, ultrasound), histopathologic assessment of the imaged tissue has seldom been reported in the published studies. As in the case of animal studies, antibody fragments rather than intact immunoglobulins have been utilized with improved imaging quality (Chatal et al., 1984; Moscatelli et al., 1986; Paganelli et al., 1986; Rogers, 1986; Vanderick et al., 1986). However, there are several major problems that require resolution before RIL can become a routine medical procedure. High uptake by normal liver tissue when ^{111}In-labeled antibodies are employed limits the usefulness of such agents. New technetium labeling kits, however, might have a great impact on RIL primarily as a result of low cost and simplicity of labeling, and lower liver uptake.

One of the most interesting observations is the high uptake of radiolabeled MAb against CEA by normal mesenteric lymph nodes (Duda et al., 1986) and testis (Beatty et al., 1986b). These problems also require resolution before full clinical utility of radiolabeled anti-CEA antibody procedures will be possible. A major perplexing issue is the very low antibody accumulation in tumors in comparison with the amount of antibody injected, which results in poor contrast between cancerous and normal tissues.

Different isotopes and different methods of imaging, such as positron emission tomography (PET) (Berche et al., 1982) and single-photon emission computed tomography (SPECT) (Henze et al., 1987; Abdel-Nabi et al., 1988; Goldenberg et al., 1990), have been employed to increase tumor/normal tissue image contrast. These techniques, however, are primarily methods for improving the sensitivity of detection and do not influence antibody accumulation.

A recent report on effects of hyperthermia on tumor CEA expression indicate that hyperthermia might increase the antigen membrane expression and shedding, and thus have clinical implications for RIL (Wong et al., 1989).

Preliminary studies have demonstrated that combinations of antibodies to different epitopes of CEA increase the rate of detection of tumors, presumably reflecting increased uptake of the injected preparations (Ichiki et al., 1986). Alternatively, increased amounts of antibody to the same epitope may produce similar results. One would expect that extremely large injected doses might be necessary to saturate the circulating and tissue epitopes. High doses of mouse anti-CEA MAbs may evoke some allergic side effects owing to foreign protein, or lead to the development of anti-murine antibodies, which could inactivate or eliminate the administered antibody, precluding sequential imaging procedures. The presence of antibodies against murine immunoglobulin, as well as antiidiotypic antibodies after injection of murine MAbs in humans, has been reported (Pimm et al., 1985b; Schrool et al., 1985; Traub et al., 1988).

Circulating CEA poses another potential problem for the RIL process. The CEA antigen shed into the circulation was shown in early studies to bind to administered anti-CEA antibodies (Hagan et al., 1985; Pimm et al., 1985b). So far, the clinical evidence described above indicates that there is no correlation between serum CEA and quality of the image or rate of detection, whereas there is a direct relationship between tumor size and tumor CEA expression and sensitivity of RIL. Tumors not expressing membrane CEA and those smaller than 1.5 cm are not imaged effectively.

On the basis of the foregoing information, it may be concluded that:

1. Primary tumors with a high CEA content have the best anti-CEA antibody uptake and are most easily imaged.
2. Hepatic metastases have a high CEA content and high antibody uptake but may not image well because of the relatively high uptake of the conjugate by normal liver.
3. Apical and intraluminal staining of tumors with anti-CEA antibody by immunochemistry correlates well with high uptake of labeled antibody.
4. Large, fungating tumors accumulate a higher proportion of the injected labeled antibody in contrast to ulcerative tumors with poorer vascularity.
5. There is no correlation between serum CEA concentration and antibody uptake by a CEA-producing tumor.

Thus, the successful clinical use of monoclonal antibodies against CEA for tumor imaging (and possible therapy) will require careful selection of patients for a number of antigen-related parameters, including CEA tumor content and distribution, immunohistopathology, gross morphology, and serum CEA quantitation.

Successful tumor imaging with labeled monoclonal antibodies will depend on further work on the pharmacokinetics of labeled antibodies and a better understanding of the immunobiology of CEA-producing tumors. Only when these parameters are understood will this promising technique complement other established methods of tumor detection and play a more important role in patient management.

7. Immunotherapy of Tumors Expressing CEA

Adenocarcinoma of the colon and rectum is the second most prevalent cancer in the United States (Silverberg, 1983). Relatively early diagnosis results in surgical cures in about 50% of the patients. To date, adjuvant chemotherapy has not been very successful in those patients whose tumors have been resected but who have a high risk for recurrence (i.e., Duke's Stages B_2 and C). Thus, new agents and different approaches to treatment must be developed.

The ability to detect tumors by RIL raises the possibility of treating such tumors by targeting with the same technology. Immunotherapy of human CEA-producing cancers may be carried out by involving several modalities, such as radioimmunotherapy (RIT), using anti-CEA antibodies to target high doses of cytotoxic radionuclides; chemoimmunotherapy, utilizing anti-CEA antibodies and drugs, toxins, or pro-drugs; active immunization with purified CEA, autologous cancer cells, or anti-CEA antiidiotypic antibodies; or photodynamic therapy. A previous review (Sikorska et al., 1988) described these modalities in detail.

Acknowledgments

We thank Angela Arseneau and Vénus Jean-Louis for their excellent technical assistance in preparation of the manuscript.

References

Aabo, K., H. Pedersen, and M. Kjaer (1986), *Eur. J. Cancer Clin. Oncol.* **22,** 211–217.

Abdel-Nabi, H. H., A. N. Schwartz, C. S. Higano, D. G. Wechter, and M. W. Unger (1987), *Radiology* **164,** 617–621.

Abdel-Nabi, H. H., A. N. Schwartz, G. Goldfogel, J. A. Ortman-Nabi, D. M. Matsuoka, M. W. Unger, and D. G. Wechter (1988), *Radiology* **166,** 747–752.

Ahlemann, L. M., H. J. Stabb, and F. A. Anderer (1980), *Biomedicine* **32,** 194–199.

Ahneen, D. I., P. K. Nakane, and W. R. Brown (1982), *Cancer* **49,** 2077–2080.

Allum, W. H., F. MacDonald, P. Anderson, and J. W. L. Fielding (1986a), *Br. J.* **53,** 203–210.

Allum, W. H., H. J. Stokes, F. MacDonald, and J. W. L. Fielding (1986b), *J. Clin. Pathol.* **39,** 610–614.

Andrew, S. M., M. V. Pimm, A. C. Perkins, and R. W. Baldwin (1986), *Eur. J. Nucl. Med.* **12,** 168–175.

Armitage, N. C., A. Davidson, D. Tsikos, and C. B. Wood (1984a), *Clin. Oncol.* **10,** 141–147.

Armitage, N. C., A. C. Perkins, L. G. Durrant, I. O. Ellist, K. C. Ballantyne, R. C. Harrison, A. M. L. Riley, R. A. Robins, M. L. Wastie, and J. D. Hardcastle (1986), *Br. J. Surg.* **73,** 965–969.

Arnaud, J. P., C. Kohl, and M. Adloff (1980), *Dis. Colon Rectum* **23,** 141–144.

Aroney, R. S., W. C. Dermody, P. Aldenderfer, P. Parsons, K. McNitt, P. J. Marangos, M. Y. Whitacre, R. W. Ruddon, P. H. Wiernik, and J. Aisner (1984), *Cancer Treat. Rep.* **68,** 859–866.

Barnett, T., S. Goebel, and J. Elting (1987), *Int. Soc. Oncodev. Biol. Med: XVth Annu.* Québec, abstr. 150.

Barone, C., A. Astone, A. Cassano, C. Garufi, P. Astone, A. Gieco, M. R. Noviello, E. Ricevuto, C. Albanese, and G. Gambassi (1990), *Oncology* **47,** 128–132.

Bates, S. E. and D. L. Longo (1987), *Semin. Oncol.* **14,** 102.

Baylin, S. B., W. R. Weisberger, J. C. Eggleston, G. Mendelsohn, M. A. Beaven, M. D. Abeloff, and D. S. Ettinger (1978), *N. Engl. J. Med.* **299,** 105–110.

Beart, R. W. Jr. and M. J. O'Connell (1983), *Mayo Clin. Proc.* **58,** 361–363.

Beart, R. W. Jr., P. P. Metzger, M. J. O'Connell, and A. I. Schutt (1981), *Dis. Colon Rectum* **24,** 585–588.

Beatty, B. G., R. J. Paxton, K. Sheibani, R. B. Duda, L. E. Williams, J. E. Shively, and J. D. Beatty (1986b), *Cancer Res.* **46,** 6503–6508.

Beatty, J. D., C. Romero, P. W. Brown, W. Lawrence, Jr., and J. J. Terz (1979), *Arch. Surg.* **114,** 563–567.
Beatty, J. D. and J. J. Terz (1982), *Prog. Clin. Cancer* **8,** 9–29.
Beatty J. D., R. B. Duda, L. E. William, K. Sheibani, R. J. Paxton, B. G. Beatty, V. J. Philben, J. L. Werner, J. E. Shively, W. G. Vlahos, W. A. Kokal, D. U. Riihimaki, J. J. Terz, and L. D. Wagman (1986a), *Cancer Res.* **46,** 6494–6502.
Beauchemin, N., S. Benchimol, D. Cournoyer, A. Fuks, and C. P. Stanners (1987), *Mol. Cell. Biol.* **7,** 3221–3230.
Beauchemin, N., C. Turbide, D. Afar, J. Bell, M. Raymond, C. P. Stanners, and A. Fuks (1989), *Cancer Res.* **49,** 2017–2021.
Beaudonnet, A., G. Gounon, J. Pichot, and M. C. Revenant (1981), *Clin. Chem.* **27,** 771.
Beaumier, P. L., K. A. Krohn, J. A. Carrasquillo, J. Eary, I. Hellström, K. E. Hellström, W. G. Nelp, and S. M. Larson (1985), *J. Nucl. Med.* **26,** 1172–1179.
Begent, R. H. J. (1984), *Ann. Clin. Biochem.* **21,** 231–238.
Benchimol, S., A. Fuks, S. Jothy, N. Beauchemin, K. Shirota, and C. P. Stanners (1989), *Cell* **57,** 327–334.
Beplev, G., M. Ostholt, K. Neumann, R. Holle, G. Jaques, K. Havemann, and H. Kalbfleisch (1989), *Anticancer Res.* **9,** 1525–1530.
Berardi, R. S., R. Ruiz, W. E. Becknell, Jr., and Y. Keonin (1977), *Geriatrics* **32,** 86–88.
Berche, C., J.-P. Mach, J. D. Lumbroso, C. Langlais, F. Aubry, F. Buchegger, S. Carrel, P. Rougier, C. Parmentier, and M. Tubiana (1982), *Br. Med. J.* **285,** 1447–1451
Bernhard, M. I., K. M. Hwang, K. A. Foon, A. M. Keenan, R. M. Kessler, J. M. Frincke, J. J. Tillam, M. G. Hanna, Jr., I. Peters, and R. K. Odham (1983), *Cancer Res.* **43,** 4429–4433.
Bezwoda, W., D. Derman, T. Bothwell, P. MacPhil, J. Levin and N. De Moor (1981), *Cancer* **48,** 1623–1628.
Böcker, W., G. Schweikhart, K. Pollow, R. Kreienberg, A. Klaubert, S. Schröder, M. Mitze, J. Bahnsen, and H. Stegner (1985), *Pathol. Res. Pract.* **180,** 490–497.
Boey, J., H. C. Cheung, C. K. Lai, and J. Wong (1984), *World J. Surg.* **8,** 279–286.
Booth, S. N., J. King, J. Leonard, G. C. Jamieson, G. D. Oates, and P. W. Dykes (1974), *Br. Med. J.* **4,** 183–187.
Bordes, M., R. Michiels, and F. Martin (1973), *Digestion* **9,** 106–115.
Börmer, O. P. and K. Nustad (1990), *J. Immunol. Methods* **127,** 171–178.
Borthwick, N. M., D. W. Wilson, and P. A. Bell (1977), *Eur. J. Cancer* **13,** 171–176.

Bosslet, K., A. Steinsträsser, A. Schwarz, H. P. Harthus, G. Lüben, L. Kuhlmann, and H. H. Sedlacek (1988), *Eur. J. Nucl. Med.* **14,** 523–528.
Bradwell, A. R., D. S. Fairweather, P. W. Dykes, A. Keeling, A. Vaughan, and J. Taylor (1985), *Immunol. Today* **6,** 163–169.
Breborowicz, J., G. C. Easty, M. Birbeck, D. Robertson, R. Nery, and A. M. Neville (1975), *Br. J. Cancer* **31,** 559–569.
Breslin, B. K. and J. B. Healy (1981), *Med. J.* **74,** 203–204.
Buchegger, F., C. M. Haskell, M. Schreyer, B. R. Scazziga, S. Randin, S. Carrel, and J.-P. Mach (1983), *J. Exp. Med.* **158,** 413–427.
Bullen, A. W., M. S. Losowsky, S. Carter, S. Patel, and A. M. Neville (1977), *Gastroenterology* **73,** 673–678.
Burgess, R. E. (1986), *Ann. Intern. Med.* **104,** 888.
Cantwell, B., M. J. Duffy, J. J. Fennelly, M. Jones and G. Duffy (1980), *Irish J. Med. Sci.* **149,** 469–474.
Carrasquillo, J. A., K. A. Krohn, P. L. Beaumier, R. W. McGuffen, J. P. Brown, K. E. Hellström, I. Hellström, and S. M. Larson (1984), *Cancer Treat.. Rep.* **68,** 317–328.
Castelli, M., S. Guadagni, A. Bagnato, M. A. Pistoia, M. Carboni, and E. Sega (1986), *Oncology* **43,** 149–153.
Chakrabaity, S., A. Tobon, J. Varani, and M. G. Brattain (1988), *Cancer Res.* **48,** 4059–4064.
Charpin, C., A. K. Bhan, V. R. Zurawski, Jr., and R. E. Scully (1982), *Int. J. Gynecol. Pathol.* **1,** 231–245.
Chatal, J. F., F. Chupin, G. Ricolleau, J. L. Tellier, A. Le Mevel, P. Fumoleau, O. Godin, and B. P. LeMevel (1981), *Eur. J. Cancer Clin. Oncol.* **17,** 233–238.
Chatal, J. F., J. C. Saccavini, P. Fumoleau, J. Y. Doullard, C. Curtet, M. Kremer, B. LeMevel, and H. Koprowski (1984), *Clin. Sci.* **25,** 307–314.
Chu, T. and T. Nemoto (1973), *J. Natl. Cancer Inst.* **51,** 1119–1122.
Chu, T. M., P. Lavin, J. Day, J. T. Evans, A. Mittleman, E. D. Holyoke, and R. Vincent (1979), in *Carcino-embryonic Antigen,* vol. 1 (Lehmann, F. G., ed.), Elsevier, Amsterdam, p. 55.
Cillari, E., A. Bellavia, G. C. Romano, G. Di Gesu, S. Palmeri, A. Norato, A. Salerno, and P. di Voti (1981), *Am. J. Reprod. Immunol.* **1,** 269–271.
Clarke, C., K. R. Hine, P. W. Dykes, T. P. Whitehead, and A. G. W. Whitefield (1980), *J. R. Coll. Phys. Lond.* **14,** 227-228.
Concannon, J. P., M. H. Dalbow, and J. C. Frich, Jr. (1973), *Radiology* **108,** 191–193.
Concannon, J. P., M. H. Dalbow, S. E. Hodgson, J. J. Headings, E. Markopoulos, J. Mitchell, W. J. Cushing, and G. A. Liebler (1978), *Cancer* **42,** 1477–1483.
Coombes, R. C., J. C. Gazet, H. T. Ford, A. G. Nash, A. McKinna, and A. M. Neville (1980), *Lancet* **1,** 296–299.

Coombes, R. C., T. J. Powles, J. C. Gazet, H. T. Ford, A. McKinna, M. Abbot, C. W. Gehrke, J. W. Keyser, P. E. G. Mitchell, S. Patel, W. H. Stimson, M. Worwood, M. Jones, and A. M. Neville (1981), *Cancer* **48,** 310–315.
Cooper, M. J., C. R. Mackie, D. B. Skinner, and A. R. Moossa (1979), *Br. J. Surg.* **66,** 120–123.
Cooper, E. H. and J. O'Quigley (1982), *Recent Results Cancer Res.* **83,** 67–76.
Cournoyer, D., N. Beauchemin, D. Boucher, S. Benchimol, and A. Fuks (1988), *Cancer Res.* **48,** 3153–3157.
Cunningham, L., B. Stocking, S. A. Halter, and G. Kalemeris (1986), *Dis. Colon Rectum* **29,** 111–116.
Davidson, B. R., V. R. Sams, J. Styles, C. Dean, and P. B. Boulos (1989), *Gut* **30,** 1260–1265.
De Jong-Bakker, M., A. M. Hart Au, J.-P. Persijn, and F. J. Cleton (1981), *Eur. J. Cancer Clin. Oncol.* **17,** 1307–1313.
DeLellis, R. A. and A. K. Lee (1984), *J. Clin. Immunoassay* **7,** 125.
Deleriche, R., N. Zamcheck, and N. Marcin (1973), *Cancer* **31,** 328–330.
Del Favero, G., C. Fabris, M. Plebani, A. Panucci, A. Piccoli, L. Perobelli, S. Pedrazzoli, U. Baccaglini, A. Burlina, and R. Naccarato (1986a), *Cancer* **57,** 1576–1579.
Del Favero, G., C. Fabris, A. Panucci, D. Basso, M. Plebani, U. Baccaglini, G. Leandro, A. Burlina, and R. Naccarato (1986b), *Bull. Cancer (Paris),* **73,** 251–255.
Denk, H., G. Tappeiner, R. Eckerstorfer, and J. H. Holzner (1972), *Int. J. Cancer* **10,** 262–272.
Denstman, F., L. Rosen, I. T. Khubchandani, J. A. Sheets, J. J. Staski, and R. D. Riether (1986), *Cancer* **58,** 2089–2095.
Dillman, R. O., J. C. Beauregard, R. E. Sobol, I. Roystom, R. M. Bartholomew, P. S. Hagan, and S. E. Halpern (1984), *Cancer Res.* **44,** 2213–2218.
Dittrich, C., R. Jakesz, L. Havelec, R. Lenzhofer, S. Breyer, and K. Moser (1985), in *Tumor Markers in Cancer Control* (Nieburgs, H. E., J. H. Holzner, and V. E. Valli, eds.), Liss, New York, pp. 181–187.
Doerr, R. J., H. Abdel-Nabi, and B. Merchant (1990), *Arch. Surg.* **125,** 226–229.
Dowling, G. P. and J. K. Kelly (1986), *Cancer* **58,** 1702–1708.
Doyle, P. J., R. I. Nicholson, G. V. Groome, and R. W. Blamey (1981), *Clin. Oncol.* **7,** 53–58.
Duda, R. B., J. D. Beatty, K. Sheibani, L. E. Williams, R. J. Paxton, B. G. Beatty, J. E. Shively, W. G. Vlahos, J. L. Werner, M. M. Kemeny, W. A. Kokal, D. U. Riihimaki, L. D. Wagman, and J. J. Terz (1986), *Arch. Surg.* **121,** 1315–1319.
Duewell, S., W. Horst, and G. Westera (1986), *Cancer Immunol. Immunother.* **23,** 101–106.

Duk, J. M., H. de Bruijn, K. H. Groenier, G. J. Fleuren, and J. G. Aalders (1990), *Cancer* **65,** 1830–1837.
Dykes, P. W., K. R. Hine, A. R. Bradwell, J. C. Blackburn, T. A. Reeder, Z. Drolc, and S. N. Booth (1980), *Br. Med. J.* **280,** 220–222.
Edington, H. D., C. G. Watson, G. Levine, W. N. Tauxe, S. A. Yousem, M. Unger, and C. D. Kowal (1988), *Surgery* **104,** 1004–1010.
Ellis, D. J., C. Speirs, R. D. Kingston, V. S. Brookes, and L. J. Dykes (1978), *Cancer* **42,** 623–625.
Endo, Y., M. Fujino, T. Kodama, T. Oda, and P. Burtin (1979), in *Carcinoembryonic Proteins,* vol. 1 (Lehmann, F. G., ed.), Elsevier, Amsterdam, pp. 91–98.
Engvall, E., J. E. Shively, and M. Wrann (1978), *Proc. Natl. Acad. Sci. USA* **75,** 1670–1674.
Evans, J. T., A. Mittelman, M. Chu, and D. Holyoke (1978), *Cancer* **42,** 1419–1421.
Fairweather, D. S., A. R. Bradwell, P. W. Dykes, A. T. Vaughan, S. F. Watson-James, and S. Chandler (1983), *Br. Med. J.* **287,** 167–170.
Falkson, H. C., J. J. van der Watt, M. A. Portugal, M. J. Pitout, and G. Falkson (1978), *Cancer* **42,** 1308–1313.
Falkson, H. C., G. Falkson, M. A. Portugal, J. J. van der Watt, and H. S. Schoeman (1982), *Cancer* **49,** 1859–1865.
Fischbach, W., J. Mössner, H. Seyschab, and H. Höhn (1990), *Cancer* **65,** 1820–1824.
Fitzgerald, P. J., J. G. Fortner, R. C. Watson, M. K. Schwartz, P. Sherlock, R. S. Benua, A. L. Cubilla, D. Schottenfeld, D. Miller, S. J. Winawer, C. J. Lightdale, S. D. Leidner, J. S. Nisselbaum, C. J. Menendez-Botet, and M. H. Poleski (1978), *Cancer* **41,** 868–879.
Fletcher, R. H. (1986), *Ann. Intern. Med.* **104,** 66–73.
Fleuren, G. J. and M. Nap (1983), Second European Conference on Clinical Oncology, Amsterdam, November 2–5.
Fritsche, R. and J.-P. Mach (1977), *Immunochemistry* **14,** 119–127.
Fuks, A., J. Shuster, and P. Gold (1980), in *Cancer Markers* (Sell, S., ed.), Humana, Clifton, NJ, pp. 315–327.
Garrett, P. E. and S. R. Kurtz (1986), *Med. Clin. North Am.* **70,** 1295–1306.
Gasparini, M., M. Ripamonti, E. Seregni, E. Regalia, and G. L. Buraggi (1988), *Int. J. Cancer (Suppl.),* **2,** 81–84.
Gilchrist, K. W., M. A. Kalish, V. E. Gould, S. Hirschl, J. E. Imbriglia, W. M. Levy, A. S. Patchefsky, J. Pickren, J. A. Roth, R. A. Schinella, I. A. Schwartz, J. E. Wheeler, and D. C. Tormey (1985), *Cancer* **56,** 351–355.
Gold, P. and S. O. Freedman (1965), *J. Exp. Med.* **121,** 439–462.
Gold, P., S. O. Freedman, and J. Shuster (1979), in *Immunodiagnosis of*

Cancer (Herberman, R. B. and K. R. McIntire, eds.), Dekker, New York, pp. 147–165.

Goldberg, M. E., L. M. Simunovic, S. L. Drake, W. F. Mueller, and H. L. Verrill (1989), *Hybridoma* **8,** 569–575.

Goldenberg, D. M., D. F. Preston, F. J. Primus, and H. J. Hansen (1974), *Cancer Res.* **34,** 1–9.

Goldenberg, D. M., F. Deland, E. Kim, S. Bennett, F. J. Primus, J. R. van Nagell, N. Estes, P. DeSimone, and P. Raybu (1978a), *N. Engl. J. Med.* **298,** 1384–1388.

Goldenberg, D. M., R. M. Sharkey, and F. J. Primus (1978b), *Cancer* **42,** 1546–1553.

Goldenberg, D. M., E. E. Kim, F. H. Deland, S. Bennett, and F. J. Primus (1980), *Cancer Res.* **40,** 2984–2992.

Goldenberg, D. M., M. Neville, A. C. Carter, V. L. W. Go, E. D. Holyoke, K. J. Isselbacher, P. S. Schein, and M. Schwartz (1981), *Ann. Intern. Med.* **94,** 407–409.

Goldenberg, D. M., H. Goldenberg, R. M. Sharkey, E. Higginbotham-Ford, R. E. Lee, L. C. Swayne, K. A. Burger, D. Tsai, J. A. Horowitz, T. C. Hall, C. M. Pinsky, and H. J. Hansen (1990), *Cancer Res. (Suppl.)* **50,** 909S–921S.

Goodyear, M. D. E., D. J. Sutherland, A. Malkin, and et al. (1984), *Rev. Endocr. Rel. Cancer* **14,** 149–153.

Goslin, R., M. J. O'Brien, G. Steele, R. Mayer, R. Wilson, J. M. Corson, and N. Zamcheck (1981), *Am. J. Med.* **71,** 246.

Goslin, R., G. Steele, J. Macintyre, R. Mayer, P. Sugarbaker, K. Cleghorn, R. Wilson, and N. Zamcheck (1980), *Ann. Surg.* **192,** 747–751.

Goslin, R. H., M. J. O'Brien, A. T. Skarin, and N. Zamcheck (1983), *Cancer* **52,** 301–306.

Gray, B. (1984), *Aust. NZJ Surg.* **54,** 1–2.

Gropp, C., K. Havemann, and F.-G. Lehmann (1978), *Cancer* **42,** 2802–2808.

Grunert, F., N. AbuHarfeil, K. Schwarz, and S. von Kleist (1985), *Int. J. Cancer* **36,** 357–362.

Haagensen, D. E. Jr., S. J. Kister, J. P. Vandevoorde, J. B. Gates, E. K. Smart, H. J. Hansen, and S. A. Wells (1978a), *Cancer* **42,** 1512–1519.

Haagensen, D. E. Jr., S. J. Kister, J. Panick, J. Giannola, H. J. Hansen, and S. A. Wells (1978b), *Cancer* **42,** 1646–1652.

Hagan, P. L., S. E. Halpern, A. Chen, L. Krishnen, J. Frincke, R. M. Bartholomew, G. S. David, and D. J. Carlo (1985), *J. Nucl. Med.* **26,** 1418–1423.

Hagan, P. L., S. E. Halpern, R. O. Dillman, D. L. Shawler, D. E. Johnson, A. Chen, L. Krishnan, J. Frincke, R. M. Bartholomew, G. S. David, and D. Carlo (1986), *J. Nucl. Med.* **27,** 422–427.

Haines, A. P., A. G. Levin, and H. A. Fritsche (1979), *Lancet* **2,** 969.
Halpern, S. E., P. Hagan, P. Garver, J. A. Koziol, A. W. N. Chen, J. M. Frincke, R. M. Bartholomew, G. S. David and T. H. Adams (1983b), *Cancer Res.* **43,** 5347.
Halpern, S. E., P. H. Stern, P. L. Hagan, A. Chen, G. S. David, W. J. Desmond, T. H. Adams, R. M. Bartholomew, J. M. Frincke, and C. E. Brautigan (1981), *Clin. Nucl. Med.* **6,** 453.
Halpern, S. E., P. H. Stern, P. L. Hagan, A. Chen, J. Frincke, R. Bartholomew, G. David, and T. Adams (1983a), in *Radioimmuno-imaging and Radioimmunotherapy* (Burchiel, S. W. and B. A. Rhodes, eds.), Elsevier, New York.
Hamada, Y., M. Yamamura, K. Hioki, M. Yamamoto, H. Nagura, and K. Watanabe (1985), *Cancer* **55,** 136–141.
Harwood, P. J., J. Boden, R. B. Pedley, G. Rawlins, G. T. Rogers, and K. D. Bagshawe (1985a), *J. Cancer Res. Clin. Oncol.* **21,** 1515–1522.
Hedin, A., S. Hammarström, and A. Larsson (1982), *Mol. Immunol.* **19,** 1641–1648.
Hefta, L. J. F., H. Schrewe, J. A. Thompson, S. Oikawa, H. Nakazato and J. E. Shively (1990), *Cancer Res.* **50,** 2397–2403.
Hefta, S. A., L. J. F. Hefta, T. D. Lee, R. J. Paxton, and E. Shively (1988), *Proc. Natl. Acad. Sci. USA* **85,** 4648–4653.
Henze, E., R. Kübel, J. Waitzinger, M. Büchler, W. E. Adam, and H. G. Beger (1987), *Eur. J. Nucl. Med.* **13,** 125–129.
Herbeth, B. and A. Bagrel (1980), *Oncodev. Biol. Med.* **1,** 191–198.
Herrera, M. A., T. M. Chu, and E. D. Holyoke (1976), *Ann. Surg.* **183,** 5–9.
Herrera, M. A., T. M. Chu, E. D. Holyoke, and A. Mittelman (1977), *Ann. Surg.* **185,** 23–30.
Hinoda, Y., M. Neumaier, S. A. Hefta, Z. Drzeniek, C. Wagener, L. Shively, L. J. F. Hefta, J. Shively, and R. J. Paxton (1988), *Proc. Natl. Acad. Sci. USA* **85,** 6959–6963
Holyoke, E. D., T. M. Chu, and G. P. Murphy (1975), *Cancer* **35,** 830–836.
Holyoke, E. D., H. O. Douglass, M. H. Goldrosen, and T. M. Chu (1979), *Semin. Oncol.* **6,** 347–356.
Holzheimer R. G. E., K. H. Muhrer, H. Muller, and K. Bosslet (1986), *Br. J. Cancer* **54,** 537–538.
Hostetter, R. B., L. B. Augustus, R. Mankarious, K. Chi, D. Fan, C. Toth, P. Thomas, and J. M. Jessup (1990), *J. Natl. Cancer Inst.* **82,** 380–385.
Ichiki, S., M. Kuroki, A. Matsunaga, F. Arakawa, N. Okamoto, and Y. Matsuoka (1986), *Cancer Res.* **77,** 1005–1011.
Jetha, N., M. L. Woo, and A. A. Nanji (1986), *Am. J. Clin. Pathol.* **85,** 255.
Jubert, A. V., T. M. Talbott, and T. M. Maycroft (1978), *Cancer* **42,** 635–639.
Kairemo, K. J. A. (1990), *Cancer Res. (Suppl.),* **50,** 949S–954S.

Kalser, M. H., J. S. Barkin, D. Redhammer, and A. Heal (1978), *Cancer* **42,** 1468–1471.

Kamarck, M. E., J. J. Elting, J. T. Hart, S. J. Goebel, P. M. M. Rae, M. A. Nothdrift, J. J. Nedwin and T. R. Barnett (1987), *Proc. Natl. Acad. Sci. USA* **84,** 5350–5354.

Kessler, M. J., J. E. Shively, D. G. Pritchard, and C. W. Todd (1978), *Cancer Res.* **38,** 1041–1048.

Khan, W. N. and S. Hammarström (1989), *Biochem. Biophys. Res. Commun.* **161,** 525–535.

Khan, W. N. and S. Hammarström (1990), *Biochem. Biophys. Res. Commun.* **168,** 214–225.

Khan, W. N., A. Osterman, and S. Hammarström (1989), *Proc. Natl. Acad. Sci. USA* **86,** 3332–3336.

Khoo, S. K., N. L. Warner, J. T. Lie, and I. R. Mackay (1973), *Int. J. Cancer* **11,** 681–687.

Klavins, J. V., Y. T. Cho, and R. Pampin (1985), *Bull. Mol. Biol. Med.* **10,** 25–31.

Klemenz, R., S. Hoffmann, and A. K. Werenskiold (1989), *Proc. Natl. Acad. Sci. USA* **86,** 5708–5712.

Koch, M., A. H. G. Paterson, and T. A. McPherson (1980), *Clin. Oncol.* **6,** 323–327.

Kodelja, V., K. Lucas, S. Barnert, S. von Kleist, J. A. Thompson, and W. Zimmermann (1989), *J. Biol. Chem.* **264,** 6906–6912.

Kohler, J. P., D. Simonowitz, and D. Paloyan (1980), *Am. Surg.* **46,** 449–452.

Kojima, O., T. Kurimoto, Y. Uehara, and et al. (1983), *J. Exp. Clin. Cancer Res.* **4,** 389–392.

Krejcarek, G. E. and K. L. Tucker (1977), *Biochem. Biophys. Res. Commun.* **77,** 581–585.

Krischke, W., N. Niederle, J. Schütte, R. Pfeiffer, and H. Hirche (1988), *Cancer* **62,** 1348–1354.

Krohn, K. A., L. Sherman, and N. L. Welch (1972), *Biochem. Biophys. Acta* **285,** 404–413.

Kuroki, M., M. Kuroki, Y. Koga, and Y. Matsuoka (1984), *J. Immunol.* **133,** 2090–2097.

Ladenson, J. H. and J. M. McDonald (1980), *Clin. Chem.* **26,** 1213–1220.

Lamki, L. M., T. P. Haynie, J. L. Murray, R. Babaian, Y. Z. Patt, and B. Merchant (1986), *Br. J. Cancer* **54,** 535.

Lang, B. A., A. Kocent, M. Nekulova, and J. Hlakova (1984), *Neoplasma* **31,** 79–87.

Larson, S. M., J. A. Carrasquillo, K. A. Krohn, J. P. Brown, J. P. McGuffin, J. M. Perens, M. M. Graham, L. D. Hill, P. L. Beaumier, K. E. Hellström, and I. Hellström (1983a), *J. Clin. Invest.* **72,** 2101–2116

Larson, S. M., J. A. Carrasquillo, K. A. Krohn, J. P. Brown, J. P. McGuffin, J. M. Perens, M. M. Graham, L. D. Hill, P. L. Beaumier, K. E. Hellström, and I. Hellström (1983b), *J. Nucl. Med.* **24,** 123–129.
Laurence, D. J. R., U. Stevens, R. Bettelheim, D. Darcy, C. Leese, C. Tuberville, P. Alexander, E. W. Johns, and A. M. Neville (1972), *Br. Med. J.* **9,** 605–609.
Lavin, P. T., J. Day, E. D. Holyoke, A. Mittelman, and T. M. Chu (1981), *Cancer* **47,** 823–826.
Lazorthes, F., P. Chiotasso, J. Roques, and J.-P. Vinel (1986), *Cancer du Rectum* **36,** 2389–2395.
Leusch, H. G., S. A. Hera, Z. Drzeniek, K. Hummel, Z. Markos-Pusztai and C. Wagener (1990), *FEBS Lett.* **261,** 405–409.
Lewi, H., L. H. Blumgart, D. C. Carter, C. R. Gillis, D. Hole, J. G. Ratcliffe, C. B. Wood, and C. S. McArdle (1984), *Br. J. Surg.* **71,** 206–208.
Lind, H. M. and P. Haghighi (1986), *Am. J. Clin. Pathol.* **86,** 538–540.
Livingstone, A. S., L. G. Hampson, J. Shuster, and E. J. Hinchey (1974), *Arch. Surg.* **109,** 259–264.
Lokich, J. J. (1982), *Cancer* **50,** 2154–2156.
Lokich, J. J., N. Zamcheck, and M. Lowenstein (1978), *Ann. Intern. Med.* **89,** 902–906.
LoGerfo, P. and F. P. Hester (1975), *Ann. Surg.* **181,** 81–84.
LoGerfo, P., J. Krupey, and H. J. Hansen (1972), *Ann. Surg.* **175,** 495–500.
Loprinzi, C. L. and D. L. Ahmann (1986), *Arch. Intern. Med.* **146,** 2125–2126.
Lowenstein, M. S. and N. Zamcheck (1977), *Gastroenterology* **72,** 161–166.
Lowenstein, M. S. and N. Zamcheck (1978), *Cancer* **42,** 1412–1418.
Lunde, O. C. H. and O. Havig (1982), *Acta Chir. Scand.* **148,** 189–193.
Mach, J.-P., P. Jaeger, and M.-M. Bertholet (1974a), *Lancet* **7,** 535–540.
Mach, J.-P., S. Carrel, C. Merenda, B. Sordat, and J. C. Cerottini (1974b), *Nature* **248,** 704–706.
Mach, J.-P., H. Vieny, P. Jaeger, B. Haldemann, R. Egely, and J. Pettavel (1978), *Cancer* **42,** 1439–1447.
Mach, J.-P., M. Forni, J. Ritschard, F. Buchegger, S. Carrel, S. Widgren, A. Donath, and P. Alberto (1980a), *Oncodev. Biol. Med.* **1,** 49–69.
Mach, J.-P., F. Buchegger, M. Forni, J. Ritschard, A. Donath, and P. Alberto (1980b), *N. Engl. J. Med.* **303,** 5–10.
Mach, J.-P., F. Bucheggar, M. Forni, J. Ritschard, , C. Berche, J.-D. Lumbroso, C. Girardet, R. S. Accolla, and S. Carrel (1981) *Immunol. Today* **2,** 239–249
Mach, J.-P., F. Bucheggar, M. Forni, J. Ritschard, S. Carrel, R. Egley, A. Donath, and A. Rohner (1983a), *Curr. Top. Microbiol. Immunol.* **104,** 49–55.
Mann, B., M. Cohen, R. Saxton, D. L. Morton, W. F. Benedict, E. L. Korn, L. Spotter, L. S. Graham, C. C. Chang, and M. W. Burk (1984), *Cancer* **54,** 1319–1327.

Mansour, E. G., M. Hastert, C. H. Park, K. A. Koelher, and M. Petrelli (1983), *Cancer* **51,** 1243–1248.
Martin, E. W. Jr., W. E. Kibbey, L. DiVecchia, G. Anderson, P. Catalano, and J. P. Minton (1976), *Cancer* **37,** 62–81.
Martin, K. W. and S. E. Halpern (1984), *Cancer Res.* **44,** 5475–5481.
Martinez, V. and J. G. Azzopardi (1979), *Histopathology* **3,** 467–488.
Marx, J. (1989), *Science* **246,** 1386–1388.
Matsuoka, Y., K. Endo, Y. Kawamura, T. Yoshida, T. Saga, Y. Watanabe, M. Koizumi, T. Nakashima, J. Konishi, N. Yamaguchi, and R. Yatain (1990), *Cancer* **65,** 506–510.
Mayer, R. J. (1988), in *Scientific American Medicine* vol. **12,** (Rubenstein, E. and D. D. Federman, eds.), Scientific American, New York, pp. 9–15.
Mayer, R. J., M. B. Garnick, G. D. Steele, and N. Zamcheck (1978), *Cancer* **42,** 1428–1433.
McLenachan, T. and B. Mansfield (1989), *Biochem. Biophys. Res. Commun.* **162,** 1486–1493.
Medical Research Council Tumour Products Committee: Clinical Subgroup (1980), *Br. J. Cancer* **41,** 976–979.
Meeker, W. R., R. Kashmire, L. Hunter, W. Clapp, and W. O. Griffen, Jr. (1973), *Arch. Surg.* **107,** 266–274.
Merril, W. W., M. Goodman, R. A. Matthay, G. P. Naegel, J. P. Vandevoorde, A. D. Myl, and H. Y. Reynolds (1981), *Am. Rev. Respir. Dis.* **123,** 29–31.
Midiri, G., C. Amanti, F. Consorti, M. Benedetti, S. Del Buono, U. Di Tondo, G. Castagna, L. Peronace, and M. Di Paola (1983), *J. Surg. Oncol.* **22,** 257–260.
Moertel, C. G., A. J. Schutt, and V. L. W. Go (1978), *JAMA* **239,** 1065–1066.
Mori, M., K. Ambe, Y. Adachi, Y. Yakeishi, K. Nakamura, Y. Hachitanda, M. Enjoli, and K. Sugimachi (1988), *Cancer* **62,** 534–540.
Moscatelli, G., M. Agostini, S. Benini, G. Paganelli, P. Riva, and V. Tison (1986), *Br. J. Cancer* **54,** 554.
Mughal, A. W., G. N. Hortobagyi, H. A. Fritsche, A. U. Buzdar, H. Y. Yap, and G. R. Blumenschein (1983), *JAMA* **249,** 1881–1886.
Myers, R. E., D. J. A. Sutherland, J. W. Meakin, J. A. Kellen, D. G. Malkin, and A. Malkin (1978), *Cancer (Suppl.),* **42,** 1520–1526.
Myers, R. E., D. J. A. Sutherland, J. W. Meakin, D. G. Malkin, J. A. Kellen, and A. Malkin (1979a), *Recent Results Cancer Res.* **67,** 26–32.
Nanbu, Y., S. Fujii, I. Konishi, H. Nonogaki, and T. Mori (1988), *Cancer* **62,** 2580–2588.
Nap, M. (1986), *Bull. Cancer* **73,** 325–331.
Nap, M., H. Keuning, P. Burtin, J. W. Oosterhuis, and G. J. Fleuren (1984), *Am. J. Clin. Pathol.* **82,** 526–534.
Nap, M., K. Mollgard, P. Burtin, and G. J. Fleuren (1985), Abstract of XIII

Annual Meeting of the International Society for Oncodevelopmental Biology and Medicine, Paris, France, September 10–13.

Nap, M., K. Mollgard, P. Burtin, and G. J. Fleuren (1988), *Tumor Biology* **9,** 145–153.

Nasierowska-Guttmejer, A. and A. Szawlowski (1989), *Int. J. Biol. Markers* **4,** 8–12.

National Institute of Health Consensus Development Conference (1981), *Ann. Intern. Med.* **94,** 407–409.

Neumaier, M., W. Zimmermann, L. Shively, L. Hinoda, Y. Riggs, and J. E. Shively (1988), *J. Biol. Chem.* **263,** 3202–3207.

Neville, A. M., S. Patel, M. Capp, D. J. R. Laurence, E. H. Cooper, C. Turberville, and R. C. Coombes (1978), *Cancer* **42,** 1448–1451.

Neville, A. M. (1981), *Br. Med. J. (Clin. Res.),* **282,** 373–375.

Northover, J. (1986), *Gut* **27,** 117–122.

Oikawa, S., H. Nakazato, and G. Kosaki (1987a), *Biochem. Biophys. Res. Commun.* **142,** 511–518.

Oikawa, S., S. Imajo, T. Noguchi, G. Kosaki, and H. Nakazoto (1987b), *Biochem. Biophys. Res. Commun.* **144,** 634–642.

Ona, F. V., N. Zamcheck, P. Dhar, T. Moore, and H. Z. Kupchik (1973), *Cancer* **31,** 324–327.

Onetto, M., M. Paganuzzi, G. B. Secco, R. Fardelli, F. Santi, S. Rovida, and G. B. Ferrara (1985), *Biomed. Pharmacother.* **39,** 392–395.

Paganelli, G., P. Riva, G. Sarti, V. Tison, G. Cacciaguerra, G. Fiorentini, G. Moscatelli, S. Benini, and M. Agostini (1986), *Br. J. Cancer* **54,** 542–543.

Pagé, M., I. Dalifard, G. Bertrand, P. G. Bocquillon, and A. Daver (1986), *Anticancer Res.* **6,** 893–896.

Palazzo, S., V. Liquori, B. Molinari, L. M. Greco, and V. Mancini (1986), *Tumori* **72,** 57–59.

Palazzo, S., V. Liquori, and B. Molinari (1984), *Tumori* **70,** 57.

Patt, Y. Z., L. M. Lamki, T. P. Haynie, M. W. Unger, M. G. Rosenblum, A. Shirkhoda, and J. L. Murray (1988), *J. Clin. Oncol.* **6,** 1220–1230.

Pavelic, Z. P., N. Petrelli, L. Herrera, M. M. Vaughan, J. S. Poecock, and L. Pavelic (1990), *J. Cancer Res. Clin. Oncol.* **116,** 51–56.

Paxton, R. J., J. G. Jakowatz, J. D. Beatty, B. G. Beatty, W. G. Vlahos, L. E. Williams, B. R. Clark, and J. E. Shively (1985), *Cancer Res.* **45,** 5694–5699.

Paxton, R. J., G. Mooser, H. Pande, T. D. Lee and J. E. Shively (1987), *Proc. Natl. Acad. Sci. USA* **84,** 920–924.

Persijn, J. P. (1980), *Neth. J. Med.* **23,** 1–3.

Persijn, J. P. and C. B. Korsten (1977), *J. Clin. Chem. Clin. Biochem.* **15,** 553–556.

Philben, V. J., J. G. Jakowatz, B. G. Beatty, W. G. Vlahos, R. J. Paxton, L. E. Williams, J. E. Shively, and J. D. Beatty (1986), *Cancer* **57,** 571–576.
Pimm, M. V. and R. W. Baldwin (1986), *J. Nucl. Med.* **27,** 1788–1789.
Pimm, M. V., A. C. Perkins, N. C. Armitage, and R. W. Baldwin (1985b), *J. Nucl. Med.* **26,** 1011–1023.
Podolsky, D. K., M. S. McPhee, E. Alpert, A. L. Warshaw, and K. Isselbaker (1981), *N. Engl. J. Med.* **304,** 1313–1318.
Pompecki, R., G. Schroder, M. Garbrecht, and H. Frahn (1978), *Dtsch. Med. Wochenschr.* **103,** 620–622.
Pressman, D. and L. Korngold (1953), *Cancer* **6,** 619–623.
Primus, F. J., C. A. Clark, and D. M. Goldenberg (1981), in *Diagnostic Immunochistohemistry,* (DeLellis, R. A., ed.), Masson, New York, pp. 263–276.
Primus, F. J., W. J. Kuhns, and D. M. Goldenberg (1983b), *Cancer Res.* **43,** 693–697.
Primus, F. J., R. J. Wang, D. M. Goldenberg, and H. J. Hansen (1973), *Cancer Res.* **33,** 2977–2982
Proceedings of the First International Conference on the Clinical Use of Carcinoembryonic Antigen (1978), *Cancer* **42,** 1397.
Pusztaszeri, G. and J.-P. Mach (1973), *Immunochemistry* **10,** 197–204.
Quetmeler, A., P. Möller, V. Schwartz, U. Abel, and P. Schlag (1987), *Cancer* **60,** 2261–2266.
Rainsbury, R. M. (1984), *Br. J. Surg.* **71,** 805–812.
Reif, A. E., L. E. Curtis, R. Duffield, and I. A. Shauffer (1974), *J. Surg. Oncol.* **6,** 133–150.
Rhodes, B. A., P. O. Zamoa, K. D. Newell, and E. F. Valdez (1986), *J. Nucl. Med.* **27,** 685–693.
Rimstein A, H.-O. Adami, B. Wahren, and B. Nordin (1979), *Br. J. Cancer* **39,** 109–115.
Riva, P., G. Moscatelli, G. Paganelli, S. Benini, and A. Siccardi (1988), *Int. J. Cancer (Suppl.),* **2,** 114–120.
Riva, P., G. Paganelli, G. Riciputi, G. Pasini, S. Benini, M. Agostini, G. Moscatelli, G. Cacciaguerra, V. Tison, P. Morigi, and V. Stancanelli (1986), *Br. J. Cancer* **54,** 538.
Robertson, J. F. R., I. O. Ellis, J. Bell, J. H. Todd, A. Robins, C. W. Elston, and R. W. Blamey (1989),*Cancer* **64,,** 1638–1645.
Rogers, G. T. (1986) *Br. J. Cancer Clin. Oncol.* **22,** 1127–1133
Rognum, T., K. Elgio, P. Brandtzaeg, H. Orjasaeter, and A. Bergan (1982), *J. Clin. Pathol.* **35,** 922–933.
Sato, C., M. Miyaki, S. Oikawa, H. Nakazato, and G. Kosaki (1988), *Jpn. J. Cancer Res. (Gann),* **79,** 433–437.
Savoie, S. and H. Sikorska (1991), *Anticancer Res.* **11,** 1–12.

Scheele, P. M., R. W. Bendon, and B. R. Mukunda (1989), *Arch. Pathol. Lab. Med.* **113,** 1142–1146.

Schrool, R.W., K.A. Foon, S.M. Beatty, R.K. Oldham, and A. Morgan (1985), *Cancer Res.* **45,** 879–885.

Schwarz, A. and A. Steinsträsser (1987), *J. Nucl. Med.* **28,** 721.

Sculier, J.P., J.J. Body, D. Jacobowitz, and J. Fruhling (1987), *Eur. J. Cancer Clin. Oncol.* **23,** 1091–1093.

Scully, R.E. (1978), in *Atals of Tumor Pathology,* Second series, AFIP, Hartmann, Washington, DC.

Sehested, M., F. R. Hirsch, and K. Hou-Jensen (1981), *Clin. Oncol.* **17,** 1125–1131.

Shani, A., J. O'Connell, C. G. Moertel, A. J. Schutt, A. Silvers, and V. L. M. Go (1978), *Ann. Intern. Med.* **88,** 627–630.

Sharkey, R. M., D. M. Goldenberg, H. Goldenberg, R. E. Lee, C. Ballance, D. Pawlyk Varga, and H. J. Hansen (1990), *Cancer Res.* **50,** 2823–2831.

Shek, P. N. (1984), in *Immunotoxicity* (P. Mullen, ed.), Springer-Verlag, Heidelberg, pp. 103–125.

Shi, Z. R., D. Tsao, and Y. S. Kim (1983), *Cancer Res.* **43,** 4045–4059.

Shimizu, M., Y. Saitoh, H. Ohyanagi, and H. Hoh (1990), *Arch. Pathol. Lab. Med.* **114,** 195–200.

Shinkai, T., M. Saijo, K. Tominaga, K. Eguchi, E. Shimizu, Y. Sasaki, J. Fujita, H. Futami, H. Ohkura, and K. Suemasu (1986), *Cancer* **57,** 1318–1323.

Shively, J. E. and J. D. Beatty (1985), *CRC Crit. Rev. Oncol. Hematol.* **2,** 355–399.

Shousha, S. and T. Lyssiotis (1978), *Histopathology* **2,** 433–447.

Shousha, S., T. Lyssiotis, V. M. Godefrey, and P. J. Sheuer (1979), *Br. Med. J.* **1,** 777–779.

Shuster, J. D., M. P. Thompson, A. Fuks, and P. Gold (1980), *Prog. Exp. Tumor Res.* **25,** 89–139.

Siccardi, A. G., G. L. Buraggi, L. Callegaro, A. Centi Colella, P. G. De Filippi, G. Galli, G. Mariani, R. Masi, R. Palumbo, P. Riva, M. Salvatore, G. A. Scassellati, K. Scheidhauer, G. L. Turco, P. Zaniol, S. Benini, G. Deleide, M. Gasparini, S. Lastoria, L. Mansi, G. Paganelli, E. Salvischiani, E. Seregni, G. Viale, and P. G. Natali (1989), *Cancer Res.* **49,** 3095–3103.

Sikorska, H., J. Shuster, and P. Gold (1988), *Cancer Detect. Prev.* **2,** 321–355.

Silva, J. S., G. S. Leight, D. E. Haagensen, P. B. Tallos, E. B. Cox, and S. A. Wells (1982), *Cancer* **49,** 1236–1242.

Silverberg, E. (1983), *Cancer Stat.* **3,** 9–25.

Smets, G., F. Warson, M.-F. Dehou, G. Storme, R. Sacré, S. van Belle, G. Somers, W. Gepts, and G. Klöppel (1990), *Virchows Arch. [A]* **416,** 539–543.

Sorokin, J. J., P. H. Sugarbaker, N. Zamcheck, M. Pisick, H. Z. Kupchik, and T.D. Moore (1974), *JAMA* **228,** 49–53.

Stabb, H. J., F. A. Anderer, T. Brummendorf, E. Stumpf, and R. Fisher (1981), *Br. J. Cancer* **44,** 652–662.

Stamatiadis, A. P., M. St. Toumanidou, G. P. Vyssoulis, A. J. Manouras, and N. S. Apostolidis (1990), *Cancer* **65,** 2055–2057.

Steele, G. Jr., S. Ellenberg, K. Ramming, M. O'Connell, C. Moertel, H. Lessner, H. Bruckner, J. Horton, P. Schein, N. Zamcheck, and J. Novak (1982), *Ann. Surg.* **196,** 162–169.

Stern, P., P. Hagan, S. E. Halpern, and et al. (1982), in *Hybridomas in Cancer Diagnosis and Treatment,* vol. 21, Raven, New York, pp. 245–253.

Stevens, D. P. and I. R. Mackay (1973), *Lancet* **ii,** 1238–1239.

Stevens, D. P., I. R. Mackay, and K. J. Culllen (1975), *Br. J. Cancer* **32,** 147–151.

Steward, A. M., D. Nixon, N. Zamcheck, and A. Aisenberg (1974), *Cancer* **33,** 1246–1252.

Stockley, R. A., J. Shaw, A. G. W. Whitfield, T. P. Whitehead, C. A. Clarke, and D. Burnett (1986), *Thorax* **41,** 17–24.

Stokes, T. C., J. F. S. Stevens, P. Long, E. Lockey, and A. L. Miller (1980), *Br. J. Dis. Chest* **74,** 390–394.

Streydio, C., K. Lacka, S. Swillens, and G. Vassart (1988), *Biochem. Biophys. Res. Commun.* **154,** 130–137.

Sugamo, K., H. Ohkura, S. Hirohashi, Y. Shimosato, Y. Sakurai, S. Kodaira, and O. Abe (1989), *Cancer Res.* **80,** 1156–1160.

Sugarbaker, P. H., W. D. Bloomer, E. D. Corbett, and J. T. Chaffey (1976), *AJR* **127,** 641–644.

Sugarbaker, P. H., W. D. Bloomer, E. D. Corbett, and J. T. Chaffey (1978), *Cancer* **42,** 1434–1436.

Sullivan, D. C., J. S. Silva, C. E. Cox, D. E. Gaagensen, Jr., C. C. Harris, W. H. Briner, and W. A. Wells, Jr. (1982), *Invest. Radiol.* **17,** 350–355.

Summary of an NIH Consensus Statement (1981), *Br. Med. J.* **282,** 373–375.

Szymendera, J. J., M. P. Nowacki, A. W. Szawlowski, and J. A. Kaminska (1982), *Dis. Colon Rectum* **25,** 46–52.

Tabor, E., R. J. Gerety, C. F. Needy, B. L. Elisberg, A. R. Colon, and R. Jones (1981), *Eur. J. Cancer* **17,** 257–258.

Tatsuta, M., H. Iishi, H. Yamamura, and S. Okuda (1988), *Oncology* **45,** 30–34.

Tawaragi, Y., S. Oikawa, Y. Matsuoka, G. Kosaki, and H. Nakazato (1988), *Biochem. Biophys. Res. Commun.* **150,** 89–96.

Te Velde, E. R., Y. P. Persi, R. E. Ballieux, and Y. Faber (1982), *Cancer* **49,** 1866–1875.

Thompson, J. and W. Zimmermann (1988), *Tumor Biol.* **9,** 63–83.

Thompson, J. A., H. Pande, R. J. Paxton, L. Shively, A. Padma, R. L. Simmer, C. W. Todd, A. S. Rissi, and J. E. Shively (1987), *Proc. Natl. Acad. Sci. USA* **84,** 2965–2970.

Tomoda, H. and M. Furusawa (1981), *Jpn. J. Surg.* **11,** 33–38.
Tormey, D. C., T. P. Waalkes, D. Ahmann, C. W. Gehrke, R. W. Sumwatt, J. Snyder, and H. Hansen (1975), *Cancer* **35,** 1095–1100.
Tormey, D. C., T. P. Waalkes, J. J. Snyder, and R. M. Simon (1977), *Cancer* **39,** 2397–2404.
Tormey, D. C. and T. P. Waalkes (1978), *Cancer* **42,** 1507–1511.
Tormey, D. C., T. E. Davis, and T. P. Waalkes (1982), in *Principles of Cancer Treatment* (Carter, S. J., E. Glatstein, and R. B. Livingston, eds.), McGraw-Hill, New York, pp. 170–177.
Touitou, Y., J. Proust, E. Klinger, J. P. Nakache, D. Huard, and A. Sachet (1984), *Eur. J. Cancer Clin. Oncol.* **20,** 369–374.
Traub, U. C., R. L. DeJager, J. Primus, M. Losman, and D. M. Goldenberg (1988), *Cancer Res.* **48,** 4002–4006.
Tsutsumi, Y., H. Nagura, and K. Watanabe (1984), *Am. J. Clin. Pathol.* **82,** 535–542.
Vanderick, J., N. Leners, A. Ferrant, C. Deckers, and G. Schulz (1986), *Br. J. Cancer* **54,** 534–535.
Van der Linden, J. C., J. P. A. Baak, J. Lindeman, A. W. M. Smeulders, and C. J. L. M. Meyer (1985), *Histopathology* **9,** 1051–1059.
Varnavides, L. A., N. J. O'Higgens, and C. G. Clark (1978), *Clin. Oncol.* **4,** 329–337.
Vest, S. L. and J. K. Roche (1982), *Dig. Dis. Sci.* **27,** 289–296.
Vider, M., R. Kashmiri, L. Hunter, B. Moses, W. R. Meeker, J. F. Utler, and Y. Maruyama (1974), *Oncology* **30,** 257–272.
Von Kleist, S., C. Wittekind, E. Sandritter, and H. Gropp (1982), *Pathol. Res. Pract.* **173,** 390–401.
Waalkes, T. P., M. D. Abeloff, K. B. Woo, D. S. Ettinger, R. W. Ruddon, and P. Aldenderfer (1980), *Cancer Res.* **40,** 4420–4427.
Waalkes, T. P., J. P. Enterline, and J. H. Shaper (1984), *Cancer* **53,** 644–651.
Waalkes, T. P., C. W. Gehrke, D. C. Tormey, K. B. Woo, K. C. Kuo, J. Snyder, and H. Hansen (1978), *Cancer* **41,** 1871–1881.
Wagener, C., Y. H. I. Yang, F. G. Crawford, and J. F. Shively (1983), *J. Immunol.* **130,** 2308–2315.
Wahl, R. L., C. W. Parker, and G. W. Philpott (1983), *J. Nucl. Med.* **24,** 316–325.
Wahren, B., E. Lidbrink, A. Wallgren, P. Eneroth, and J. Zajicek (1978), *Cancer* **42,** 1870–1878.
Walker, R. A. (1980), *J. Clin. Pathol.* **33,** 356–360.
Wanebo, H. J., B. Rao, C. M. Pinsky, R. G. Hoffman, M. Stearns, M. K. Schwartz, and H. F. Oettgen (1978a), *N. Engl. J. Med.* **299,** 448–451.
Wanebo, H. J., M. Stearn, and M. K. Schwartz (1978b), *Ann. Surg.* **188,** 481–493.

Wang, D. Y., R. D. Bulbrook, J. L. Hayward, J. C. Hendricks, and P. Franchimont (1975), *Eur. J. Cancer* **11,** 615–618.
Wang, D. Y., R. E. Knyba, R. D. Bulbrook, R. R. Millis, and J. L. Hayward (1984), *Eur. J. Cancer Clin. Oncol.* **20,** 25–31.
Watanabe, S., and J. Y. Chou (1988a) *J. Biol. Chem.* **263,** 2049–2054.
Watanabe, S., and J. Y. Chou (1988b) *Biochem. Biophys. Res. Comun.* **152,** 762–768
Williams, A. F. (1987), *Immunol. Today* **8,** 298–303.
Williams, R. R., K. R. McIntire, T. A. Waldmann, M. Feinleib, V. L. W. Go, W. B. Kannel, T. R. Dawber, W. P. Castelli, and P. M. McNamara (1977), *J. Natl. Cancer Inst.* **58,** 1547–1551.
Wittekind, C., S. von Kleist, and W. Sandritter (1981), *Oncodev. Biol. Med.* **2,** 381–390.
Wolmark, N., B. Fisher, H. S. Wieand, and R. S. Henry (1981), *Ann. Surg.* **199,** 375–382.
Wood, C. B., J. G. Ratcliffe, R. W. Burt, A. J. H. Malcolm, and L. H. Blumgart (1980), *Br. J. Surg.* **67,** 46–48.
Wong, A. and H. M. Yazdi (1990), *Acta Cytologica* **34,**192–196.
Wong, J. Y. C., N. F. Mivechi, R. J. Paxton, L. E. Williams, B. G. Beatty, J. D. Beatty, and J. E. Shively (1989), *Int. J. Rad. Oncol. Biol. Phys.* **17,** 803–808.
Yap, B. S., H. Y. Yap, H. A. Fritsche, G. Blumenschein, and G. P. Bodey (1980), *JAMA* **244,**1601–1603.
Zamcheck, N., T. L. Moore, P. Dhar, and H. Kupchik (1972), *N. Engl. J. Med.* **286,** 83–86.
Zamcheck, N., W. G. Doos, R. Prudente, B. B. Lurie, and L. S. Gottlieb (1975), *Hum. Pathol.* **6,** 31–45.
Zamcheck, N. (1978), *Excerpta Medica* **439,** 64–79.
Zamcheck, N. (1981a), *Cancer Bull.* **33,** 141–151.
Zamcheck, N. and E. W. Martin (1981b), *Cancer* **47,** 1620–1627.
Zimmermann, W., B. Ortlieb, R. Friedrich, and S. Von Kleist (1987a), *Proc. Natl. Acad. Sci. USA* **84,** 2960–2964.
Zimmermann, W., B. Ortlieb, F. Rudert, S. Barnett, M. Weiss, S. Von Kleist, B. Weber, J. E. Shively, and J. Thompson (1987b), Abstract Book and Program for the XV Annual Meeting of the International Society for Oncodevelopment Biology and Medicine, Quebec, Canada, August 30–September 3, 1987, Abstract 134, p. 125.
Zimmermann, W., B. Weber, B. Ortlieb, F. Rudert, W. Schempp, H. H. Fiebig, J. E. Shively, S. Von Kleist, and J. A. Thomson (1988), *Cancer Res.* **48,** 2550–2554.

Chapter 5

Prostate-Specific Antigen

T. Ming Chu

1. Introduction

The single most important development in clinical cancer markers since the early 1970s, when carcinoembryonic antigen (CEA) was approved by the Food and Drug Administration, is the approval of a prostate-specific antigen (PA or PSA) as a cancer-marker test for adenocarcinoma of the prostate in 1985. In fact, whatever CEA can do for gastrointestinal cancer, PSA can do, and do it better, for prostate cancer. The clinical application of PSA in diagnosis, prognosis, and monitoring of prostate cancer is the subject of this chapter. Basic characteristics of this marker of prostate cancer also will be reviewed. Reviews of similar topic are available elsewhere (Wang et al., 1982; Chu, 1985, 1990; Chu and Murphy, 1986; Brawer and Lange, 1989; Catalona et al., 1989; Killian and Chu, 1990). It should be noted that PSA is not a neoantigen of prostate cancer or a prostate cancer specific antigen; rather, it is expressed equally, but exclusively, by normal, benign hyperplastic and cancerous prostate glands (Wang et al., 1979; Papsidero et al., 1981).

From: *Serological Cancer Markers* Edited by Stewart Sell ©1992 The Humana Press, Totowa, NJ

2. Molecular and Biological Characteristics

The existence of various prostate-specific antigens has been reported for some time (Flocks et al., 1960; Ablin et al., 1970). PSA, the specific marker used for the detection and diagnosis of prostate cancer discussed here, was identified, purified, and characterized initially in 1979 by Wang et al. Purified PSA is a glycoprotein with a mol wt of 34 kDa and isoelectric point of 6.9, consisting of approx 93% peptide and 7% carbohydrate (Wang et al., 1979, 1983). The peptide backbone of 240 amino acid residues has been completely sequenced, with proline and isoleucine as the C- and N- terminal amino acid, respectively (Watt et al., 1986). Asparagine-45 for N- linkage and serine-69, theonine-70, and serine-71 for O-linkage have been postulated as the possible locations of carbohydrate side chains, yet the sequence of oligosaccharide is to be determined. Other physicochemical parameters of PSA include a Stoke's radius of 24Å, a sedimentation coefficient of 3.1 S, and a partial specific volume of 0.73 mL/g (Wang et al., 1983).

Possibly because of its unique primary and/or three-dimensional structure, specific polyclonal antibodies and monoclonal antibodies have been generated against PSA (Wang et al., 1979; Papsidero et al., 1983; Chu et al., 1989). A cluster of two epitopes that are spatially related or in close topographical proximity representing a prostate-specific antigenic domain has been identified by monoclonal antibodies (Chu et al., 1989). However, the exact amino acid sequence or residues of this antigenic domain remain unknown. The existence of other prostate-specific antigenic determinants is also possible.

Purified PSA is shown to express a mild protease activity, distinct from any other known proteases (Ban et al., 1984). A high degree of amino acid sequence homology is shared between PSA and serine protease of the kallikrein family (Watt et al., 1986). Extending from this finding, PSA has been claimed to be a glandular kallikrein, and the gene for this kallikrein-PSA, sometimes called kallikrein-I, has been cloned and shown to be situated at chromosome 19 (Lilja, 1988; Henttu and Vihko, 1989; Lundwall, 1989;

Reigman et al., 1989). Although molecular biology work of kallikrein-PSA has been reported, there are no direct data unequivocally linking the identity between PSA/PA and human glandular kallikrein. Therefore, the validity and usefulness of this information should be reserved at this time. The proteolytic activity of PSA is claimed to be associated with liquefaction of seminal clots and with the structural protein of human seminal coagulum as a potential physiological substrate (Lilja, 1988). Yet a recent report has challenged this claim (Dube et al., 1989).

Some workers have claimed the identify of PSA with p30, a semen-specific protein (Sensabaugh, 1978). However, physicochemical characteristics of p30 and PSA, including homogeneity of purified protein, binding and elution profile on ion-exchange column, immunoelecrophoretic migration pattern, isoelectric point, and molecular weight, clearly indicate that PSA is distinctly different from p30. Some investigators have also claimed the identity of PSA with γ-seminoprotein (Hara et al., 1971). Yet the molecular weight and amino acid composition reported initially for γ-seminoprotein also clearly distinguish PSA from γ-seminoproein.

One aspect of PSA's protease activity is of practical interest in clinical oncology/urology, i.e., autodigestion of PSA (Ban et al., 1984). The possible locations of three endoproteolytic cleavages (lysine-148, lysine-185, and arginine-85) have been identified (Watt et al., 1986). The addition of protease inhibitors to PSA assay specimens and reagent kits should therefore be considered in order to avoid this possible autohydrolysis of PSA in solution.

3. Initial Serum Assay and Clinical Evaluation

Subsequent to the 1979 report of PSA, sera from patients with prostate cancer were detected to contain PSA immunochemically identical to that of the prostate gland (Papsidero et al., 1980). A quantitative and reproducible sandwich-type enzyme-linked immunosorbent assay (ELISA) with sensitivity of 0.1 ng PA/mL using a specific rabbit polyclonal antiserum was developed

(Kuriyama et al., 1980). The clinical potential of this ELISA for diagnosis, prognosis, and monitoring of prostate cancer was soon realized.

In this first ELISA for PSA, normal male controls were found to contain serum PSA ranging from <0.1 to 2.6 ng/mL (mean 0.47). No circulating PSA was found in normal female controls or female patients with cancer. Male patients with cancers other than prostate cancer were found to exhibit a level of PSA similar to that of male controls.

An elevated serum PSA level (>1.8 ng/mL) was found in patients with prostatic cancer. In patients with various clinical stages of prostate cancer, the mean values were 4.8 ng/mL for stage A, 5.0 for B, 10.1 for C, and 24.2 for stage D. Many patients with stage C and D prostate cancer were found to contain highly elevated serum PSA. Patients with benign prostatic hyperplasia (BPH) exhibited a mean of 3.4 ng/mL, which was statistically different from that of normal male controls. A suggestive difference in the mean PSA levels was found beween stage A prostate cancer and BPH, and a highly significant difference was found between stage C or D and BPH.

In an initial double-blind study with the National Prostatic Cancer Project Treatment Group, patients with advanced prostate cancer (D_2) in whom previous hormonal therapy had failed, and who were then randomized to receive adjuvant chemotherapies, were evaluated by serum PSA assay for their treatment response and survival (Kuriyama et al., 1981). An excellent correlation between serum PSA levels and patient's clinical status was detected: PSA levels increased as disease progressed, decreased as disease regressed, and remained fluctuating when patients had stable disease; i.e., PSA is a monitoring indicator for prostate cancer. Another significant finding was that the patient's survival, regardless of treatment regimen, was proportionally and inversely related to the pretreatment serum PSA levels; i.e., PSA is a prognostic indicator for prostate cancer.

These two classic papers of ours (Kuriyama et al., 1980, 1981) reported essentially the same information that has been reported in over hundreds of papers since 1981. This provided the basis for eventual clinical application of PSA as the most effective tumor marker to date for the management of prostate cancer.

Since our initial ELISA, improved immunoassay systems, especially with the use of monoclonal antibody reagents, have been available commercially. The assay kit manufactured by Hybritech Corporation (San Diego, CA) was approved by the Food and Drug Administration in 1985. Hopefully, others will follow soon.

4. Stability of Circulating Prostate-Specific Antigen

As determined by the assay kit of Hybritech, serum PSA is stable at room temperature for 2 d, at 4°C for 7 d, and at –20 or –80°C for longer periods of time (up to 9 mo). Thawing and freezing (at –20 and –80°C) of serum specimens eight times over a 6-mo period does not affect the PSA level (Killian et al., 1988).

Serum PSA levels in vivo show no circadian rhythmic variation (Shirbiny et al., 1990). A minimum daily or hourly random fluctuation has been reported (Maatman, 1989).

5. Screening and Early Detection of Prostate Cancer

Our initial results indicating some degrees of overlapping between BPH and early prostate cancer would suggest that serum PSA alone is of limited use as a general screening tool for early detection of prostate cancer (Kuriyama et al., 1980). In a recent study involving 321 patients (220 controls, 30 BPH, and 71 with carcinoma), a conclusion essentially identical to ours was reached, i.e., it is misleading to use PSA alone as a means of cancer screening for the general public (Caty et al., 1988).

However, when used in combination with transrectal ultrasound (TUS) technique, PSA is of practical clinical value in early detection of prostate cancer. In a study in which 256 patients with hypoechoic lesions of prostate found at ultrasound were further evaluated with PSA and digital rectal examination (DRE) (Lee et al., 1989), positive predictive value for prostate cancer for TUS alone was 41%; it increased to 61% if the patient had a positive result from DRE, to 51% if the PSA level was elevated, and to 71% if both the DRE result and the PSA level were abnormal. On the other hand, the positive predictive value for TUS decreased to 24% if DRE results were normal, to 12% if the PSA was normal, and to 5% if both DRE and PSA were normal. No cancers were detected in lesions 1.0 cm or less if DRE and PSA were normal. These data indicated that PSA is a valuable complement to TUS examination.

Another study assessing the ability of PSA and TUS to diagnose persistent prostate cancer in 26 patients following an I-125 seed implant also provided some interesting information (Lee et al., 1988). The positive predictive values for cancer were 91% by TUS, 100% by DRE, and 89% by PSA. The negative predictive values were 13% for DRE and 0% for PSA. The overall detection rates for 26 patients were 81% for TUS, 27% for DRE, and 62% for PSA. The clinical value of serum PSA, the most simple and cost-effective tool, as shown in these two studies is very impressve.

The largest and perhaps most interesting study so far involving TUS, DRE, and PSA in the search for prostate cancer was reported by Cooner et al. (1988). In that study 225 men out of 415, 50–89 yr of age, were followed by DRE yearly for 2–21 yr, and had no findings of abnormality to warrant biopsy. TUS-suspected areas were found in 96 (43%) of the 225 patients, and biopsies were performed on each of them, and detected 28 (29%) carcinoma. Among these 28 men with prostate cancer, 7 (25%) had PSA of <4 ng/mL, 11 (39%) had 4–10 ng/mL, and 10 (36%) had >10 ng/mL. Of these 225 patients, 164 had PSA <4 ng/mL, of which 157 had benign disease and 7 (4.3%) had malignancy upon prostate biopsy. Forty-three patients had PSA of 4–10 ng/mL, of which 32 (74%) had presumably benign disease and 11 (26%) had cancer. Eighteen patients had PSA >10 ng/mL, of which 8 (44%) had presumably benign and 10 (56%) had malignant disease. These encouraging data on PSA, when combined with TUS and DRE, should be pursued, and systematically and prospectively evaluated in well-controlled and documented subjects in long-term study (Anderson and Dunnick, 1989).

Therefore, no single test is ideal for screening. The study did recommend baseline PSA and TUS examination at age 50 followed by annual DRE and PSA determination (Cooner et al., 1988). If either becomes abnormal, TUS is then recommended. At the present stage of development and technology, TUS examination and PSA assay, with or without DRE, appear to be effective for screening the high-risk population for prostate cancer.

6. Staging of Prostate Cancer

As discussed above, serum PSA levels are elevated in some patients with BPH and overlap with the early stage of prostate cancer. To avoid this potential diagnostic difficulty, the use of a higher cutoff point has been applied, e.g., 10 ng/mL. With this adjustment, in one report an elevated PSA was found in 43% of 91 untreated patients with localized prostate cancer, 92% of 60 untreated patients with advanced disease, and none of 10 patients with BPH (Ercole et al., 1987). In fact, elevation of PSA in BPH patients generally is only slight and would not interfere with clinical interpretation of the data. A recent paper reported that the degree of concanavalin A binding can be used to differentiate serum PSA of benign disease from that of malignant lesions (Barak et al., 1989b).

Serum PSA is associated with stage of prostate cancer. In a study of 60 patients with prostate carcinoma, an elevated PSA was found in 16 of 24 (67%) with localized disease (M0) and 34 of 36 (85%) of those with metastatic spread (M1) (Ferro et al., 1987). Additionally, PSA assay from 230 patients with untreated adenocarcinoma of the prostate revealed that PSA level was directly proportional to advanced clinical stage. Serum PSA was able to distinguish stages C plus D_1 from A_2 plus B_1 (Stamey and Kabalin, 1989).

In a study involving 74 patients undergoing radical prostatectomy, PSA levels were abnormal (>10 ng/mL) in 26/44 (59%) of the patients with extracapsular disease and in only 2/30 of those without extracapsular disease (Ercole et al., 1987). Overall, an elevated PSA was found in stage B_2 (2/6), C_1, (2/13), C_2 (4/6), C_3 (8/8), and D_2 (12/17). None of the 10 patients with A_1, 4 with A_2, or 10 with B_1 tumors was found to exhibit an elevated PSA.

Recently available data reveal the association between serum PSA level and prostate size/weight of BPH. The increase in serum PSA level in BPH has been shown in one study to correlate well to the prostate mass ($\gamma = 0.794$) (Barak et al., 1989a). No patient with a prostate weight of >30 g had a PSA of <5 ng/mL, and all patients with PSA of <4 ng/mL had prostate weight of <10 g. Another study reported a more defined association: Serum PSA correlated to prostate size and also to the quantity of prostate epithelia (Weber et al., 1989).

7. Monitoring of Prostate Cancer

The most effective clinical value of PSA is its use as a simple laboratory parameter for monitoring treatment response and predicting disease recurrence in patients with prostate cancer. In a study of 152 patients, serum PSA either reflected or predicted clinical status in almost all (>97%) of the patients (Ercole et al., 1987). PSA was a significant prognosticator before and during endocrine therapy in 49 patients with advanced disease (D_2), and of predictive value in determining clinical status in 6 patients with progression and 35 patients with no progression. Also, in a recent study in which high-dose intravenous estrogen therapy was shown to be effective in relieving bone pain caused by metastatic disease in 22 of 29 patients with advanced hormone-resistant prostate cancer, a significant decrease in serum PSA was detected (Ferro et al., 1989), suggesting that the clinical benefit is a result of a direct inhibitory effect of estrogen on prostate tumor cells, as reflected by its diminished synthesis and secretion of PSA.

PSA is an effective indicator for response to radiotherapy and predictor for disease recurrence. Serial serum PSA was determined in a total of 163 men who had received external beam radiotherapy or had been implanted with ^{125}I seeds. PSA levels after radiotherapy were directly related to initial clinical stage and Gleason grading before treatment. Increasing PSA levels after radiotherapy were correlated to progression to metastatic disease, and residual cancer (Stamey et al., 1989).

In another study of 71 patients with regionally confined prostate cancer, who were irradiated with aim to cure, PSA levels were measured before, during, and after radiotherapy. PSA was found to correlate well to estimated clinical tumor stage. PSA levels that failed to normalize 6 mo after the resumption of treatment indicated a high risk of recurrence (Landmann and Hunig, 1989).

For patients treated with radical prostatectomy, serum PSA assay is a simple and most reliable monitoring tool (Ahmann and Schifman, 1987; Oesterling et al., 1988). Preoperatively, PSA levels were found to correlate to capsular penetration, lymph node involvement, and seminal vesicle involvement. Postoperatively, of the 101 patients who had favorable pathological findings at surgery, 91% (15/20 of patients with capsular penetration and 77/81 of those with organ-confined cancer) had a follow-up PSA level between 0 and 0.2, whereas only 19% (5/26) with either seminal vesicle or lymph node involvement had a PS level <0.2 ng/mL. An elevated follow-up PSA level was found in all patients with documented clinical recurrence.

In a recent study that involved 10 consecutive patients who underwent radical prostatectomy, PSA levels before and after surgery were evaluated (Lange et al., 1989). Preoperative PSA levels tended to increase with the increasing severity of pathological stage. However, the positive (78%) and negative (61%) predictive values of PSA to predict extracapsular disease were not sufficient to make this test alone useful for staging. Among men whose PSA was <0.4 ng/mL (sensitivity of the assay), only 9% demonstrated recurrence as documented by positive bone scan or progressively elevated PSA levels within 6–50 mo. Significantly, in men whose 3- to 6-mo PSA level was >0.4 ng/mL, there was evidence of recurrence in 100% within 6–49 mo. Progressively elevated PSA levels preceded recurrence from 12 to 43 mo in all 6 patients who had positive bone scans, and increasing PSA levels since radical prostatectomy have continued for 9–65 mo in the 11 patients who have no radiological evidence of recurrent disease at the time of this report. Overall, this long-term follow-up study revealed that PSA level 3–6 mo after radical prostatectomy is a sensitive and reliable indicator of persistent disease after surgery and often precedes other evidence of the disease by many months or years. This critical new finding may alter concepts about surgical results, and possibly shorten and sharpen clinical studies involving adjuvant therapy after radical prostatectomy.

In a large study involving both regionally confirmed and metastatic prostate cancer, a long-term (1–8 yr) follow-up revealed that, regardless of therapy received by the patients, PSA is a significant and reliable marker for prognoses of disease progression and disease-free survival time (Killian et al., 1986).

8. Comparison Between Prostate-Specific Antigen and Prostatic Acid Phosphatase

Data available from extensive clinical evaluation of PSA and prostatic acid phosphatase (PAP) generally have concluded that PSA is more sensitive and reliable than PAP as a serum marker for prostate cancer (Chu, 1990). Three recent studies are briefly discussed here to further support this conclusion.

In one study blood samples from 500 patients with clinical prostatic symptoms were assayed for both PSA and PAP. On the basis of histologic data, 200 prostate adenocarinomas, 276 BPH, 16 cases of prostatitis, 5 cancers of the bladder, and 3 prostatodynias were diagnosed. All the serum samples from prostate carcinoma patients showed elevated PSA at diagnosis, whereas 70% of these showed normal PAP levels. The sensitivity of the PSA assay is 100% when 2.5 ng/mL is selected as the upper limit of normal. Yet the specificity (97%) and the positive predictive value (79%) are better at 10 ng/mL. In the follow-up, PSA is a better marker than PAP for detecting disease progression and appears to constitute an evolutive tumor-mass index (Guillet et al., 1988).

In one study dealing with monitoring and staging of early prostate cancer (Ercole et al., 1987) with extracapsular disease, 93% were shown to have a PSA of >10 ng/mL, whereas an elevated PAP (>24 ng/mL) was detected in 59% of patients (the elevated values in both assays were calculated from the 97th percentile among BPH patients). In 86 patients with advanced disease, 98% had an elevated PSA, and 78% showed elevated PAP. Significantly, in 76% of the patients who had both elevated PSA and PAP, the PSA level was more elevated in 94%.

In fact, some investigators have proposed the discontinued use of PAP, since it is so inferior to PSA (Buamah et al., 1988). In one study PSA and PAP were compared in 232 patients with prostate cancer, 21 of whom had metastatic disease and 111 of whom had intracapsular cancer. Seventy percent had an elevated PSA and only 27% had increased PAP. All with metastatic prostate carcinoma had elevated PSA, but only 62 had elevated PAP. The authors advocated that, since the PAP test is much less efficient than the PSA test, it should be discontinued.

9. Radioimmunodetection

Radioimmunodetection of metastatic prostate cancer with ^{111}In-labeled monoclonal antibody directed against PSA has been reported in a pilot study. The ^{111}In-labeled antibody was injected into 10 patients, 9 with metastatic disease. The results were comparable with those of the standard technetium bone scan (Meyers et al., 1989). Although this initial study revealed interesting data, at this stage of the technology development of radioimmunodetection of cancer, the use of this time-consuming and expensive approach in general would not provide any new or additional information compared to PSA serum assay as described, or immunohistochemical examination, described in the following section.

10. Immunohistopathology of Prostate Cancer

In addition to serum assay, PSA also is a most reliable cancer marker for the immunohistopathological examination of tumors involving the prostate, and for identification of prostate origin of metastasis in various tissues and organs. Because of its unique and stable antigenicity, the specific molecular determinants of PSA are preserved in conventionally prepared, formalin-fixed, paraffin-embedded tissue specimens. Its prostate-specificity makes PSA the most simple and reliable marker in the identification of secondary prostate tumor cells.

The clinical application was first reported in 1981 by Nadji et al. using a selected and specific rabbit polyclonal antiserum to PSA for the examination of 19 primary prostate carcinomas and 49 metastatic prostate carcinomas, along with 78 nonprostate specimens. Without exception, all 68 primary and secondary prostate carcinoma specimens showed distinctive positive stain. The intensity of immunostain reaction varied from cell to cell, from area to area, and from primary to metastatic tumor in the same patient. The positive stain was confined to cytoplasm of epithelia, with greater concentration in the paranuclear area of the luminal aspects of the cells. None of the 78 nonprostate specimens was stained positively. Of clinical interest was the finding that 17 tumors of the urinary bladder with extension to the prostate all stained negatively. This initial report firmly established the clinical value of PSA as an immunohistopathological marker for prostate carcinoma. It provided a simple means for the differential diagnosis of metastatic adenocarcinoma in male patients; for example, the identification of secondary tumor cells in the lymph nodes, distant organs, and bone marrow. PSA was further shown to be a tissue marker for the histological classification of tumor involving prostate gland and adjuvant tissues, and for solving a most common diagnostic problem in histopathology.

Reagents made in a kit form commonly used for tissue examination are readily available from commercial sources. In fact, more than 300 publications dealing with PSA in the area of immunohistopathological examination have appeared in literature since 1981. Only a very few examples are mentioned here.

Using a murine anti-PSA monoclonal antibody, F5, the initial report on the application of PSA expression in identifying metastatic tumors was confirmed with a panel of 98 tissue specimens, 25 of prostate origin and 73 of nonprostate origin (Papsidero et al., 1985). All metastatic tumors secondary to prostate adenocarcinoma were identified positively, regardless of the site of dissemination. In the meantime, all nonprostate metastases were stained negatively, including many originating from other genitourinary tracts. These results confirmed the initial report, indicating a perfect score in both specificity and sensitivity (Nadji et al., 1981). The key reason for these perfect results is the fine specificity of antigenic determinants expressed by the PSA molecule (Chu et al., 1989).

The most common clinical application of PSA in immunohistopathology is its use in differential diagnosis of bladder carcinoma from prostate carcinoma. One of the more interesting reports, as described in detail here, is a prospective study involving 21 patients in whom the tumors of the head and neck of the bladder could not be categorized as prostatic or urothelial in origin by conventional endoscopic or histopathological examinations (Ford et al., 1985). In eight of 21 of the patients with lesions of the bladder neck, four had a past history of prostate tumor, two had urothelial tumors, and the other two had both. PSA stain was positive in three of the four patients with a previous prostate neoplasm and in one of the two with a previous history of transitional cell carcinomas. In the two patients who had had both prostatic and transitional cell carcinomas in the past, the bladder neck lesion was PSA-positive in one and negative in the other. All patients with PSA-positive lesions were treated as having prostate carcinomas and all negative ones as having transitional cell carcinomas of the bladder. The tumors of the bladder neck occurred *de novo* in the remaining 13 patients, of which eight were PSA-positive, indicating a prostate origin, and seven of these were treated for prostate carcinoma. In the remaining patient, PSA stain was focal and only weakly positive. He underwent radiotherapy and radical cystoprostatectomy, since the endoscopic appearance and histological results, showing an anaplastic carcinoma, were considered more indicative of a urethelial than a prostate tumor. Subsequent examination of the surgical specimen confirmed this to be a positive prostate tumor. In five patients the bladder neck tumor was PSA-negative. Four were treated appropriately for urothelial tumor and one, with a history of rectal cancer, was treated for recurrence of rectal carcinoma. In two additional patients, the origin of lymph node metastases with atypical tumor morphology (cervical nodes in one and retroperitoneal node in the other) was detected by PSA-positive stain in the absence of a clinically apparent primary carcinoma. The primary carcinomas were subsequently confirmed on prostate biopsies.

11. Concluding Remarks

The clinical application of PSA as a prostate cancer marker has been briefly reviewed. Although PSA alone cannot be used in general screening for early detection of prostate cancer, its combined use with transrectal ultrasound is a potentially effective clinical tool. After a decade of practical use, PSA is shown unequivocally to be more sensitive and reliable than PAP. PSA is most useful in staging and monitoring prostate cancer, particularly in following up treatment response and clinical status, and in detecting early disease recurrence. PSA also is an effective immunohistological marker for differential diagnosis of metastatic carcinomas, especially in the identification of metastatic prostate carcinoma in distant organs and tissues, and for the differential diagnosis of primary prostate carcinoma from poorly differentiated transitional cell carcinoma of the bladder. With its definitive use as both serum and tissue markers, PSA represents the most successful example of human cancer markers to date.

(Note added in proof: Catalona et al. [1991] just reported that the combined serum PSA assay DRE, with TUS performed in patients with abnormal findings, provides a better method of early detection of prostate cancer than DRE alone.)

Acknowledgments

The author thanks his students and colleagues at Roswell Park Memorial Institute and National Prostatic Cancer Treatment Project for contributions to our work on PSA, which was supported by the National Cancer Institute.

References

Ablin, R. J., P. Bronson, W. A. Soanes, and E. Witebsky (1970), *J. Immunol.* **104,** 1329–1339.

Ahmann, F. R. and R. B. Schifman (1987), *J. Urol.* **137,** 431–434.

Anderson, S. and N. R. Dunnick (1989), *Invest. Radiol.* **24,** 257–259.

Ban, Y., M. C. Wang, K. W. Watt, R. M. Loor, and T. M. Chu (1984), *Biochem. Biophys. Res. Commun.* **123,** 482–488.

Barak, M., Y. Mecz, A. Lurie, and N. Gruener (1989a), *J. Lab. Clin. Med.* **113,** 598–603.

Barak, M., Y. Mecz, A. Lurie, and N. Gruener (1989b), *Oncology* **46,** 375–377.

Brawer, M. R. and P. H. Lange (1989), *Urology* **33,** S11–S16.

Buamah, P. K., P. Johnson, and A. W. Skiller (1988), *Br. J. Urol.* **62,** 581–583.

Catalona, W. J., D. S. Coffey, and J. Karr, eds. (1989), *Clinical Aspects of Prostate Cancer: Assessment of New Diagnostic and Management Procedures,* Elsevier, New York.

Catalona, W. J., D. S. Smith, T. L. Ratliff, K. M. Dodds, D. E. Coplen, J. J. Yuan, J. A. Petros, and G. L. Andriole (1991), *N. Engl. J. Med.* **324,** 1156–1161.

Caty, A., P. Gosselin, J. Cazin, J. M. Dehaut, and L. Adenis (1988), *Am. J. Clin. Oncol.* **11,** S63–S64.

Chu, T. M. (1985), in *Monoclonal Antibodies in Cancer* (Sell, S. S. and R. A. Reisfeld, eds.), Humana, Clifton, NJ, pp. 309–324.

Chu, T. M. (1990), in *Immunodiagnosis of Cancer* (Mercer, D. W. and R. Herberman, eds.), Marcel Dekker, New York, pp. 339–356.

Chu, T. M. and G. P. Murphy (1986), *Urology* **27,** 487–491.

Chu, T. M., E. Kawinski, N. Hibi, G. Croghan, J. Wiley, C. S. Killian, and D. Corral (1989), *J. Urol.* **141,** 152–156.

Cooner, W. H., B. R. Mosley, C. L. Rutherford, J. H. Beard, H. S. Pond, N. B. Bass, and W. J. Terry (1988), *J. Urol.* **139,** 758–761.

Dube, J. Y., D. Gaudreault, and R. Tremblay (1989), *Andrologia* **21,** 136–139.

Ercole, C. J., P. H. Lange, M. Mathiesen, R. K. Chiou, P. K. Reddy, and R. L. Vessella (1987), *J. Urol.* **138,** 1181–1184.

Ferro, M. A., I. Barnes, J. B. Roberts, and P. J. Smith (1987), *Br. J. Urol.* **60,** 69–73.

Ferro, M., D. Gillatt, M. Symes, and P. J. Smith (1989), *Urology* **34,** 135–138.

Flocks, R. H., V. C. Urich, C. A. Patel, and J. M. Optiz (1960), *J. Urol.* **84,** 134–135.

Ford, T. F., D. Butcher, J. R. W. Masters, and M. C. Parkinson (1985) *Br. J. Urol.* **57,** 50–55.

Guillet, J., C. Role, A. T. Duc, and H. Francis (1988), *Am. J. Clin. Oncol.* **11,** S61–S62.

Hara, M., Y. Koyanagi, T. Inoue, and T. Fukuyama (1971), *Jpn. J. Leg. Med.* **25,** 322–324.

Henttu, P. and P. Vihko (1989), *Biochem. Biophys. Res. Commun.* **160,** 903–910.

Killian, C. S. and T. M. Chu (1990), *Cancer Invest.* **8,** 27–37.

Killian, C. S., F. P. Vargas, and T. M. Chu (1988), *Clin. Chem.* **34,** 1296.

Killian, C. S., L. J. Emrich, F. P. Vargas, N. Yang, M. C. Wang, R. Priore, G. P. Murphy, and T. M. Chu (1986), *J. Natl. Cancer Inst.* **76,** 179–185.

Kuriyama, M., M. C. Wang, C. L. Lee, L. D. Papsidero, C. S. Killian, H. Inaji, N. S. Slack, G. P. Murphy, and T. M. Chu (1981), *Cancer Res.* **41,** 3874–3876.

Kuriyama, M., M. C. Wang, L. D. Papsidero, C. S. Killian, T. Shimano, L. A. Valenzuela, T. Nishiura, G. P. Murphy, and T. M. Chu (1980), *Cancer Res.* **40,** 4658–4662.

Landmann, C. and R. Hunig (1989), *Int. J. Radiat. Oncol. Biol. Phys.* **17,** 1073–1076.

Lange, P. H., C. J. Ercole, D. J. Lightner, E. E. Fraley, and R. Vessella (1989), *J. Urol.* **141,** 873–879.

Lee, F., S. T. Pederson, L. Meilsman, D. B. Siders, P. Littrup, R. P. Dorr, and F. J. Pauli (1988), *Int. J. Radiat. Oncol. Biol. Phys.* **15,** 1453–1459.

Lee, F., S. T. Pederson, P. Littrup, R. D. McLeary, T. A. McHigh, A. P. Smid, P. J. Stella, and G. S. Borlaza (1989), *Radiology* **170,** 29–32.

Lilja, H. (1988), *Scand. J. Clin. Lab. Invest. Suppl.* **191,** 13–20.

Lundwall, A. (1989), *Biochem. Biophys. Res. Commun.* **161,** 1151–1159.

Maatman, T. J. (1989), *J. Urol.* **141,** 1378–1380.

Meyers, F. J., S. J. Denardo, D. Macey, R. D. White, and M. Unger (1989), *Prostate* **14,** 209–220.

Nadji, M., S. Z. Tabei, A. Castro, T. M. Chu, M. C. Wang, G. P. Murphy, and A. R. Morales (1981), *Cancer* **48,** 1229–1232.

Oesterling, J. E., D. W. Chan, J. I. Epstein, A. W. Kimball, D. J. Bruzek, R. C. Rock, C. B. Brendler, and P. C. Walsh (1988), *J. Urol.* **139,** 766–772.

Papsidero, L. D., M. C. Wang, L. A. Valenzuela, G. P. Murphy, and T. M. Chu (1980), *Cancer Res.* **40,** 2428–2432.

Papsidero, L. D., G. A. Croghan, J. Asirwatham, J. Gaeta, P. Abenoza, L. Englander, and L. Valenzuela (1985), *Am. J. Pathol.* **121,** 451–454.

Papsidero, L. D., G. A. Croghan, M. C. Wang, M. Kuriyama, E. A. Johnson, L. A. Valenzuela, and T. M. Chu (1983), *Hybridoma* **2,** 139–147.

Papsidero, L. D., M. Kuriyama, M. C. Wang, J. S. Horoszewicz, S. S. Leong, L. A. Valenzuela, G. P. Murphy, and T. M. Chu (1981), *J. Natl. Cancer Inst.* **66,** 37–44.

Riegman, P. H., R. J. Ulietstra, J. A. van der Korput, J. C. Romijn, and J. Trapman (1989), *FEBS Lett.* **247,** 123–126.

Sensabaugh, G. F. (1978), *J. Forensic Sci.* **23,** 106–115.

Shirbiny, A. M., T. Nielson, and H. N. Pawar (1990), *Urology* **35,** 88–92.

Stamey, T. A. and J. N. Kabalin (1989), *J. Urol.* **141,** 1070–1075.

Stamey, T. A., J. N. Kabalin, and M. Ferrai (1989), *J. Urol.* **141,** 1084–1087.

Wang, M. C., R. M. Loor, S. L. Li, and T. M. Chu (1983), *IRCS Med. Sci.* **11,** 327–328.

Wang, M. C., L. Valenzuela, G. P. Murphy, and T. M. Chu (1979), *Invest. Urol.* **17,** 159–163.

Wang, M. C., M. Kuriyama, L. D. Papsidero, R. M. Loor, L. A. Valenzuela, G. P. Murphy, and T. M. Chu (1982), in *Methods of Cancer Research* vol. 19 (Busch, H., and L. C. Yeoman, eds.), Academic, New York, pp. 179–197.

Watt, K. W. K., P. J. Lee, T. M' Timkulu, W. P. Chan, and R. M. Loor (1986), *Proc. Natl. Acad. Sci. USA* **83,** 3166–3170.

Weber, J. P., J. E. Oesterling, C. A. Peters, A. W. Partin, D. W. Chan, and P. W. Walsh (1989), *J. Urol.* **141,** 987–992.

Chapter 6

Enzyme Markers

Doris Balinsky

1. Introduction

It has been known for many years that the enzyme complement of a tumor cell differs in many ways from that of its normal counterpart, reflecting its altered metabolism. Certain enzyme activities may be increased or decreased, or different forms (isozymes) of an enzyme may occur in the tumor. Some of these isozymes may be related to forms normally found in the fetus or placenta (oncodevelopmental forms), or occurring in nonmalignant tissues of the body unrelated to the tissue from which the tumor originated. Attempts to exploit this information clinically have led to the assay of a wide variety of enzymes in the search for both serum and tissue tumor markers. Enzymes, like other tumor markers, enter the circulation if they are shed from the tumor surface, are secreted by the tumor, or are released as a result of cell death.

Serum enzyme assays have proven most useful for monitoring the effects of therapy and to detect recurrence of tumors. Elevated enzyme levels in cancer patients frequently decrease to normal levels following successful treatment; unchanged or rising

From: *Serological Cancer Markers* Edited by Stewart Sell ©1992 The Humana Press, Totowa, NJ

serum levels indicate lack of response. Patients who have been successfully treated can be monitored by periodic assays of serum enzymes; in some cases, increases in serum enzymes have been shown to predate clinical evidence of tumor recurrence. Serum enzymes may also have prognostic value, as the level frequently reflects tumor burden. Unfortunately, enzyme assays have not proven useful for early detection of tumors, mainly because of the wide range of values found in the normal healthy population and the considerable overlap with values in diseased patients. Diagnostic applications also have proved disappointing. Despite extensive study, no unique, cancer-specific enzyme has been found. Unless an organ-specific enzyme is being examined, the source of the elevated enzyme activity is not easy to identify; moreover, many of the enzyme changes occur both in benign and in malignant disease. Enzymes have also been examined as tumor markers in tissue, where they can be used to detect heterogeneity of tumor tissue, to help indicate tumor margins, or to locate metastases; such applications will probably be expanded in the 1990s.

In this chapter, no attempt is made to discuss all the enzymes that have been studied as potential tumor markers. Instead, I have selected representative examples that have been extensively evaluated and that illustrate some of the potential applications and limitations of the use of enzymes for clinical evaluation of cancer patients.

2. Neuron-Specific Enolase (NSE)

The enolase gamma–gamma isozyme known as NSE occurs in cells of neuronal or neuroendocrine origin. Although not a tumor-specific enzyme, it appears to be useful as a marker for tumors derived from cells of the neuroendocrine system, such as small cell lung cancer (SCLC). NSE has been widely recognized as a tumor marker for SCLC since Carney et al. (1982) first showed its elevation in serum of patients with this disease. Although these early studies and several others showed correlation of serum activities with extent of disease, review of data from several laboratories led Carney and Teeling (1988) to caution that it should not be used for either diagnosis or prognosis, for two reasons. First, in addition to its elevation in SCLC, it is also frequently raised in a significant percentage of patients with nonsmall cell lung cancer, thus, it cannot be used to distinguish these two diseases. Second, although many researchers find correlation of serum level with extent of disease, there is considerable overlap between serum values for patients with limited and with extensive disease, so it cannot be used to predict stage or extent of disease. They consider that initial NSE levels do not provide information additional to that obtained by standard staging techniques and procedures. It should be noted that serum NSE is also elevated in a small percentage of patients with tumors that are not of neuroendocrine or neuronal origin, including prostate cancer and hypernephroma (Burghuber et al., 1990).

Its usefulness for monitoring response to therapy of patients with SCLC was recently assessed by several groups of British and Dutch investigators (Splinter et al., 1989). Their studies led them to recommend that NSE levels should be monitored at six-weekly intervals—this assay alone was considered adequate to monitor response to therapy, and to supersede the use of radiological and radionuclide imaging methods. These recommendations are based on results of a study in which NSE was assayed in serum samples collected from 115 patients with SCLC prior to each course of chemotherapy, and during follow-up. It was found that decreasing or increasing levels of serum NSE accurately predicted major response or lack of it and correlated with independent clinical assessments; no false positive elevations in NSE level were observed. However, this conclusion is counter to that reached by others who show several cases in which radiological evidence of tumor recurrence predated elevation of serum enolase, and who thus consider that NSE should only be used as an adjunct to radiological assessment (Nou et al., 1990).

Owing to high NSE levels in neuroblastoma cells, serum NSE has been evaluated as a prognostic indicator for children with neuroblastoma. It was indeed found to have prognostic value, but only in patients with advanced disease; elevated levels correlated with poor prognosis, successful therapy was indicated by decreased levels, and relapse led to increasing levels in some cases (Zeltzer et al., 1986). However, in children with early stage disease, the NSE levels were not found to be predictive of relapse. At a recent consensus conference held to standardize international criteria for diagnosis, staging, and response to treatment of neuroblastoma patients, NSE was not included among the markers currently recommended because of limitations of standardization and availability (Brodeur et al., 1988).

3. Acid Phosphatase

The prostate-specific form of acid phosphatase (PAP) (also known as tartrate-resistant acid phosphatase) has long been studied as a marker of prostate cancer. Its elevation in bone metastases of prostate cancer was first noted more than 50 years ago (Gutman et al., 1936). Serum levels of this enzyme are elevated in late stage cancer, but the sensitivity for detection of early stage cancer is low, so it cannot be used for screening. Moreover, as often occurs when assaying an organ-specific marker, elevated serum enzyme levels cannot distinguish benign from malignant disease. Thus, benign prostatic hypertrophy can also lead to elevated serum PAP (Daver et al., 1988). Since the discovery by Wang et al. (1979) of the serine protease, prostate-specific antigen (PSA) (*see* Chapter 5 in this book), the latter organ-specific marker has largely superseded PAP assay for management of prostate cancer patients, although some clinicians have found measurement of both markers useful to improve the clinical evaluation of patients suspected of having prostate cancer (Daver et al., 1988). Unfortunately, many of the problems noted above for PAP also hold for PSA (Daver et al., 1988).

A more promising application of PAP may be for prognosis. Patients whose prostate tumor tissues showed intense staining for PAP appeared to be more responsive to hormone therapy than those with lower values (Hammond et al., 1989). The staining intensity was found to be unrelated to Gleason grade or to serum levels. Additional studies will be required to substantiate these observations. Another use of this organ-specific enzyme may be as a tissue marker for identifying metastases, using diagnostic imaging techniques. Radiolabeled monoclonal antibodies to PAP have been used to determine lymph node invasion by prostatic cancer; preliminary studies have confirmed that those nodes that were positive by this noninvasive technique were also positive on histologic examination (Leroy et al., 1989). Again, confirmatory studies of this interesting observation are required.

4. Alkaline Phosphatase

Alkaline phosphatase is widely distributed in mammalian tissues, and has been used clinically as a serum marker for over 60 years, especially for diagnosing bone and liver disease (*see* review by Moss, 1987). It exists in a number of isozymic forms, derived from at least four separate genes, one coding for the bone and liver forms, one for the intestinal form, one for a placental form, and one for a placental-like form. The latter three genes all appear to be located on chromosome 2q37 (Martin et al., 1989). The bone and liver forms have been used to monitor metastases to those organs, usually in association with other markers. For example, hydroxyproline has been used to help distinguish hyperparathyroidism from bone metastases (Stepan et al., 1989), and 5'-nucleotidase has been used to help identify liver metastases.

The unexpected discovery that the serum and tumor tissue of a male lung cancer patient contained a form of alkaline phosphatase resembling an isozyme normally only occurring in placenta (Regan isozyme, PLAP) (Fishman et al., 1968) led to a flurry of studies in a search for other "oncodevelopmental" markers. A closely-related form, the Nagao isozyme ("PLAP-like"), was found in another lung cancer patient (Nakayama et al., 1970). This form occurs in small amounts in normal testis and thymus. Another tumor-related form, the Kasahara isozyme (Warnock and Reisman, 1969) is found in hepatoma and is related to a form occurring in fetal intestine.

Despite these discoveries, PLAP has not been widely used as a tumor marker in clinical laboratories. The early assays involving heat inactivation or inhibition by L-phenylalanine to identify the tumor-specific form had low specificity. With the advent of monoclonal antibodies, more sensitive and specific assays may be attainable. In a recent multicenter study, sera from patients with a variety of cancers were evaluated using commercially available monoclonal antibodies to PLAP (De Broe and Pollet, 1988). PLAP was found to be a useful marker for testicular cancer, especially seminoma (72% sensitivity). It was also elevated in 49% of sera from ovarian cancer patients, but, when assayed in association with the ovarian cancer marker CA 125, it identified few additional cases. It should be considered only for monitoring; diagnostic use is hampered by 9% false positivity in benign disease, and by its elevation in the sera of heavy smokers without overt lung disease. Combination of PLAP with a new marker for mucinous ovarian tumors, CA 54/61, is reported to be a more sensitive marker combination than PLAP plus CA 125 (Nozawa et al., 1989). These authors found only 35% sensitivity for ovarian cancer with PLAP alone, confirming that it is not a useful marker for diagnosis. At this stage, PLAP is unlikely to replace current markers for ovarian and testicular cancer. PLAP may have some value in diagnostic imaging. Monoclonal antibodies to PLAP, labeled with ^{111}Indium, have been used to localize small tumors and lymph node metastases by immunoscintigraphy (Epenetos et al., 1985).

5. Ornithine Decarboxylase (ODC)

Polyamines, including spermidine, spermine, and putrescine, are essential for growth and proliferation of tissues. The first and the rate-limiting enzyme of the polyamine biosynthetic pathway is an inducible enzyme, ODC, whose activity appears to be elevated in developing, proliferating, and neoplastic tissues. For this reason, it has been evaluated as a potential tumor marker in colonic mucosa. Studies with small numbers of subects showed statistically significant increases of ODC activity in dysplastic colonic polyps relative to normal flat colonic mucosa; adenomatous polyps had intermediate activity (Luk and Baylin, 1984). Elevated activities were shown in both primary and metastatic colorectal cancers

(Herrera and Petrelli, 1988). ODC activity in colonic adenomas was intermediate between that of normal colonic mucosa and colorectal cancer (Rohzin et al., 1984), in line with the postulated progression of the disease via adenomatous polyps to frank cancer. ODC thus appears to be a marker of the relative proliferative activity of colonic mucosa at various stages of progression from normal to carcinoma. A more recent study aimed at determining whether ODC could be used for screening showed that ODC activity in normal-appearing rectal mucosa was elevated in patients with both benign and malignant neoplasia; however, it could not distinguish these conditions (Koo et al., 1988).

Of more interest is ODC's possible prognostic value in identifying persons at risk of developing colonic cancer, especially those carrying the genotype for familial polyposis. This is an inherited autosomal dominant disease in which affected subjects develop numerous polyps that progress to colorectal cancer if not treated. Morphologically normal mucosa from patients with polyps had higher activity than that from normal control subjects (Luk and Baylin, 1984); this elevated activity could indicate predisposition to polyp formation. Normal-appearing mucosa from asymptomatic family members showed a biphasic distribution of ODC levels, with approximately half the subjects having the same levels as control subjects from unaffected families, and the other half having higher activities. Follow-up data are needed to determine whether the persons with higher mucosal activities were more susceptible to polyposis than those with normal levels; initial follow-up showed polyp formation in 1 of the 14 individuals with high ODC levels (Luk et al., 1988).

6. Glycosyltransferases and Sialyltransferases

Many tumor-associated antigens appear to be glycolipids, glycoproteins, or mucins located on the cell surface, or secreted into the circulation. They differ structurally from their counterparts associated with related normal tissues, the differences usually being attributable to incomplete or altered carbohydrate side chains on the tumor forms (*see* Chapter 11 in this book). This has led scientists to examine in detail the activities and properties of the transferases responsible for catalyzing attachment of terminal glycosyl and sialyl moieties to the carbohydrate side chains. Specific substrates have been synthesized for some of these enzymes in the hope that they might help distinguish tumor and normal forms. More recently, the genes for some of these enzymes have been cloned, which should allow scientists to understand their regulation better.

The Lewis a and Lewis X blood group antigens, which occur in many tumors, have a terminal galactosyl group on the antigenic side chain. The enzyme catalyzing its attachment to the carbohydrate side chain, galactosyltransferase, has been assayed in tumors and in sera from cancer patients. Serum galactosyltransferase activity was found to have little value for diagnosis, as it was elevated in only one-third of cancer patients. However, it may have some prognostic value, as patients with elevated activities appeared to have significantly poorer prognosis (Davey et al., 1986b). Elevated levels were found to occur more frequently in patients with metastasis, especially in the liver (Davey et al., 1986a). More recent attempts to improve the specificity of tumor detection by use of a synthetic substrate for this enzyme were not successful, as there was considerable overlap of activities between sera from patients with malignancy and those from healthy controls (Madiyalakan et al., 1987).

Some years ago, the occurrence of an electrophoretically distinct tumor-associated isozyme, galactosyltranferase II, was shown in sera of 71% of cancer patients studied (Weiser et al., 1976), leading to hopes that it might become a useful diagnostic tool. More recent studies have confirmed that significant elevations of this isozyme occur in cancer patients, but the sensitivity was only 55%, even though all the patients had advanced cancer (Uemura et al., 1988). Moreover, isoelectric focusing has shown tremendous heterogeneity of this enzyme (Davey et al., 1986a), making analysis of isozymes even more complicated. The presently available assay systems are too cumbersome for clinical laboratory use, hence this isozyme is not currently in routine use as a tumor marker.

Unusual fucosylated forms of tumor-associated antigens have been observed, e.g., the Lewis X antigen, hence, serum fucosyltransferases have been evaluated as tumor markers. Early studies showed elevations of fucosyltransferase in sera from cancer patients (Ronquist and Nou, 1983), with decreases following successful surgery (Bauer et al., 1978). In an attempt to improve the specificity of the assay, these studies were repeated using synthetic substrates for α-(1→3)-L-fucosyltransferase (Yazawa et al., 1988). These latter studies showed increases in patients with advanced disease, but less clear-cut increases in many patients with early disease. As with many tumor markers, there is overlap with some cases of non-neoplastic disease and healthy controls, making this more useful for monitoring patients than for diagnosis.

Increased sialylation of tumor-associated antigens has been observed in many cases, leading to study of circulating sialyltransferase. Several studies showed elevation of this enzyme in plasma of patients with cancers of various types, with reduction of enzyme activity following successful therapy (Papadopoulou-Boutis et al., 1985; Dao et al., 1986; Dwivedi et al., 1988). This enzyme may have prognostic value, since a few node-negative breast cancer patients whose high serum levels did not decrease following surgery were later found to develop metastases (Dao et al., 1986). Further work is required to determine the usefulness of this enzyme as a tumor marker.

7. Proteases

A very important goal in cancer diagnosis is the ability to predict whether or not a tumor will metastasize to other sites. Many studies have examined the possible role of proteases in tumor metastasis, postulating that proteases could facilitate the escape of tumor cells from the site of the primary tumor and their entry into a new location (*see* review by Liotta and Stetler-Stevenson, 1989). The presence of proteases in tumors was indicated by early observations of the dissolution of plasma clots on which pieces of tumor tissue were grown. The most widely-studied proteases include plasminogen activators, collagenases, and cathepsins.

7.1. Plasminogen Activator

Plasminogen activator is a serine protease occurring in at least two genetically distinct isozymic forms: tissue-type plasminogen activator (t-PA) and urokinase-type plasminogen activator (u-PA). Its name derives from its action in catalyzing the conversion of plasminogen to the active protease plasmin. U-PA is elevated in tumors (*see* reviews by Dano et al., 1985; Markus, 1988). Patients with very high levels tend to have a poorer prognosis than those with lower levels (Duffy et al., 1988a). Colonic polyps have levels of both u-PA and t-PA intermediate between those for normal tissue and for adenocarcinoma, correlating with the possible premalignancy of these polyps (de Bruin et al., 1987). Significant correlation between messenger RNA levels for u-PA and presence of regional lymph node metastases has been shown for lung cancer, consistent with a possible role of u-PA in tumor invasiveness. However, in breast cancer, there was no correlation of u-PA mRNA with lymph node status (Sappino et al., 1987). T-PA, on the other hand, is decreased in tumors (de Bruin et al., 1987), and breast cancer patients with high levels of this enzyme appear to have significantly longer disease-free intervals than those with low levels; this has suggested use of t-PA levels as prognostic indicators (Duffy et al., 1988b). It should be noted that t-PA is present in endothelial cells and may be elevated in highly vascularized tumors. These enzymes require further evaluation before their clinical usefulness can be assessed.

7.2. Collagenase

One of the major components of the basement membrane separating the tumor from its surrounding tissues is type IV collagen. Recent studies have shown correlation of metastatic potential with levels of collagenase IV, the protease degrading Type IV collagen (*see* review by Liotta and Stetler-Stevenson, 1990). Type IV collagenase activity has been studied in gastric and colorectal carcinomas (Garbisa et al., 1990). The enzyme occurred in all the invasive gastric carcinomas and in most of the invasive colorectal carcinomas studied. Low-grade colonic cancers rarely showed the presence of this enzyme, but most gastric carcinomas, even when confined to the mucosa, stained for the enzyme. This may reflect the observation that even gastric cancers apparently still confined to the mucosa have frequently already metastasized. Normal gastric and colorectal mucosa, and adenomatous polyps did not stain. Measurements of this enzyme thus may have potential as prognostic indicators of tumor metastasis in gastric and colorectal cancers, although further evaluation is required. Type IV collagenase distribution has also been examined in normal, benign, and malignant human breast tissues (Monteagudo et al., 1990). In normal breast tissue, it was confined to myoepithelial cells; in benign hyperplasia, it frequently occurred in epithelial cells as well. Strong immunostaining occurred in a high percentage of carcinomas; the staining was stronger than in benign hyperplasia, but there were no significant differences in staining intensity between *in situ* and invasive carcinomas. However, further studies with larger numbers of tumors have indicated that a higher percentage of cells stain positively in invasive carcinoma tissues compared to *in situ* carcinomas (D'Errico et al., 1991). This suggests that the enzyme may have potential as a marker of tumor aggressiveness in breast tumors as well as in gastrointestinal tumors.

7.3. Cathepsins

Cathepsins are papain-like cysteine proteases occurring in mammalian tissues. Cathepsin B- and L-like activities appear to be significantly elevated in colorectal cancer tissues compared to apparently normal mucosa from the same patient. Levels were significantly higher in patients with low-grade tumors (Duke's A) compared with more advanced tumors (Duke's B, C, and D), suggesting a role for these enzymes in early progression of colorectal cancer (Sheahan et al., 1989).

Early studies aimed at identifying proteins inducible by estrogens in hormone-dependent human breast cancer cell lines led to discovery of a 52-kDa protein with mitogenic and proteolytic activity. This molecule was subsequently shown to be a precursor of the lysosomal protease cathepsin D (Augereau et al., 1988). Its occurrence in primary breast cancers was shown by immunohistochemical staining of frozen tissue sections with monoclonal antibodies to procathepsin D (Garcia et al., 1987). Although it occurred in 64% of biopsies from 232 primary breast cancers, the staining was very heterogeneous, affecting only 1–30% of the epithelial cells. Moreover, staining was more intense in benign mastopathies and in cells bordering the lumen of large cysts than in tumors, suggesting it is a marker of proliferation rather than of malignancy (Garcia et al., 1987).

Several groups of investigators have evaluated cathepsin D as a prognostic indicator for breast cancer patients. Two approaches have been used for determining cathepsin D content of breast tumors. One approach is to assess the intensity of immunohistochemical staining of tumor sections; the second is to quantitate cathepsin D immunologically in cytosolic tumor extracts. Different conclusions have been reached by use of the different techniques. Immunohistochemical staining allows the investigators to determine the cathepsin D content only in the tumor cells; by this technique high levels of cathepsin D in estrogen receptor-positive breast tumor tissues were found to be correlated with *increased* disease-free and overall survival in lymph node-positive patients (Henry et al., 1990). Cathepsin D assay in cytosol of tumor extracts measures the enzyme in all components of the tissue specimen, including tumor cells, and associated stromal and inflammatory cells. This type of assay has been evaluated by two groups of investigators, using different antibodies and different techniques (Thorpe et al., 1989; Tandon et al., 1990). Both groups showed that high cathepsin D levels appeared to be predictive of *reduced* time to recurrence and reduced overall survival, though one group (Tandon et al., 1990) found that the data were only statistically significant in lymph node-negative patients. Multivariate analyses indicated that cathepsin D was the most valuable predictive indicator among those tested, similar in value to lymph node status. If these observations are confirmed in clinical trials of larger scale, they could be important in affecting therapy of breast cancer patients. The National Cancer

Institute recently published a "clinical alert" recommending that all patients with breast cancer, even those with no lymph node involvement, be considered for aduvant therapy. Since 70% of node-negative breast cancer patients will have no recurrence of disease, it would be helpful if oncologists could identify these patients and thus spare them the toxicities associated with chemotherapy.

These studies indicate the importance of evaluating not only a specific tumor marker, but also the technique that will be most consistent and useful clinically. At this stage, it is not possible to determine which of these approaches will be most valuable. It should be noted that the three studies dealing with prognostic evaluation (Thorpe et al., 1989; Tandon et al., 1990; Henry et al., 1990) have only been published very recently, thus further evaluation must be awaited.

8. Terminal Deoxynucleotide Transferase (TdT)

All the enzymes discussed above have been evaluated as markers of solid tumors. The only enzyme that has shown some clinical value in the study of leukemias is TdT (*see* review by Bollum and Chang, 1986). TdT is a DNA polymerase that catalyzes the addition of terminal nucleotides to a growing nucleotide chain. The enzyme occurs in normal thymus and in a small percentage of cells in normal bone marrow. It appears to be a marker of immature lymphoid cells. Since the first observation of its elevation in circulating blast cells of a patient with childhood T-cell acute leukemia (McCaffrey et al., 1973), it has been extensively evaluated as an aid to classification of leukemias. It is elevated in cells from a high percentage of patients with acute lymphocytic leukemia, but more recent studies using more sensitive techniques show it also to be elevated in a large number of patients with acute myelogenous leukemia, as well as during blast crisis in some patients with chronic myelogenous leukemia (Drexler et al., 1986). It is absent in most mature B- and T-cell malignancies, and in chronic leukemias except during blast crisis. In addition to its application to leukemia classification, it appears to have some prognostic value, as patients with higher levels have shorter remission time than those with lower levels.

9. Other Enzymes

A number of other enzymes have been evaluated over the years as tumor markers and have been reviewed extensively in the past (e.g., Balinsky, 1980; Schwartz, 1989). Lactate dehydrogenase and its isozymes have been widely used clinically as serum markers for heart and liver disease, as well as for cancer. Increases in LDH_5, the most cathodic form, occur in many tumor tissues. Since total LDH activity is commonly assayed as part of a routine serum work-up, its activity is often monitored as an adjunct to other tests, and has been shown to be related to tumor burden. Serum creatine kinase and its isozymes too have been used to monitor a number of diseases, including cancer, but are not routinely used for cancer evaluation. Serum amylase has been used to monitor pancreatic cancer, but cannot distinguish pancreatitis from malignant pancreatic disease, thus cannot be used for diagnosis. Many clinical laboratories include these enzymes in their menus and will provide assays at physicians' request.

10. Concluding Remarks

The examples cited indicate that serum levels of some enzymes are useful for monitoring patient response to therapy and for detection of tumor recurrence. They may have prognostic value as indicators of extensive disease. However, because of low sensitivity and specificity of most assays, they are presently not useful for diagnosis of specific tumors, or for detection of tumors at early stages to screen asymptomatic persons. Tissue assays may have prognostic value in determinations of aggressiveness of tumors. They can also be used to indicate heterogeneity of tumors and extent of disease, and to locate metastases. In general, enzyme assays are used as adjuncts to other clinical parameters, and in this way, can be helpful to the physician in evaluating a patient's disease status.

References

Augereau, P., M. Garcia, M. G. Mattei, V. Cavailles, F. Depadova, D. Derocq, F. Capony, P. Ferrara, and H. Rochefort (1988), *Mol. Endocrinol.* **2,** 186–192.

Balinsky, D. (1980), in *Cancer Markers: Diagnostic and Developmental Significance* (Sell, S., ed.), Humana, Clifton, NJ, pp. 191–224.

Bauer, C. H., W. G. Reutter, K. P. Erhart, E. Koettgen, and W. Gerok (1978), *Science* **201,** 1232–1233.

Bollum, F. and L. Chang (1986), *Adv. Cancer Res.* **47,** 37–61.

Brodeur, G. M., R. C. Seeger, A. Barrett, F. Berthold, R. P. Castleberry, G. D'Angio, B. De Bernardi, A. E. Evans, M. Favrat, A. I. Freeman, G. Haase, O. Hartmann, F. A. Hayes, L. Helson, J. Kemshead, F. Lampert, J. Ninane, H. Ohkawa, T. Philip, C. Pinkerton, J. Pritchard, T. Sawada, S. Siegel, E. I. Smith, Y. Tsuchida, and P. A. Voute (1988), *J. Clin. Oncol.* **6,** 1874–1881.

Burghuber, O. C., B. Worofka, G. Scherthaner, N. Vetter, M. Neumann, R. Dudczak, and R. Kuzmits (1990), *Cancer* **65,** 1386–1390.

Carney, D. N., D. C. Ihde, M. H. Cohen, P. J. Marangos, P. A. Bunn, Jr., J. D. Minna, and A. F. Gazdar (1982), *Lancet* **1,** 583–585.

Carney, D. N., and M. Teeling (1988), *Eur. J. Cancer Clin. Oncol.* **24,** 825–828.

Dano, K., P. Andreasen, J. Grondahl-Hansen, P. Kristensen, L. S. Nielsen, and K. Skriver (1985), *Adv. Cancer Res.* **44,** 139–266.

Dao, T. L., C. Ip, J. K. Patel, and G. S. Kishore (1986), in *Tumor Markers and Their Significance in the Management of Breast Cancer,* Alan R. Liss, NY, p. 31–43.

Daver, A., J. Y. Soret, Y. Coblentz, Y. M. Allain, P. Cellier, and P. Chaveau (1988), *Am. J. Clin. Oncol.* **11** (Suppl. 2), S53–S60.

Davey, R., R. Harvie, J. Cahill, and J. Levi (1986a), *Br. J. Cancer* **53,** 211–215.

Davey, R. A., S. T. Milliken, R. M. Harvie, E. J. Cahill, L. J. Morgan, Z. Kerestes, and J. A. Levi (1986b), *Cancer Res.* **46,** 5973–5975.

De Broe, M. E., and D. E. Pollet (1988), *Clin. Chem.* **34,** 1995–1999.

de Bruin, P. A. F., G. Griffioen, H. W. Verspaget, J. H. Verheijen, and C. B. H. W. Lamers (1987), *Cancer Res.* **47,** 4654–4657.

D'Errico, A., S. Garbisa, L. A. Liottta, V. Castronovo, W. G. Stetler-Stevenson, and W. F. Grigioni, (1991), *Modern Pathol.* **4,** 239–246.

Drexler, H. G., M. Menon, and J. Minowada (1986), *Acta Haematol. (Basel)* **75,** 12–17.

Duffy, M. J., P. O'Grady, D. Devaney, L. O'Siorain, J. J. Fennelly, and H. R. Lijnen (1988a), *Cancer* **62,** 531–533.

Duffy, M. J., P. O'Grady, D. Devaney, L. O'Siorain, J. J. Fennelly, and H. R. Lijnen (1988b), *Cancer Res.* **48,** 1348–1349.

Dwivedi, C., M. Dixit, and R. E. Hardy (1988), *Cancer Detect. Prev.* **11,** 191–196.

Epenetos, A. A., D. Snook, G. Hooker, R. Begent, H. Durbin, R. T. D. Oliver, W. F. Bodmer, and J. P. Lavender (1985), *Lancet* **2,** 350–353.

Fishman, W. H., N. R. Inglis, L. L. Stolbach, and M. J. Kraut (1968), *Cancer Res.* **28,** 150–154.

Garbisa, S., A. D'Errico, W. F. Grigioni, G. Biagini, C. Caenazzo, G. Fastelli, W. Stetler-Stevenson, and L. Liotta (1990), in *Genetic Mechanisms in Carcinogenesis and Tumor Progression* (Harris, C. C. and Liotta, L. A., eds.), Wiley-Liss, New York, pp. 203–212.

Garcia, M., M. J. Lacombe, H. Duplay, V. Cavailles, D. Derocq, J. C. Delarue, B. Krebs, G. Contesso, H. Sancho-Garnier, G. Richer, J. Domergue, M. Namer, and H. Rochefort (1987), *J. Steroid Biochem.* **27,** 439–445.

Gutman, E. B., E. E. Sproul, and A. B. Gutman (1936), *Am. J. Cancer* **28,** 485–495.

Hammond, M. E., W. T. Sause, K. L. Martz, M. V. Pilepich, S. O. Asbell, P. Rubin, R. P. Myers, and G. M. Farrow (1989), *Cancer* **63,** 461–466.

Henry, J. A., A. L. McCarthy, B. Angus, B. R. Westley, F. E. B. May, S. Nicholson, J. Cairns, A. L. Harris, and C. H. W. Horne (1990), *Cancer* **65,** 265–271.

Herrera, L. and N. Petrelli (1988), *Dis. Colon Rectum* **31,** 352–354.

Koo, H. B., E. R. Sigurdson, J. Daly, M. Berenson, S. Groshen, and J. DeCosse (1988), *J. Surg. Oncol.* **38,** 240.

Leroy, M., P. Teillac, J. Rain, J. C. Saccavini, A. Le Duc, and Y. Najean (1989), *Cancer* **64,** 1–5.

Liotta, L. A. and W. Stetler-Stevenson (1989), in *Cancer: Principles & Practice of Oncology,* vol. 1 (de Vita, V. T. Jr., S. Hellman, and S. A. Rosenberg, eds.), J. B. Lippincott, Philadelphia, PA, pp. 98–115.

Liotta, L. A. and W. Stetler-Stevenson (1990), in *Seminars in Cancer Biology,* vol. 1 (Gottesman, M. M., ed.), W.B. Sanders, Philadelphia, PA, pp. 99–106.

Luk, G. D. and S. B. Baylin (1984), *N. Engl. J. Med.* **311,** 80–83.

Luk, G. D, J. A. Moshier, and M. N. Ehrenpreis (1988), *Prog. Clin. Biol. Res.* **279,** 227–239.

Madiyalakan, R., C. F. Piskorz, M. S. Piver, and K. L. Matta (1987), *Eur. J. Cancer Clin. Oncol.* **23,** 901–906.

Markus, G. (1988), *Enzyme* **40,** 158–172.

Martin, D., D. Tucker, I. Campbell, and J. Trowsdale (1989), *Clin. Chim. Acta* **186,** 165–170.

McCaffrey, R. A., D. Smoler, and D. Baltimore (1973), *Proc. Natl. Acad. Sci. USA* **70,** 521–525.

Monteagudo, C., M. J. Merino, J. San-Juan, L. A. Liotta, and W. G. Stetler-Stevenson (1990), *Am. J. Pathol.* **136,** 585–592.

Moss, D. W. (1987), *Clin. Biochem.* **20,** 225–230.
Nakayama, T., M. Yoshida, and M. Kitamura (1970), *Clin. Chim. Acta* **30,** 546–548.
Nou, E., L. Steinholz, J. Bergh, K. Nilsson, and S. Pahlman (1990), *Cancer* **65,** 1380–1385.
Nozawa, S., Y. Udagawa, H. Ohkura, Y. Negishi, K. Akiya, N. Inaba, H. Takamizawa, E. Kimura, and Y. Terashima (1989), *Clin. Chim. Acta* **186,** 275–284.
Papadopoulou-Boutis, A., A. Kortsaris, L. Boutis, O. Antonoglou, T. Karemphyllis, D. Mouratidou, S. Koukourikos, and A. S. Trakatellis (1985), *Cancer Detect. Prev.* **8,** 141–150.
Ronquist, G. and E. Nou (1983), *Cancer* **52,** 1679–1683.
Rozhin, J., P. S. Wilson, A. W. Bull, and N. D. Nigro (1984), *Cancer Res.* **44,** 3226–3230.
Sappino, A.-P., N. Busso, D. Belin, and J.-D. Vassali (1987), *Cancer Res.* **47,** 4043–4046.
Schwartz, M. K. (1989), *Clin. Lab. Med.* **9,** 757–765.
Sheahan, K., S. Shuja, and M. Murname (1989), *Cancer Res.* **49,** 3809–3814.
Splinter, T. A., D. N. Carney, M. Teeling, M. D. Peake, G. S. Kho, R. Oosterom, and E. H. Cooper (1989), *Cancer Res. Clin. Oncol.* **115,** 400–401.
Stepan, J. J., M. Mickulecky, V. Bek, P. Broulik, and V. Pacovsky (1989), *Neoplasma* **36,** 495–501.
Tandon, A. K., G. M. Clark, G. C. Chamness, J. M. Chirgwin, and W. L. McGuire (1990), *N. Engl. J. Med.* **322,** 297–302.
Thorpe, S. M., H. Rochefort, M. Garcia, G. Freiss, I. B. Christensen, S. Khalaf, F. Paolucci, B. Pau, B. B. Rasmussen, and C. Rose (1989), *Cancer Res.* **49,** 6008–6014.
Uemura, M., R. C. Winant, and A. E. Brandt (1988), *Cancer Res.* **48,** 5335–5341.
Wang, M. C., L. A. Valenzuela, G. P. Murphy, and T. M. Chu (1979), *Invest. Urol.* **17,** 159–163.
Warnock, M. L. and R. Reisman (1969), *Clin. Chim. Acta* **24,** 5–11.
Weiser, M. M., D. K. Podolsky, and K. J. Isselbacher (1976), *Proc. Natl Acad. Sci.USA* **73,** 1319–1322.
Yazawa, S., R. Madiyalakan, H. Izawa, T. Asao, K. Furukawa, and K. L. Matta (1988), *Cancer* **62,** 516–520.
Zeltzer, P. M., P. J. Marangos, A. E. Evans, and S. L. Schneider (1986), *Cancer* **57,** 1230–1234.

Chapter 7

Alkaline Phosphatases as Tumor Markers

Torgny Stigbrand and Britta Wahren

1. Introduction

Human alkaline phosphatase (ALP), ortophosphoric-monoester phosphohydrolase (alkaline optimum), EC 3.1.3.1, consists of at least four genetically different isozymes, the tissue-unspecific alkaline phosphatase (AP), the intestinal alkaline phosphatase (IAP), the placental alkaline phosphatase (PLAP), and the PLAP-like alkaline phosphatase, an isozyme that is very similar to PLAP (Stigbrand and Fishman, 1984). These four isozymes are encoded by separate but related genes (Kam et al., 1985; Weiss et al., 1986; Berger et al., 1987; Millán and Manes, 1988). It is generally considered that the genes involved have descended from a common ancestral gene, which was duplicated during the course of the evolution. Mutations and further duplications might then explain the ocurrence of this complex multiple enzyme system in humans (Stigbrand et al., 1982).

The abundance in nature of alkaline phosphatases indicates an involvement in fundamental biochemical processes (McComb et al., 1979). Phosphate metabolism is of vital importance to many

From: *Serological Cancer Markers* Edited by Stewart Sell ©1992 The Humana Press, Totowa, NJ

cell functions, and inorganic phosphate plays a central role in the intermediate metabolism. Both the exchange of metabolic energy by the ATP system and the activation/inactivation of enzymes by phosphorylation/dephosphorylation reactions exemplify this. Furthermore, phosphate is an essential part of membrane lipids, nucleotides, coenzymes, and a number of metabolites. Phosphorylation and dephosphorylation reactions are controlled by specific enzymes, phosphorylases, and phosphatases, respectively.

The ALPs have several biological functions, although none of them have proven to be essential for cellular life. They have an extensive range of potential substrates and a wide spectrum of other identified activities (Harris, 1989). All ALPs exhibit phosphotransferase and phosphoprotein phosphatase activites (Huang et al., 1976; Layne and Majjar, 1977; Mellegren et al., 1977; Herraez et al., 1980; Swarup et al., 1981; Lau et al., 1982). The ALPs have been implicated to be involved in bone calcification as well as in phosphate transport in epithelial cells of the intestine (Iiizumi et al., 1983; Hirano et al., 1985). Indeed, in hypophosphatasia, which is an inborn error of metabolism, characterized by generalized deficiency in all tissues of the tissue-unspecific ALP and a characteristic pronounced deficient osteogenesis (Rathabun, 1984; Damovitch et al., 1986), a mutation in the coding region of the tissue-unspecific ALP gene was identified in a typical case of the perinatal form of the disease (Weiss et al., 1988, 1989). This finding is compelling evidence that the tissue-unspecific ALP is involved in the skeletal mineralization.

All ALPs are glycoproteins anchored in the external surface of the plasma membrane by an aspartic or glutamic acid residue at the carboxy terminal end, which is linked to a glycolipid structure containing phosphatidylinositol (Low et al., 1986; Cross, 1987; Bailey et al., 1989). The isozymes are active in a dimeric state, dependent on magnesium and zinc ions for catalytic activity and with an apparent subunit mol wt of 65–85 kDa and with pI of 4.5–4.8. The adult IAP does not, however, contain oligosaccharide chains with terminal sialic acid and this isozyme does not bind to ConA or lentil-lectin-Sepharose (Lehmann, 1980).

A number of different technologies have been introduced for the quantitative determination of the different phosphatase isozymes, such as kinetics of heat inactivation (Whitby and Moss, 1975), urea inactivation (Bahr and Wilkinson, 1967), sensitivity to sodium thiocyanate (Hirano et al., 1983), uncompetitive inhibition by amino acids (Doellgast and Fishman, 1976), mobility at electrophoresis (Green et al., 1972), and immunochemical reactivity (Slaughter et al., 1981; Meyer et al., 1982; Millán and Stigbrand, 1983; Wahren et al., 1986). By the introduction of assays employing isozyme-specific monoclonal antibodies, the knowledge of the complex phenotypic expression of isozymes in tissue have been better known.

PLAP was the first phosphatase isozyme to be reported to be ectopically synthesized in a patient with an oat-cell carcinoma of the lung (Fishman et al., 1986), and the isozyme was named Regan after that patient. The isozyme was identified as PLAP in terms of amino acid inhibition, heat stability, and electrophoretic migration. A similar type of tumor related phosphatase, with properties similar to PLAP, was described in 1970 by Nakayama and coworkers (Nakayama et al., 1970) and named the Nagao isozyme. This isozyme later turned out to be the PLAP-like isozyme or germ-cell alkaline phosphatase. The interest for these isozymes has been significant in tumor biology, because of the reexpression eutopically or ectopically of typical normal embryonic proteins during malignant transformation. The overall incidence of elevated PLAP or PLAP-like isozymes in serum of patients with malignancies has been reported to be comparatively low. The following incidence numbers have been given for tumors derived from prostate 18% (Slack et al., 1981), stomach 36% (Muensch et al., 1986), pancreas 27–30% (Fishman et al., 1975; Muensch et al., 1986), colon 10–54% (Fishman et al., 1975; Rasmuson et al., 1984; Muensch et al., 1986), breast 5–23% (Wada et al., 1975; Stigbrand et al., 1985; Van de Voorde et al., 1985; Muensch et al., 1986), lung 9–40% (Fishman et al., 1975; Rasmuson et al., 1984; Van de Voorde et al., 1985; Pollet et al., 1985; Muensch et al., 1986), uterus 5–68% (Fishman et al., 1975; Kellen et al., 1976; McLaughlin et al., 1983; Stigbrand et al., 1985; Van de Voorde et al., 1985), ovary 35–50% (Fishman et al., 1975; McLaughlin et al., 1983; Rasmuson et al., 1984; Dass and Bagshawe, 1984; Stigbrand et al., 1985; Pollet et al., 1985; Nouwen et al., 1985; Muensch et al., 1986), and testis 36–100%. The frequency of serum elevations in these malignancies differs considerably between investigations, and relatively high frequencies have been found repeatedly only in ovarian and testicular cancers (*see* Table 1).

1.1. Phosphatase Isozymes in Testis and Testicular Tumors

Approximately 40% of all testicular germ-cell tumors are seminomas. Although the survival rate is high, the course is fatal for approx 10% of the patients. It is well known that both alfafetoprotein (AFP) and human chorionic gonadotropin (HCG) are invaluable in the monitoring of nonseminoma germ-cell tumors (NSGCT). Elevation of these two markers have been found in patients with seminomas, but the incidence was only 10–20% (Jacobsen and Norgaard-Pedersen, 1984; Yamamoto et al., 1988). It has also been suggested that elevated AFP indicates the presence of nonseminomatous components (Lange et al., 1982). No available marker for seminomas had been established until Wahren et al. (1979) presented the potentials of using PLAP as a seminoma marker. This observation has been confirmed by many other investigators.

Immunohistochemical investigation of seminomas identifies the isozyme in high frequency (75–100%) in the cell membrane and occasionally in low amounts in the cytoplasm (Wahren et al., 1979; Uchida et al., 1981; Jacobsen and Norgaard-Pedersen, 1984; Epenetos et al., 1984; Brehmer-Andersson et al., 1990). The distribution and intensity of staining vary between tumors as well as between different areas of the same tumor. Interestingly, with a panel of six MAbs investigated, differences in reactivity patterns were identified, implying heterogeneity of both the quantity of the enzyme in each tumor cell and the enzyme itself from an immunohistochemical point of view (Paiva et al., 1983).

In the normal testis, identification of this isozyme has been difficult to establish, probably because of the low levels present.

Table 1
Elevation of Serum PLAP Levels in Patients with Testicular Tumors

Author	Year	Ab	Method	Seminoma positive/total	%	NED
Wahren et al.	1979	poly	RIA	10/19	53	7/26
Lange et al.	1982	poly	ELISA	16/28	57	0/33
Javadpour	1983	poly	ELISA	12/32	40	6/49
Jeppson et al.	1983	poly	RIA	9/21	43	9/68
Dass and Bagshawe	1984	poly	RIA	31/51	61	
				22/33[a]		
Norgaard-Pederson and Millán (DATECA)	1984	poly	RIA, Stage I	94/307	31	
			RIA, Stage II	44/74	69	
Cooper et al.	1985	MAb	ELISA	25/41	61	2/11
Epenetos et al.	1985b	MAb	ELISA	11/11	100	10/70
				6/6[a]	100	
Horwich et al.	1985	MAb	ELISA	15/16	94	16/46
Pledger et al.	1985	poly	ELISA	4/7	57	
Tucker et al.	1985	MAb	ELISA	14/16	88	
				7/13[a]		
Wahren et al.	1986	MAb	ELISA	46/73	63	3/68
				5/11[a]		
Yamamoto et al.	1988	MAb	ELISA	18/21	86	
				3/6[a]		
Koshida	1990, unpubl.	MAb	ELISA	16/26	62	

[a]Mixed tumors containing seminoma component.

Chang et al. (1980) were the first to identify trace expression of PLAP in normal testis and Hirano et al. (1987a) were able, by use of specific MAbs, to establish this isozyme as the PLAP-like or germ-cell phosphatase. On the basis of the reactivity with some monoclonal antibodies and enzyme inhibitors, Millán et al. (1982) proposed an expression of new locus of phosphatases, the PLAP-like isozyme in the normal testis. Wahren et al. (1986) could distinguish six PLAP-like phenotypes in seminomas by the use of monoclonal antibodies, one of which appeared identical to placental PLAP. The majority, however, appeared immunologically distinct. These observations, taken together, indicate that the expression of the PLAP-like isozyme in seminomas in fact is a true eutopic expression of the normal phenotypic expression seen in the normal testis.

By means of sensitive discriminating assays capable of measuring each of the three major phosphatase isozymes, without any crossreactivity (Hirano et al., 1986, 1987b), it has been possible to make several basic observations on the phosphatase isozyme pattern seen in seminomas. Both AP and the PLAP-like isozyme are expressed in levels 10–100 times or folds above the levels seen in the normal testicular tissue (Hirano et al., 1987a; Koshida et al., 1989a). Another distinct feature of the enhanced expression of isozymes is the clear appearance of microheterogeneity in the translated final products as confirmed by lectin chromatographies and electrophoretic behavior (Hirano et al., 1987a; Koshida et al., 1989a,b; Koshida and Wahren, 1989b).

When sera from seminoma patients were assayed by both catalytical and immunocatalytical assays (MICAs), divergent PLAP content was observed. Similar results were obtained from seminoma tissues, whereas serum samples from pregnant females gave almost identical values in the two assays (Koshida and Wahren, 1989a). The results were interpreted as an indication of the existence of a population of tumor-derived PLAP-like isozymes, which is partially heat-sensitive, making the assay conditions for these isozymes of significant importance. A significant heterogeneity of the seminoma-derived isozyme has been verified by use of starch gel electrophoresis. Broad bands with mobility patterns not related to the common PLAP phenotypes were seen, and isoelectric focusing revealed complex patterns of isoelectric point distributions in both catalytic and immunochemical activities (Koshida et al., 1989a,b; Koshida and Wahren, 1989b). This heterogeneity was shown to be partially caused by changes in the carbohydrate moiety and by a confirmed variability in hydrophobicity of the molecule, which in turn may be related to the anchoring carboxy terminal end.

Table 2
PLAP Content in Testicular Tumors

	No. of tissues	Frequency >200 ng/g,%	Tissue level, ng/g
Seminoma pure	31	100	11,900 (900–51,000)
Seminoma component	4	50	4977
Embryonal carcinoma	8	38	412
Other testicular diseases	9	22	197
Normal testis	11	0	75

Data summarized from refs. Jeppson et al., 1984b, and Yamamoto et al., 1988.

The drastic increase in phosphatase activity of two of the major isozymes in seminomatous tissue (Yamamoto et al., 1988; Hirano et al., 1987a; Jeppson et al., 1984b) (*see* Table 2) indicates that the catalytic properties of the isozymes might be of importance to the tumor progression. Basic levels of PLAP and the PLAP-like isozymes are low in healthy, nonpregnant nonsmokers (Domar, 1987). Smokers usually present a slight increase in level, but enough to be classified as above the upper normal cutoff level (Stevens and MacKay, 1973; Alexander et al., 1976). The incidence of elevated levels in smokers has been reported to be 46–65% (Tonik et al., 1983; McLaughlin et al., 1984; Muensch et al., 1986). No biochemical characteristics differentiated the PLAP-like enzymes found in seminoma patients from that of smokers (Koshida et al., 1990). The isozyme present in human lung was recently purified and characterized and it turned out to be the PLAP-like or germ-cell alkaline phosphatase, which is also trace expressed in the human lung (Hirano et al., 1989). Smoking habits of patients thus have to be taken into account when PLAP or PLAP-like isozyme levels are evaluated. Smoking habits of the patients may also sometimes contribute to positive results in patients with no evidence of disease (NED) (Jeppson et al., 1983; Epenetos et al., 1985b; Tucker et al., 1985).

The frequency of elevated serum samples in seminoma patients varies between 36 and 100%, with an average around 70% (Koshida and Wahren, 1989a, *see also*Table 1 in this chapter). The most comprehensive investigation of PLAP-like enzyme in blood of seminoma patients is that of the Danish testicular study (DATECA). In it, the investigators clearly demonstrated a rising occurrence of markers with higher stages (Norgaard-Pedersen and Millán, 1984). The elevations usually are moderate compared to HCG. The relationship between tumor burden (stage) and serum levels is not particularly firm (Lange et al., 1982; Jeppson et al., 1983; Dass and Bagshawe, 1984; Horwich et al., 1985; Yamamoto et al., 1988), which might indicate that release and/or synthesis of the isozyme may depend on the differentiation level of the tumor. In metastasis, 75% of elevated values were reported (Jeppson et al., 1983).

1.2. Phosphatase Isozymes in Ovary and Ovarian Epithelial Tumors

Compared to the situation with testicular tumors and, especially, seminomas, a number of well-established markers exist for ovarian epithelial tumors, i.e., CA 125, OCAA, OCA, and cytokeratins (Stigbrand et al., 1990). The ovarian tumors, however, seem to follow the same pattern of phosphatase isozyme expression as the seminomas. The normal ovary presents as the dominating phosphatase isozyme the tissue-unspecific isozyme (AP) and trace expression of the PLAP-like or germ-cell alkaline phosphatase, which amounts to approx 10% of the catalytic activity (Koyama et al., 1989). This trace-expressed isozyme has been purified and characterized and is the PLAP-like isozyme (Koyama et al., 1990). Following malignant transformation, a drastic increase occurs with both these isozymes, amounting to 10–100 times the levels seen in the normal ovary. Both these isozymes, AP and the PLAP-like isozyme, are expressed in significant amounts and may be released into the circulation (Koyama et al., 1989, 1990).

Immunohistochemical staining on formalin-fixed tumor tissues used for routine histopathologic examinations indicate that all the four major groups of ovarian adenocarcinomas, i.e., serous, mucinous, endometroid, and mesonephoric tumors express the antigen in similar incidences (46–67%) (Stendahl et al., 1989). These tumors constitute 80% of all ovarian cancers. The mucinous and mesonephric tumors have been reported to present more intense staining. Besides the plasma membrane staining, granular staining also has been found in the cytoplasm, in mucinous and mesonephric carcinomas close to the luminal end, and in serous and endometroid carcinomas more diffusely distributed (Stendahl et al., 1989). A heterogenous staining pattern at the cellular level is also seen within the tumors, as was the case for the seminomas. When possible to measure, the relative content of the PLAP-like isozyme in some tumors have been shown to be around 40% elevated, indicating that almost one-half of the catalytical phosphatase activity in these tumors is derived from the PLAP-like isozyme (Koyama et al., 1989).

The purified isozyme from ovarian epithelial tumors also displays microheterogeneity as demonstrated by phenyl-Sepharose affinity chromatography and binding to the lectin Con A. In the tumor-derived population of PLAP-like isozyme molecules, 18% did not bind to Con A (Koyama et al., 1990).

The significance of the PLAP-like antigen as a monitoring serum marker for ovarian epithelial tumors has been controversial (Fishman et al., 1975; Dass and Bagshawe, 1984; Stigbrand et al., 1985; Pollet et al., 1985; Nouwen et al., 1985; Muensch et al., 1986; Koyama et al., 1989). This has been partly as a result of the different types of assays used to quantify the enzyme, i.e., catalytical, immunocatalytical, or immunochemical. The potential existence of partially heat-sensitive tumor-derived isozymes makes pure catalytical assays less accurate. By the development of isozyme-specific monoclonal antibodies, it now seems to be the consensus that 40–50% of all ovarian cancer patients have significantly elevated serum levels. Endometroid and nonmucinous adenocarcinomas are often associated with high levels of the PLAP-like isozyme, and the serum levels are positively correlated to tumor burden and outcome of the disease. Compared to CA 125, however, both the incidence and the range of values for the PLAP-like isozymes are lower. In some cases, additional information has been provided by determination of the PLAP-like isozyme level (Stigbrand et al., 1990).

An interesting observation has been made (Stendahl et al., 1989) that patients with high serum levels usually display low tumor content of the isozyme and vice versa, indicating that the release of this marker from the tumor to the circulation may, in fact, be the major mechanism gearing the relation of the serum levels and tumor levels. This information may be of significance when radioimmunolocalization and radioimmunotherapy are considered. Commercial tests for the PLAP/PLAP-like isozyme are now available and their use is slowly increasing. The low-incidence rate, however, makes this marker less used than CA 125.

1.3. Alkaline Phosphatase Isozymes in Human Colorectal Adenocarcinomas

It has recently been shown that other tumors, outside the gonadal sphere, may display significant elevations of the PLAP-like isozyme, both in the tumor tissues and in the circulation (Harmenberg et al., 1989). In a series of 20 tumors and mucosal samples from colorectal carcinomas, again, the tissue-unspecific alkaline phosphatase and the PLAP-like isozyme were significantly elevated in the tumor tissue, whereas in fact, the IAP isozyme, which normally constitutes the major catalytic activity in the intestine, in most cases, was shown to be lower than in the normal mucosa (Harmenberg et al., 1991). By using one monoclonal antibody, capable of discriminating between PLAP and the PLAP-like isozyme, the latter was appearing also in the colon adenocarcinomas. A PLAP-like gene was recently identified and cloned from a colon cancer cell line (Gum et al., 1990).

1.4. Radioimmunolocalization and Radioimmunotherapy Using Anti-PLAP Antibodies

Radiolabeled antibodies with specificity against tumor antigens have attracted considerable interest as a means of detecting tumors and their metastases. Both PLAP and the PLAP-like isozyme normally appear on the outer plasma membrane surface, and would then constitute suitable targets for radioimmunodetection. Both polyclonal and monoclonal antibodies against PLAP demonstrate a significant localization to experimental tumors in nude mice (Jeppson et al., 1984a; Stigbrand et al., 1989), but not to tumors in which PLAP was not measurable. With one anti-PLAP H7 monoclonal antibody, it has furthermore been demonstrated that the biological half-life of the radiolabeled antibody in vivo in nude mice is around 170 h, which was significantly longer than in the nontumorous animal (Stigbrand et al., 1989). In nude mice it has furthermore been possible to demonstrate growth-inhibiting effects of both ^{131}I- and ^{125}I-labeled anti-PLAP monoclonal antibodies (Riklund et al., 1990). The studies of patients are more limited, but Epenetos et al. (1985a) have in fact reported a clinical application of a radiolabeled MAb against PLAP for detection of tumors from the testis, ovary, and cervix. They were able to demonstrate that an indium-111-labeled MAb could localize, with a high degree of accuracy, the presence of active disease in patients with PLAP-positive tumors. This was demonstrated in cases in which the tumors could not be detected with other imaging techniques, including ultrasonography and tomography.

Acknowledgments

This investigation was supported by grants from the Swedish Cancer Society, Cancer Foundation in Stockholm, Lions Foundation in Umeå, and the Medical Faculty at the University of Umeå.

References

Alexander, J. C., N. A. Silverman, and P. B. Chretien (1976), *JAMA* **235,** 1975.
Bahr, M. and J. H. Wilkinson (1967), *Clin. Chim. Acta* **17,** 367–370.
Bailey, C. A., L. Cerber, A. D. Howard, and S. Udenfriend (1989), *Proc. Natl. Acad. Sci. USA* **86,** 22–26.
Berger, J., E. Garattini, J. C. Hua, and S. Udenfriend (1987), *Proc. Natl. Acad. Sci. USA* **84,** 695–698.

Brehmer-Andersson, E., E. Ljungdahl-Ståhle, H. Yamamoto, K. Koshida, T. Stigbrand, and B. Wahren (1990), *Acta Path. Scand.* **98,** 977–982.
Chang, C. H., D. Angellis, and W. H. Fishman (1980), *Cancer Res.* **40,** 1506.
Cooper, E. H., N. B. Pidcoch, W. G. Jones, and A. M.Ward (1985), *Eur. J. Clin. Oncol.* **21,** 525–530.
Cross, G.A.M. (1987), *Cell* **48,** 179–181.
Damovitch, S. D., P. N. Bear, and L. Laster (1986), *N. Engl. J. Med.* **278,** 1253–1260.
Dass, S. and K. D. Bagshawe (1984), in *Progress in Clinical and Biological Research* (Stigbrand, T., and W. H. Fishman, eds.), Vol. 166, Liss, New York, p. 49.
Doellgast, G. J. and W. H. Fishman (1976), *Nature* **259,** 49–51.
Domar, U. (1987), MS thesis, Umeå University, Umeå, Sweden.
Epenetos, A. A., P. Travers, K. C. Gatter, R. D. T. Oliver, D. Y. Mason, and W. F. Bodmer (1984), *Br. J. Cancer* **49,** 11.
Epenetos, A. A., D. Snook, G. Hooker, R. Begent, H. Durbin, R. T. D. Oliver, W. F. Bodmer, and J. P. Lavender (1985a), *Lancet* **II,** 350.
Epenetos, A. A., A. J. Munro, D. F. Tucker, W. Gregory, W. Duncan, R. H. MacDougall, M. Faux, P. Travers, and W. F. Bodmer (1985), *Br. J. Cancer* **51,** 641.
Fishman, W. H., N. R. Inglis, L. L. Stolback, and M. J. Krant (1986), *Cancer Res.* **28,** 150.
Fishman, W. H., N. R. Inglis, J. Vaitukaitis, and , L. L. Stolbach (1975), *Natl. Cancer Inst. Monogr.* **42,** 63–70.
Green, S., F. Cantor, N. Inglis, and W. H. Fishman (1972), *Am. J. Clin. Pathol.* **57,** 52–64.
Gum, J. R., J. W. Hicks, T. L. Sack, and K. S. Kim (1990), *Cancer Res.* **50,** 1085–1091.
Harmenberg, V.U., J.-E. Frödin, E. Ljungdahl-Ståhle, H. Mellstedt, B. Wahren, and T. Stigbrand (1989), *Tumor Biol.* **10,** 225–231.
Harmenberg, U., M. Koha, R. Mahiya, K. Koshida, B. Brismar, T. Stigbrand, and B. Wahren, (1991), *Tumor Biol.* (in press)
Harris, H. (1989), *Clin. Chim. Acta* **186,** 133–150.
Herraez, H. A., F. J. Burguillo, M. G. Roig, and J. L. Usero (1980), *Int. J. Biochem.* **11,** 511–518.
Hirano, K., K. Kusano, H. Matsumoto, H. Stigbrand, S. Iino, and K. Hayashi (1989), *Eur. J. Biochem.* **183,** 419–423.
Hirano, K., U. Domar, H. Yamamoto, E. Brehmer-Andersson, B. Wahren, and T. Stigbrand (1987a), *Cancer Res.* **47,** 2543.
Hirano, K., H. Matsumoto, T. Tanaka, S. Iino, U. Domar, and T. Stigbrand (1987b), *Clin. Chim. Acta* **166,** 265.
Hirano, K., Y. Iiizumi, Y. More, K. Toyoshi, M. Sugiura, and S. Iino (1985), *J. Biochem.* **97,** 1461–1466.

Hirano, K., Y. Iiizumi, M. Syugiura, J. Miyazaki, K. Miki, S. Iino, H. Suzuki, and T. Oda (1983), *Chem. Pharm. Bull.* **31,** 3248–3254.

Hirano, K., Y. Iiizumi, Y. Hayashi, T. Tanaha, M. Suguira, K. Mayashi, Z.-D. Lu, and S. Iino (1986), *Anal. Biochem.* **154,** 624.

Horwich, A., D. F. Tucker, and M. J. Peckman (1985), *Br. J. Cancer* **51,** 625.

Huang, K.-P., J. C. Robinson, and J. Y. Chou (1976), *Biochem. Biophys. Res. Commun.* **70,** 186–192.

Iiizumi, Y., K. Hirano, M. Sugiura, S. Inio, H. Suzuki, and T. Oda (1983), *Chem. Pharm. Bull.* **31,** 772–775.

Jacobsen, G. K. and B. Norgaard-Pedersen (1984), *Acta Pathol. Microbiol. Immunol. Scand.* **92,** 323.

Javadpour, N. (1983), *Cancer* **52,** 887.

Jeppson, A., B. Wahren, J. L. Millán, and T. Stigbrand (1984a), *Br. J. Cancer* **49,** 123.

Jeppson, A., B. Wahren, E. Brehmer-Andersson, C. Silfvervärd, T. Stigbrand, and B. Wahren (1984b), *Int. J. Cancer* **34,** 757–761.

Jeppson, A., B. Wahren, T. Stigbrand, F. Edsmyr, and L. Andersson (1983), *Br. J. Urol.* **55,** 73.

Kam, W., E. Clauser, Y. S. Kim, Y. W. Kan, and W. J. Rutter (1985), *Proc. Natl. Acad. Sci. USA* **82,** 8715–8719.

Kellen, J. A., R. S. Bush, and A. Malkin (1976) *Cancer Res.* **36,** 269.

Koshida, K. and B. Wahren (1989a), *Urol. Res.* **18,** 87–92.

Koshida, K. and B. Wahren (1989b), *Clin. Chim. Acta* **186,** 255–264.

Koshida, K., T. Stigbrand, H. Hisazumi, and B. Wahren (1989a), *Tumor Biol.* **10,** 173.

Koshida, K., T. Stigbrand, H. Hisazumi, and B. Wahren (1989b), *Tumor Biol.* **10,** 181.

Koshida, K., T. Stigbrand, E. Munck-Wikland, H. Hisazumi, and B. Wahren (1990), *Urol. Res.* **18,** 169–173.

Koyama, I., U. Stendahl, and T. Stigbrand (1989), *Clin. Chim. Acta* **186,** 295–300.

Koyama, I., K. Hirano, R. Makiya, U. Stendahl, and T. Stigbrand (1990), *Br. J. Cancer* **62,** 6–11.

Lange, P. H., J. L. Millán, T. Stigbrand, R. L. Vessella, E. Ruoslahti, and W. H. Fishman (1982), *Cancer Res.* **42,** 3244.

Lau, K. H. W., I.-I. G. Chen, and J. A. Thomad (1982), *Mol. Cell. Biochem.* **44,** 149–159.

Layne, P. P. and V. A. Majjar (1977), *Arch. Biochem. Biophys.* **180,** 328–333.

Lehmann, F. G. (1980), *Klin. Wochenschr.* **58,** 947-951.

Low, M. G., M. A. J. Ferguson, A. H. Futerman, and I. Silman (1986), *TIBS* **44,** 212–215.

McComb, R. B., G. N. Bowers, Jr., and S. Posen (1979), *Alkaline Phosphatases,* Plenum, New York and London.

McLaughlin, P. J., H. Gee, and P. M. Johnson (1983), *Clin. Chim. Acta* **130,** 199.
McLaughlin, P. J., A. M. Twist, C. C. Evans, and P. M. Johnson (1984), *J. Clin. Pathol.* **37,** 826.
Mellegren, R. L., G. R. Slaughter, and J. A. Thomas (1977), *J. Biol. Chem.* **252,** 6082–6089.
Meyer, L., M. A. Lafferty, M. G. Raducha, C. J. Foster, K. J. Gogolin, and H. Harris (1982), *Clin. Chim. Acta* **126,** 109–117.
Millán, J. L. and T. Manes (1988), *Proc. Natl. Acad. Sci. USA* **85,** 3024–3028.
Millán, J. L., A. Eriksson, and T. Stigbrand (1982), *Hum. Genet.* **62,** 293.
Millán, J. L. and T. Stigbrand (1983), *Eur. J. Biochem.* **136,** 1–7.
Muensch, H. A., W. C. Maslow, F. Azama, M. Bertrand, P. Dewhurst, and B. Hartman (1986), *Cancer* **58,** 1689–1692.
Nakayama, T., M. Yodhida, and M. Kitamura (1970), *Clin. Chim. Acta* **30,** 546.
Norgaard-Pederson, B. and J. L.Millán (1984), *l'Inserm* **123,** 463–482.
Nouwen, E. J., D. E. Pollet, J. B. Schelstraete, M. W. Ederdekens, C. Hänsch, A. Van de Voorde, and M. E. de Broe (1985), *Cancer Res.* **45,** 892.
Paiva, J., I. Damjanov, P. H. Lange, and H. Harris (1983), *Am. J. Pathol.* **111,** 156.
Pledger, D. R. and J. B. Mahon (1985), *Clin. Biochem.* **18,** 213–216.
Pollet, E. D., E. J. Nouwen, J. B. Schelstraete, J. Renard, A. Van de Voorde, and M. E. de Broe (1985), *Clin. Chem.* **31,** 41.
Rasmuson, T., A. Jeppson, and T. Stigbrand (1984), *Progress in Clinical and Biological Research,* (Stigbrand, T. and W. H. Fishman, eds.), vol. 166, Liss, New York, p. 309.
Rathabun, R. C. (1984), *Am. J. Dis. Child.* 75, 822–831.
Riklund, K.E., R. Makiya, B. Sundström, L.-E. Thornell, and T. Stigbrand (1990), *Anticancer Res.* **10,** 379–384.
Slack, N. H., T. M. Chu, L. Z. Wajsman, and G. P. Murphy (1981), *Cancer* **47,** 146.
Slaughter, C. A., M. C. Coseo, M. P. Camcro,and H. Harris (1981), *Proc. Natl. Acad. Sci. USA* **78,** 1124–1128.
Stendahl, U., A. Lindgren, B. Tholander, R. Makiya, and T. Stigbrand (1989), *Tumor Biol.* **10,** 126–132.
Stevens, D. P. and I. R. MacKay (1973), *Lancet* **II,** 1238.
Stigbrand, T. and W. H. Fishman (1984), *Human Alkaline Phosphatases,* A. R. Liss, New York.
Stigbrand, T., J. L. Millán, and W. H. Fishman (1982), in *Isozymes: Current Topics in Biological and Medical Research,* (Rattazzi, M. C., Scandalios, Y. G., and G. S. Whitt, eds.),vol. 6, A. R. Liss, New York, pp. 93–117.
Stigbrand, T., P. Holmgren, A. Jeppsson, M. G. Damber, and B. Schoultz (1985), *Acta Obstet. Gynecol. Scand.* **64,** 99–103.

Stigbrand, T., K. Riklund, B. Tholander, K. Hirano, and O. Lalos (1990), *Eur. J. Gynaecol. Oncol.* XI, 5, 351–360.
Stigbrand, T., S-O. Hietala, B. Johansson, R. Makiya, K. Riklund, and L. Ekelund (1989), *Tumour Biol.* **10/5,** 243–251.
Swarup, G., S. Cohen, and D. L. Garbers (1981), *J. Biol. Chem.* **256,** 8197–8201.
Tonik, S. E., A. E. Ortmeyer, J. E. Shindelman, and H. H. Sussman (1983), *Int. J. Cancer* **31,** 51.
Tucker, D. F., R. T. D. Oliver, P. Travers, and W. F. Bodmer (1985), *Br. J. Cancer* **51,** 631.
Uchida, T., T. Shimoda, H. Miyata, T. Shikata, S. Iino, H. Suzuki, T. Oda, K. Hirano, and N. Sugiura (1981), *Cancer* **48,** 1455.
Van de Voorde, A., G. De Groote, P. De Waele, M. E. De Broe, D. Pollet, J. De Boever, D. Vandekerckhove, and W. Fiers (1985), *Eur. J. Cancer Clin. Oncol.* **21,** 65.
Wada, H. G., J. G. Shindelman, A. E. Ortmeyer, and H. H. Sussman (1975), *Int. J. Cancer* **23,** 781.
Wahren, B., P. Å. Holmgren, and T. Stigbrand (1979), *Int. J. Cancer* **24,** 749–753.
Wahren, B., J. Hinkula, T. Stigbrand, A. Jeppsson, L. Andersson, P. L. Esposti, F. Edsmyr, and J. L. Millán (1986), *Int. J. Cancer* **37,** 595–600.
Weiss, M. J., D. E. Cole, K. Ray, M. P. Whyte, M. A. Lafferty, R. A. Mulivor, and H. Harris (1988), *Proc. Natl. Acad. Sci. USA* **85,** 7666–7669.
Weiss, M. J., P. S. Henthorn, M. A. Lafferty, C. Slaughter, M. Raducha, and H. Harris (1986), *Proc. Natl. Acad. Sci. USA* **83,** 7182–7186.
Weiss, M. J., K. Ray, M. D. Fallon, M. P. Whyte, K. N. Fedde, M. A. Lafferty, R. A. Mulivor, and H. Harris (1989), *Am. J. Hum. Genet.* **44,** 686–694.
Whitby, L. G. and D. W. Moss (1975), *Clin. Chim. Acta.* **59,** 361–367.
Yamamoto, H., U. Ruden, P. Esposti, K. Hirano, T. Stigbrand, L. Andersson, H. Hisazumi, and B. Wahren (1988), *Urol. Res.* **16,** 31–36.

Chapter 8

Sex-Associated Hormones

Shahla Masood

1. Introduction

Experimental and clinical observations support the concept that sex steroid hormones may play a role in the development, growth, and behavior of certain tumors (Moore, 1936; McEwen et al., 1975, 1982; Noble, 1977; Trachtenberg and Walsh, 1982). It has been known for many years that prognosis of patients with various malignancies differ between males and females, and some tumors can be alleviated and partially controlled by endocrine therapy (Beatson, 1896; Huggins and Hodges, 1941; Huggins and Bergenstal, 1952; Luft et al., 1958; Bodenham and Hale, 1972; Sadoff et al., 1973; Poisson, 1984). Thus, there is no doubt that some cancers are hormone-dependent. A significant number of breast and prostatic carcinomas have been treated with various additive or ablative hormonal manipulation (Young and Kent, 1968; Mass et al., 1972; Englesman et al., 1973; Leung et al., 1973; Savlov et al., 1974). The detection of specific sex steroid hormone receptor proteins in hormone-dependent tumors has enhanced our understanding of tumor biology and the mechanism of endocrine therapy. Aside from carcinomas of prostate, breast, and the female reproductive organ, many solid organs have been tested for the presence of estrogen

From: *Serological Cancer Markers* Edited by Stewart Sell ©1992 The Humana Press, Totowa, NJ

receptor (ER) and progesterone receptor (PgR) and other steroid receptors. A fair number of these tumors have shown expression of sex steroid hormone receptors (Lee, 1984b; Poisson, 1984; Corbishley et al., 1986; Lesch and Gross, 1987; Yokozzski et al., 1988; Erdstein et al., 1989; Nagasue et al., 1989; Urba et al., 1990). This review attempts to summarize the functional characteristic and the prognostic and therapeutic significance of sex steroid hormone receptors in various tumors.

2. Historical Background

Hormone dependency of breast cancer has been known since 1896, when Beatson reported remission of metastatic breast cancer following removal of a patient's ovaries. In the 1940s, orchiectomy was introduced for the treatment of prostate cancer (Huggins and Hodges, 1941). Adrenalectomy (Huggins and Bergenstal, 1952) and hypophysectomy (Luft et al., 1958) were utilized for the treatment of metastatic breast disease in postmenopausal women.

By the early 1960s endocrine ablation became the preferred treatment for advanced breast cancer. However, only 25–30% of all patients so treated showed any clinical response. This led to development of steroid-binding test procedures in an attempt to predict which patients would respond to hormone therapy. In 1961, Folca et al. demonstrated that patients who subsequently benefited from ablative surgery had tumors that showed preferential uptake of tritiated estrogen.

In 1970, Jensen operated the first in vitro assay demonstrating a good correlation of patient response to endocrine therapy. Following the initial indication of a "receptor" for estrogen that seemed to correlate clinical responsiveness to endocrine therapy, many other investigators soon confirmed that knowledge of ER status was important for proper management of cancer (Mass et al., 1972; Englesman et al., 1973; Leung et al., 1973; Savlov et al., 1974).

It was also recognized that PgR synthesis is usually an estrogen-dependent process (Harwitz et al., 1975). Therefore, the presence of PgR might be an indicator of a fully functional ER mechanism. The assessment of PgR in addition to ER has been demonstrated to improve the predictive value of hormone receptor determination, and PgR appears to be a more important prognostic indicator than ER (Clark et al., 1983).

In the past few years, monoclonal antibodies specific to both estrogen and progesterone receptors have been developed (King and Greene, 1984; Press and Greene, 1988). In addition, human genes for the receptors have been cloned (Walter et al., 1985; Misrahi et al., 1987). The ER gene, on chromosome 6, produces two 65-kDa subunits. The PgR gene, on chromosome 11, transcribes two dissimilar subunits, of 95 and 120 kDa. Each cell contains about 10,000 ERs and 50,000–100,000 PgRs.

These important developments allow more precise study of sex steroid hormone receptor expression and may lead to improved management of hormone-dependent tumors.

3. Mechanism of Steroid Hormone Action

Sex steroid hormones interact with specific binding proteins called "receptors" modulating cell proliferation (Anderson, 1984). Receptors are macromolecular proteins normally present in breast and female reproductive organs. Although it was thought originally that estrogen binds to a cytoplasmic receptor (Noleboom and Gorski, 1965), it has since been shown that estrogen receptor (ER) proteins reside predominently within the nucleus (King and Greene, 1984; Welshons et al., 1984). According to the current model (Fig. 1), which is a modification of the "two–step" hypothesis originally proposed by Gorski et al. (1968) and Jensen et al. (1968) (Fig. 2), the steroid hormone initially associates with lower affinity type II receptors in the cytoplasm and then binds to the high-affinity receptors in the nucleus. The hormone–receptor complex then undergoes molecular changes that lead to association of receptor complex with chromatin. The chromatin–receptor complex stimulates gene expression, leading to the synthesis of new messenger RNA and proteins characteristic of the hormone's cellular effect (Martin and Sheridan, 1982). Activation of ER also stimulates transcription of

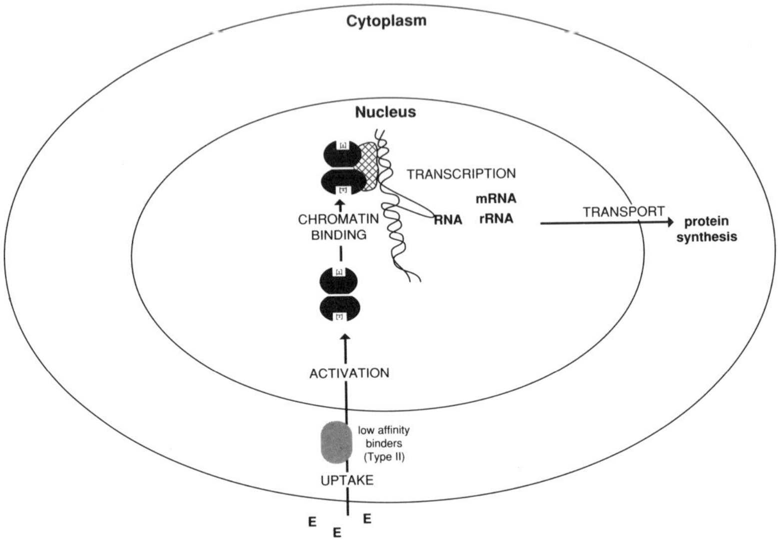

Fig. 1. New model for the sequence of events in interaction of steroid hormone with a target cell. The steroid hormone associates with low-affinity receptors in the cytoplasm and then binds to high-affinity receptors in the nucleus. Upon binding to nuclear chromatin, the estrogen/receptor complex stimulates RNA polymerase activity, which leads to production of new messenger RNA (mRNA) and synthesis of new protein characteristics.

progesterone receptors on RNA. Binding of PgR with progesterone then induces growth, mitogenic factors, and synthesis of up to 100 proteins (Meyer et al., 1989).

Several studies indicate that there are at least two estrogen receptors, each with different affinities for estrogen (Clark et al., 1978; Chamness et al., 1980). The type I "true" receptor, also known as estrophilin, is not bound to endogenous hormone and is easily extractable from tissue homogenates with buffers of low ionic strength. This is the type of ER that is routinely determined in specimens (cytosolic ER) and has the greatest affinity for estrogen. Type II "low-affinity" receptors are most likely a different group of proteins, which was first reported in the cytosol of rat uterus in 1978 (Clark et al., 1978). This second ER, although it displays similar

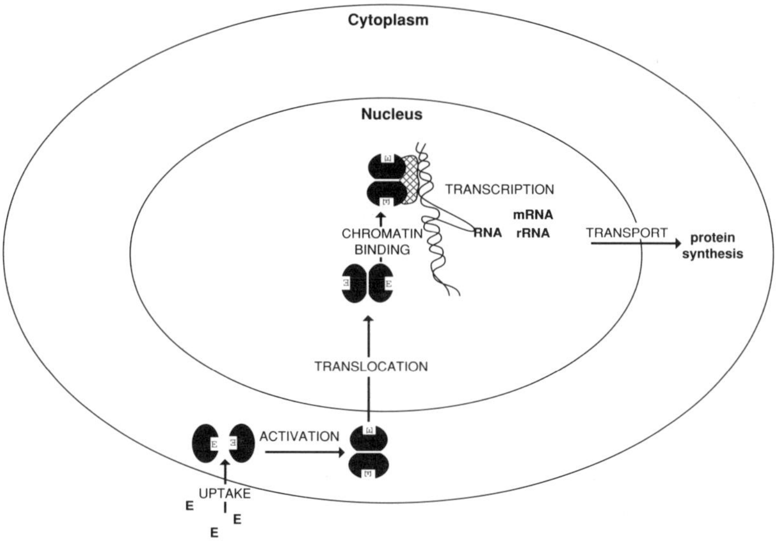

Fig. 2. Old model for the sequence of events in the mechanism of steroid hormone action on a target. The difference is in the formation of hormone/receptor complex within the cytoplasm followed by translocation into the nucleus. Within the nucleus, the rest of the events are similar to those in the new model.

steroid and tissue specificity, is distinct from the true, type I ER and has a lower estrogen affinity. Its functional significance is unclear at present.

A fair number of breast cancers fail to express ER. Gene mutation, heterogeneity of receptors in tumors, and transfection with the *ras* oncogene are the suggested mechanisms (Kasid and Lippman, 1987; Raam et al., 1988; Hill et al., 1989).

4. Methods for the Assay of Steroid Receptors

4.1. Biochemical Assays

The biochemical or steroid-binding assays are now considered the standard to which all other methods are compared. These assays employ radioligands that combine with receptor sites in a tumor extract to form a steroid–receptor complex. The bound complexes are then separated from unbound radioligands by either absorption of hormone to dextran-coated charcoal (DCC) or sucrose-gradient centrifugation, leaving the receptor-bound hormone intact. The DCC technique is more frequently employed than sucrose-gradient centrifugation (Wittliff, 1975; Clark et al., 1976).

Current biochemical assays have some inherent disadvantages (Wittliff, 1975, 1977; Raam et al., 1981; Greene and Jensen, 1982; Oxley et al., 1982; Straus et al., 1982; McClelland et al., 1986). The steroid-binding with the receptor is noncovalent, and the radiolabeled marker can be lost by dissociation. Traces of heavy-metal ions may diminish binding. Receptor protein may undergo degradation during storage and processing of the tumor specimen. In certain patients, the receptor may already be occupied by nonradioactive hormone, interfering with binding of the radiolabeled steroid markers unless an exchange step is employed. In addition, if nontumor tissue binds to the radioligand or if the steroid binding site is occupied by endogenous estradiol, false high values may be obtained. Antiestrogen therapy may result in false low values.

The biochemical methods require expensive ultracentrifugation equipment, scintillation counters, and radiolabeled chemicals, limiting employment to reference laboratories and large medical centers. Biochemical assays cannot assess tumor hormone-receptor heterogeneity. Some lesions may be too small for biochemical assay. Only 55–60% of patients with tumors classified as receptor positive by biochemical assay respond to endocrine therapy (McGuire et al., 1975). Thus, practical methods that are simpler, less expensive, and less sensitive to errors or variations than the commonly used biochemical assays are clearly needed.

4.2. Immunochemical Assays

Immunofluorescence (Nenci et al., 1976; Pertschuk, 1976; Nenci, 1978; Pertschuk et al., 1978) and immunoperoxidase (Ghosh et al., 1978; Kurzon and Sternberger, 1978; Walker et al., 1980) methods were the first immunochemical assays to be reported. These methods require incubation of tissue sections or isolated cells with estradiol and the addition of antiestradiol antibody. Either fluores-

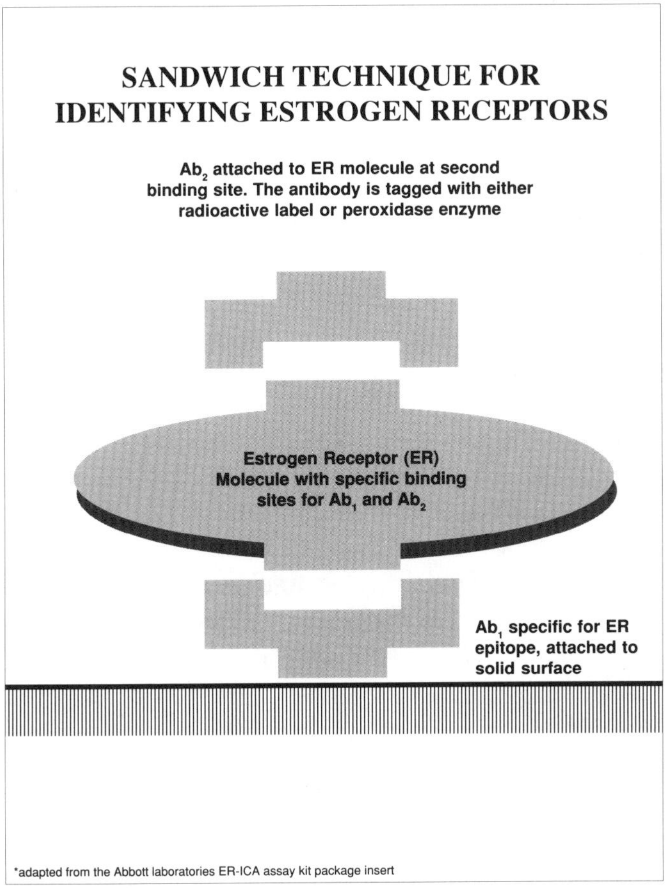

Fig. 3. Schematic presentation of immunometric and enzyme-linked immunoassay for detection of estrogen receptor.

cein-labeled anti-IgG or an unlabeled antibody that can bind to a peroxidase–antiperoxidase complex is employed to identify a positive reaction; more recently, immunoradiometric assay and enzyme-linked immunoassay methods have been completed. In both of these procedures, a polystyrene bead coated with an antiestrophilin antibody is incubated with a homogenate of the tissue sample. Binding of the tissue receptor immobolizes the receptor on the bead. After several washings, a second antibody is added, labeled with I-125 or peroxidase for detection (Fig. 3).

These techniques are relatively easy to perform and demonstrate good correlation to sucrose density gradient values (Greene and Jensen, 1982; Greene et al., 1984). However, unresolved issues remain (Pertschuk, 1976), including the availability of receptor-bound estradiol to antibody, the concentration of estradiol necessary to visualize the response, and the ability of other ligands to compete for the estradiol binding site. In addition, these procedures do not resolve the potential problem of tumor heterogeneity.

4.3. Fluorescent Technique

Cytochemical assay, introduced by Lee in 1978, is based on the assumption that if a dye is attached to a steroid hormone molecule so that the important physiological determinants of the hormone are preserved, the dye may serve as a cytochemical receptor tracer. A patented procedure called Fluoro-Cep™ (Zeus Technologies, Inc., Raritan, NJ) employs estradiol linked to bovine serum albumin (BSA), coupled to fluorescein isothiocyanate (FITC). Similarly, progesterone is linked to BSA and coupled to tetramethylrhodamine isothiocyanate (TMRITC). The fluorescent cytochemical technique compares favorably with the biochemical assay (Pertschuk et al., 1980; Jacobs et al., 1983; Lee, 1984a).

Estrogen-binding substances demonstrated by this cytochemical fluorescent technique appear to belong to the family of ERs that are heterogenous in molecular configuration and in subcellular distribution (Gardner and Wittliff, 1973; Clark et al., 1978; Pertschuk et al., 1980; Wiehle and Wittliff, 1983). Clinical response rates for the fluorescent cytochemical method are almost comparable to those obtained with the biochemical DCC assay (Henson et al., 1977; McGuire et al., 1977; Pertschuk et al., 1987; Chen et al., 1989).

In spite of these findings, the fluorescent cytochemical technique remains a subject of controversy. This technique may identify the lower affinity, type II cytoplasmic estrogen-binding proteins, rather than the high-affinity, type I nuclear ER, as measured biochemically (Nenci, 1978; Jacobs et al., 1983; Janssens et al., 1985). The fluorescent cytochemical technique may recognize hormone-specific binding sites, which may correspond to the presence of type I estrogen receptors (Mercer et al., 1980).

Coexistence of cytoplasmic and nuclear estrogen receptors was reported by Lee in 1989. Utilizing serial cryostat frozen sections from 157 human mammary carcinomas, topographical distribution of ER-positive cells by the fluorescent cytochemical method was almost identical to that found by immunoperoxidase assay utilizing monoclonal antibody to nuclear ER receptor. There was a 94–97% concordance between the two procedures, thus supporting the usefulness of the fluorescent assay.

4.4. Immunoperoxidase Technique

The immunocytochemical assay method detects receptors in frozen tissue sections, in formalin-fixed tissue, and in cytological specimens. Monoclonal antibodies are applied to tissue sections, and binding can be visualized using a peroxidase–antiperoxidase technique (Fig. 4). ER monoclonal antibodies are produced by hybridomas, utilizing rats immunized with purified receptor from MCF–7-type human breast cancer cell (Greene et al., 1980, 1984). In this procedure, the tumor section mounted on a microscope slide is incubated with a rat monoclonal antibody to human estrophilin. A goat antirat immunoglobulin fixed to horseradish peroxidase binds to the rat monoclonal antibody. After a wash step, the tumor section is exposed to a chromogenic substance, which reacts with the horseradish peroxidase to form an insoluble brown substance at the receptor site, yielding brown nuclear staining (Fig. 5).

The immunocytochemical assay depends on recognition of the receptor protein by monoclonal antibodies, rather than on steroid-binding activity. The specificity of the antibody eliminates interference by other steroid-binding proteins.

A commercially available kit for Estrogen Receptor Immunochemical Assay (ER–ICA, from Abbott Laboratories, Chicago, IL) has been shown to be highly specific and sensitive for hormone-receptor analysis of cytologic preparations and frozen human tumor tissue (King et al., 1985; Charpin et al., 1986, 1988; Flowers

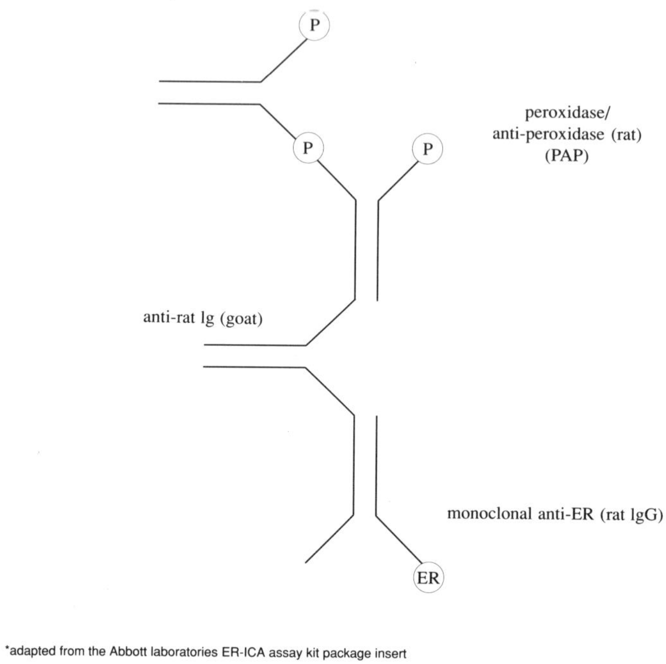

Fig. 4. Schematic presentation of peroxidase–antiperoxidase technique for identifying estrogen receptor.

et al., 1986; Jensen et al., 1986; Lozowski et al., 1987; Masood, 1988a; Allred et al., 1990; Lundy et al., 1990).

The immunocytochemical assay is also suitable for routinely prepared, paraffin-embedded tissue and offers a reliable and reproducible alternative when tissue is unavailable or is not suitable for DCC biochemical or immunocytochemical assay. This method is especially well-suited to retrospective studies on archived materials and may also provide information regarding tumor heterogeneity. Good results have been obtained using paraffin-embedded fixed tissue, with excellent correlation to the biochemical DCC assay (Anderson et al., 1986, 1988a,b; Shintaku and Said, 1987; Masood et al., 1990).

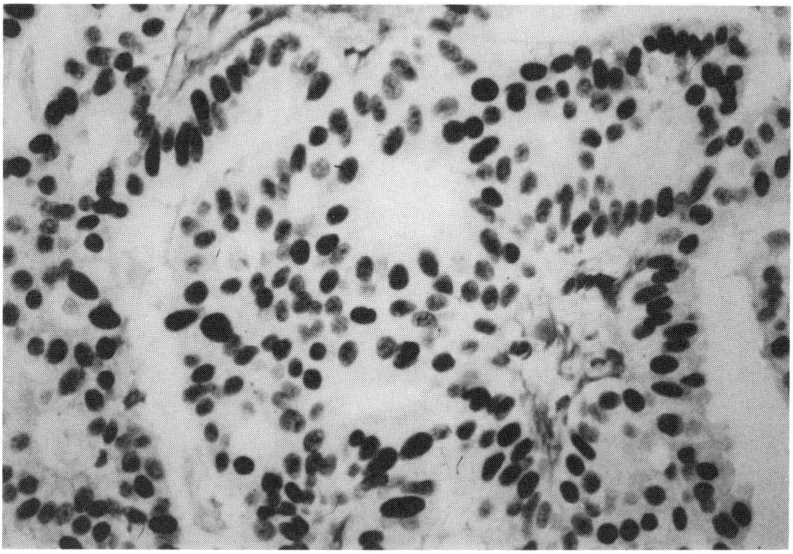

Fig. 5. Photomicrograph of papillary carcinoma of breast, demonstrating strong nuclear staining to the antiestrogen receptor monoclonal antibody (peroxidase–antiperoxidase, original magnification × 250).

Using immunocytochemical assay on formalin-fixed tissue has also permitted the study of hormone-receptor expression in *in situ* carcinoma of the breast (Barnes and Masood, 1990). The results of this study suggest that the dynamics of ER expression previously described in breast carcinoma (Meyer and Lee, 1980) may also apply to breast carcinoma *in situ.* The ER status of invasive carcinoma frequently could be predicted by observing ER status expressed in areas of carcinoma *in situ* (Fig. 6).

Monoclonal antibodies directed against PgR have recently been produced (Logeat et al., 1983; Press and Greene, 1988), permitting Progesterone-Receptor Immunocytochemical Assay (PgR-ICA). Limited data available to date show good concordance between PgR-ICA and DCC (Perrot- Applanot et al., 1987; Pertschuk et al., 1988; Masood et al., 1989a; Isola et al., 1990).

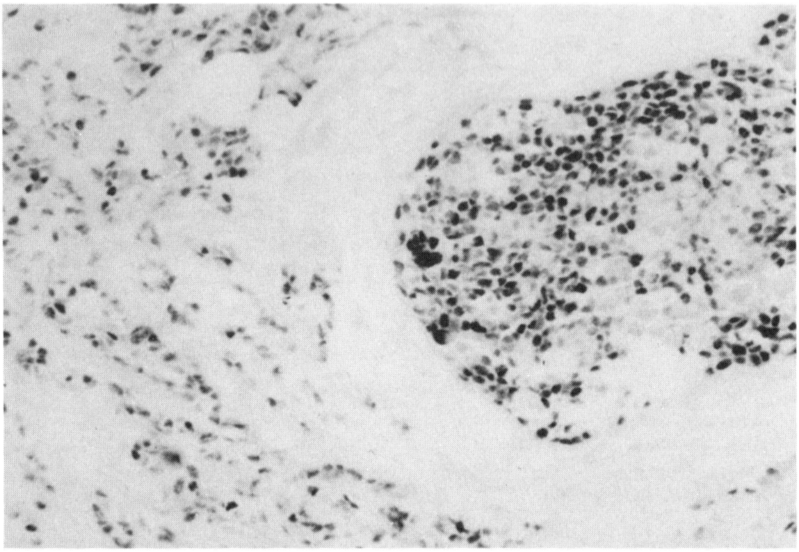

Fig. 6. Coexistence of an infiltrating duct cell carcinoma with an *in situ* component. Note similar ER expression presented by nuclear staining (peroxidase–antiperoxidase, original magnification × 250).

5. Advantages and Limitations of Cytochemical Hormone-Receptor Assays

5.1. Advantages

Compared with the biochemical DCC methods, the cytochemical method is less expensive and does not require expensive equipment. Thus, it is suitable for community hospitals (Masood and Johnson, 1987; Masood, 1988b).

The immunoperoxidase technique is less tedious than biochemical assays, but requires expensive monoclonal antibodies. The expense and time required may be greatly reduced with the use of an automated instrument, the Fisher "Code-On" System, for the assay (Masood et al., 1989c).

Cytochemical hormone-receptor assays are easy to perform and require only small amounts of tissue. This technique has been

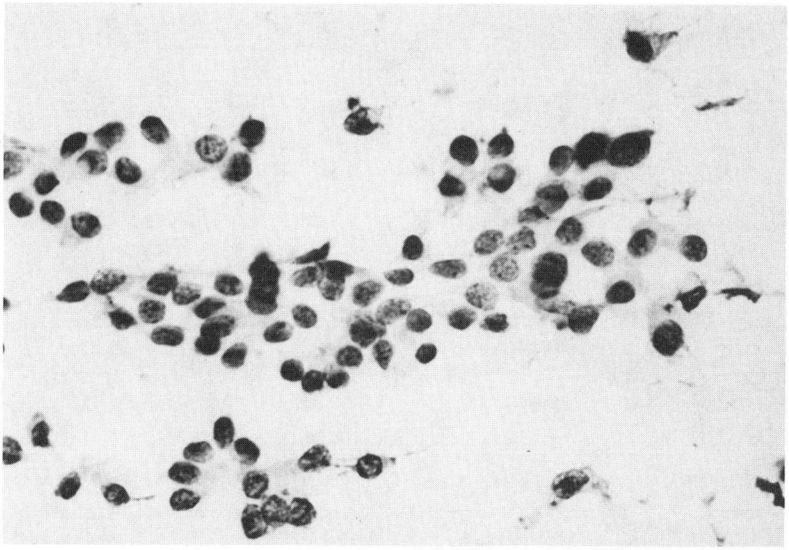

Fig. 7. Fine-needle aspirate of primary breast carcinoma. Malignant cells show loss of cohesion (Diff-Quik stain, original magnification × 250).

successfully utilized for assessment of hormone-receptor content of cytologic material in imprint preparations, fine-needle aspirates, and malignant effusions and frozen and formalin-fixed tissues (Meyer and Lee, 1980; Logeat et al., 1983; Anderson et al., 1986, 1988a,b; Flowers et al., 1986; Lozowski et al., 1987; Masood and Johnson, 1987; Perrot-Applanot et al., 1987; Shintaku and Said, 1987; Masood, 1988b, 1989, 1990a–c, 1991; Barnes and Masood, 1990; Lundy et al., 1990; Masood et al., 1990) (Figs.7, 8).

According to the reports in the literature, correlation between cytochemical and biochemical assays has been generally good. The reported discrepancies are mainly attributable to sampling error, inherent problems in the homogenization procedure in the biochemical assay, few to no tumor cells in the sample, tumor hormone-receptor heterogeneity, and the presence of mixed benign epithelial and stromal components. In situations with positive DCC and nega-

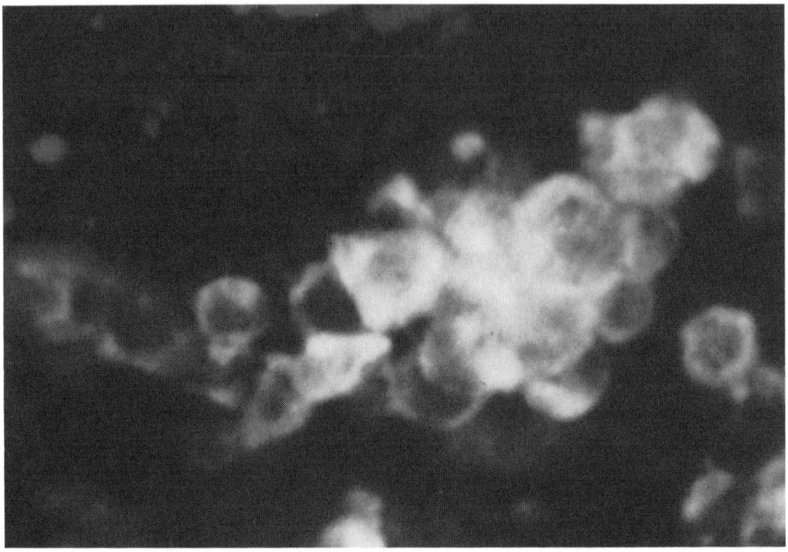

Fig. 8. Fluorescent photomicrograph of ER positive tumor cells obtained from fine needle aspirate of patient with primary breast carcinoma (Fluoro-Cep × 400).

tive immunocytochemical assay, hormone receptor expression may be present in nonmalignant components of the lesion only (Fig. 9).

Heterogeneity of tumor hormone-receptor expression is only possible by visualization of ER and PgR distribution in a tumor via cytochemical assays (Fig. 10). This information may allow identification of patients whose ER-positive tumors may contain subpopulations of hormone-unresponsive cells and ultimately explain some of the variation in the observed response to hormone therapy.

5.2. Limitation

5.2.1. Standardization

Biochemical assays have been used as a traditional assay for assessment of hormone receptors for many years. Standard reagents have been prepared, which has helped to minimize interlaboratory variability. No standardization exists for cytochemical hormone-receptor assays. Many national studies of cancer therapy protocol

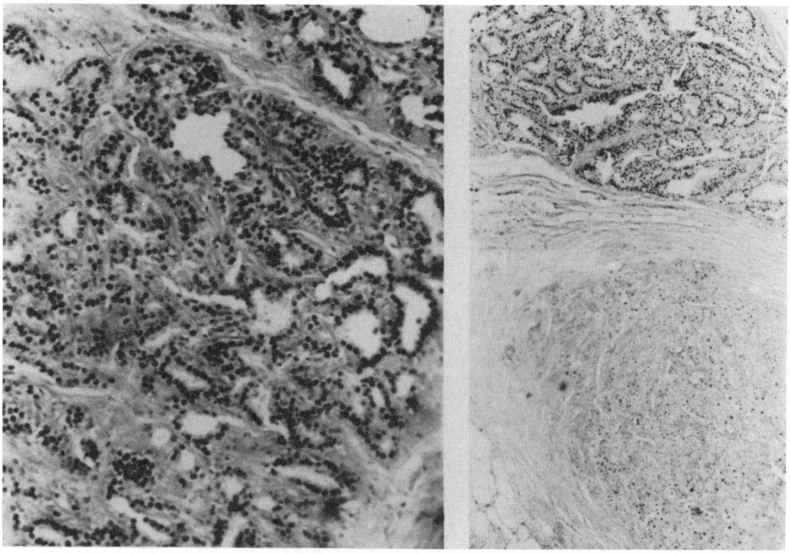

Fig. 9. Photomicrograph of an infiltrating duct-cell carcinoma of breast with adjacent benign epithelial component. Tumor cells are negative for estrogen receptor; the benign cells show strong ER expression (peroxidase–antiperoxidase, original magnification × 250).

still require biochemical assay as the measure of the hormone-receptor expression.

5.2.2. Quantitation

Biochemical assays provide quantitative values expressed as femtomole of ER and/or PgR per milligram of total sample protein. Quantitation is not yet available with cytochemical assays. It has not been shown that quantitative values beyond a defined minimum are useful for selecting treatment options. Thus, it may be adequate to initiate or withhold hormonal therapy based on positive or negative results. However, many investigators feel that quantitation of hormone receptors may have prognostic value (DeSombre and Jensen, 1980; Fujimoto et al., 1984). Visual "semiquantitative" estimates of ER-ICA staining intensity to obtain a weighted mean index for the overall cancer-cell population have correlated to DCC

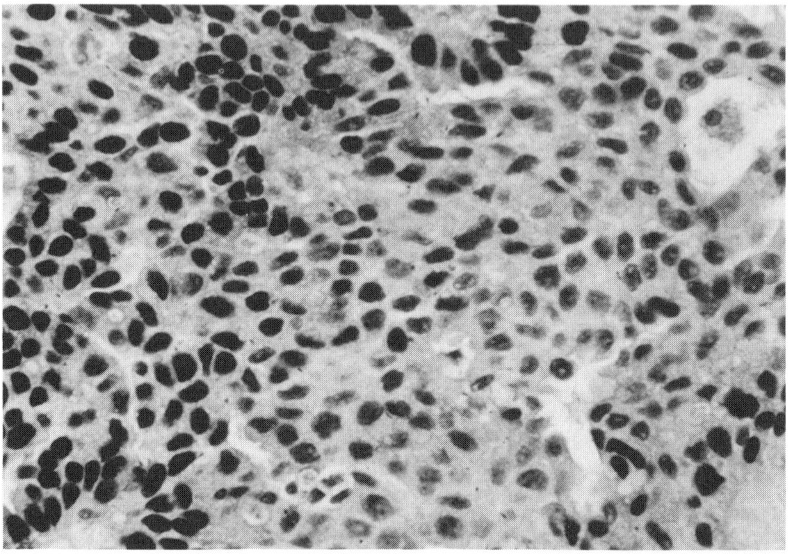

Fig. 10. Tumor hormone-receptor heterogeneity demonstrated by variation in the intensity of nuclear staining of tumor cells in an infiltrating duct-cell carcinoma of breast (peroxidase–antiperoxidase, original magnification × 250).

biochemical assays (Anderson et al., 1986; Masood, 1989; Masood et al., 1990). However, true quantitative methods are needed for distinguishing positive and negative cases and for evaluating tumor hormone-receptor heterogeneity. Standard methodology and analytical criteria have not yet been developed.

The Cell Analysis System (CAS) has been employed to analyze nuclear ER staining intensity. This computer-assisted image analysis may provide an effective means of quantitating immunocytochemical hormone-receptor assays in patients with breast cancer (Bacus et al., 1988). Other investigators also have utilized imaging systems for quantitation of hormone receptors (Charpin et al., 1986; Sklarew and Pertschuk, 1987; Cohen et al., 1988).

Sklarew and Pertschuk in 1987 reported on "receptogram analysis," which is a pattern-oriented approach to evaluating ER status and potential response to antiestrogen therapy. Recently, they

Table 1
Pattern of Hormone Receptor Expression
and the Response to Endocrine Therapy in Patients with Breast Cancer

Pattern of expression	ER^+ PgR^+	ER^+ ER^-	ER^- PgR^-	ER^-PgR^+
Frequency	40%	30%	25%	<5%
Response to endocrine therapy	70–80%	30–60%	5–20%	35–45%

reported superiority of the "receptogram analysis" to DCC assay in predicting response to hormone therapy in 58 stages III and IV breast cancer patients studied (Sklarew et al., 1990). Despite these promising results, further studies are needed to develop and clarify the role of hormone-receptor quantitation by cytochemical assay.

6. Sex Steroid Hormone Receptors in Sex-Organ Malignancies

6.1. Breast

In American women the overall frequency of ER positivity in breast cancer is about 77%; the frequency of PgR positivity is 55% (Thorpe, 1988). The frequency of ER positivity is highest among postmenopausal women, and the frequency of PgR positivity is highest among premenopausal women. This change may be attributable to a compound effect of age and menopausal status (Pedersen, 1983). In an attempt to classify different biological types of breast cancer, cancers designated as hormone-responsive have been those having an intact receptor structure characteristic of normal estrogen-responsive tissue, ER^+ PgR^+. Cancers that are hormonally nonresponsive are often ER^- PgR^- and cancers that are of a more dubious hormone-responsive nature are ER^+, PgR^- and ER^-, PgR^+ (Table 1) (Osborne and McGuire, 1984; Rose, 1986; Chevallier et al., 1988).

Basically, analysis of ER and PgR in breast cancer tissue has enhanced our understanding of the biology of tumor and provided

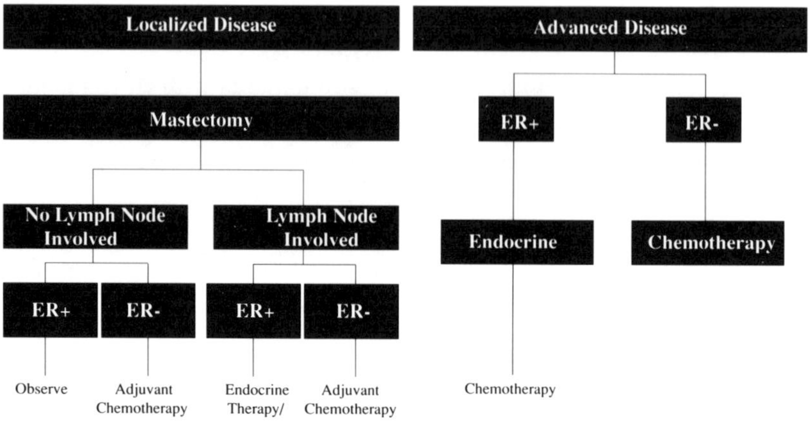

Fig. 11. Choosing the therapeutic approach.

a rationale for optimal treatment of the disease (Fig. 11). Furthermore, determination of hormone receptors is of utmost importance in predicting the outcome for patients with breast cancer. In recognition of this, at a consensus-development meeting held on "Steroid Hormone Receptors and Breast Cancer" at the National Institutes of Health (Bethesda, MD) in June, 1979, it was recommended that receptor analysis be performed on tissue from all primary breast cancer.

In addition to ER and PgR status, tumor size, grade of anaplasia, and lymph-node involvement are major prognostic factors used to classify patients into low- and high-risk groups for recurrent disease. The relationship between hormone-receptor status and the first three variables previously mentioned is well known (Rose, 1986; Mouridsen et al., 1987; Chevallier, 1988). Receptor status is significantly associated with both tumor size and grade of anaplasia. Receptor-positive tumors tend to be smaller and demonstrate a higher degree of differentiation than receptor-negative tumors. No significant relationship between receptor status and lymph-node involvement is noted (Thorpe, 1988).

Nevertheless, despite implementation of these morphologic and biochemically established prognostic factors, approx 30% of patients categorized as being at low risk for recurrent disease experience recurrent disease within five years (Mourisden et al., 1987). Thus other prognostic factors must be found. DNA ploidy study, assessment of proliferative index, and detection of epidermal growth factor have been demonstrated to be of some prognostic significance (Sainsbury et al., 1987; Dressler et al., 1988). In addition, the rapidly expanding field of molecular biology has brought at least two oncogenes into consideration: the *H–ras* (Theillet et al., 1986; Dickson et al., 1987) and *Her–2/neu* oncogenes (Slaman et al., 1987). High concentration of a protease, 52 K cathespin–D, has also been found to be associated with shorter disease-free interval in postmenopausal, primary breast cancer patients (Rochefort et al., 1988).

On the other hand, some arguments have been made that, since other prognostic factors are at least as important as hormone-receptor status in predicting tumor behavior, and since the probable hormone-receptor status can be surmised from histological features (Berger et al., 1987), there might be no need for assessment of ER and PgR after all (Barnes et al., 1989).

6.2. Ovary

Most frequently observed receptors in ovarian tumors are those for androgens (Hamilton et al., 1981; Wurz et al., 1983), glucocorticoids (Galli et al., 1981), estrogens, and progesterones (Pollow et al., 1983b; Teufel et al., 1983; Lautta, 1984; Schwartz et al., 1985). Physiochemical data indicates that the receptor proteins for sex steroid hormone receptors, i.e., ER and PgR in ovarian tumors, are similar to the receptor proteins found in breast and other female reproductive organs. Therefore, the procedure used for measurement of sex steroid hormone receptors in breast and other sites has been applied to the study of hormone receptors in ovarian tumors. This includes the use of ER and PgR immunocytochemical assay, the results of which have shown strong correlation to the biochemical results (Vinko et al., 1983; Press et al., 1985; Masood, 1988a).

It has been known for the past years that many primary ovarian carcinomas and their metastases are rich in sex steroid hormone receptors (Pollow et al., 1983b; Teufel et al., 1983; Lautta, 1984; Schwartz et al., 1985). Since then, the prognostic, diagnostic, and therapeutic implications of hormone receptors in ovarian cancers have been under intense investigation (Schwartz et al., 1982; Kauppila et al., 1983). ER expression continues in patients with advanced disease and even after chemotherapy (Teufel et al., 1983; Richman et al., 1985), whereas PgR is lower if the patient has received chemotherapy (Teufel et al., 1983). Thus it is feasible to assess ER content in tumors from patients with advanced disease who have been treated medically. This provides the basis for possible new therapeutic modalities, such as the use of radiolabeled ER ligands for imaging and the treatment of ER-rich malignant tumors (Holt et al., 1983; Lorincz et al., 1985).

Sex steroid hormone receptor proteins appear to have lower values in premenopausal than in postmenopausal patients with ovarian cancer (Masood, 1988a). Up to now, no strong relationship between the age, size, stage, node status, histopathological differentiation, and the amount of sex steroid hormone receptors in ovarian carcinomas have been found (Creasman et al., 1981; Holt et al., 1981; Schwartz et al., 1982; Press et al., 1985; Masood et al., 1989b; Harding et al., 1990).

The epithelial and sex cord stromal tumors of the ovary reportedly contain ER and PgR. The serous epithelial tumors express sex steroid hormone receptors more frequently than mucinous tumors. Germ cell tumors do not express ER and PgR (Quinn, 1984). In the study of 89 nonpretreated epithelial ovarian cancers conducted by Harding and his associates (1990), 33% were ER^+, PgR^+, and 40% ER^-, PgR^-, 20% were ER^+, PgR^-, and 7% were ER^-, PgR^+ (Table 2).

The prognostic significance of ER and PgR expression in ovarian tumors is not yet well established (Schwartz et al., 1982; Pollow et al., 1983b; Teufel et al., 1983; Vinko et al., 1983; Richman et al., 1985). Iverson et al. (1986) studied the relationship between hormone-receptor expression and patient survival. They concluded that patients with PgR^+ tumors had significantly longer survival times. The expression of ER alone was not found to be a significant prognostic factor. This observation has been confirmed by others (Vinko et al., 1983; Slotman et al., 1989). Meanwhile, some authors agree

Table 2
Pattern and Frequency of Estrogen and Progesterone Receptors in Epithelial Ovarian Cancer

Pattern	Frequency
$ER^+ PgR^+$	33%
$ER^- PgR^-$	40%
$ER^+ PgR^-$	20%
$ER^- PgR^+$	7%

with our conclusion that there are no apparent effects of receptor status on the clinical outcome for patients with ovarian cancer (Holt et al., 1981; Richman et al., 1985; Iversen et al., 1986).

Hormonal therapy in advanced carcinoma has shown mixed results. Gronroas et al. (1984) treated epithelial tumors in vitro with tamoxifen and medroxyprogesterone acetate and concluded that usefulness of sex steroid hormone receptors alone in selecting hormonal therapy is poor in predicting tumor response. Runge et al. (1986) found that in vitro inhibition of ovarian epithelial colonies was significant and dose-dependent with tamoxifen and 4-OH–tamoxifen; however, there was no significant correlation between in vitro responsiveness and level of hormonal receptors. Geisler (1985) treated 34 patients with advanced epithelial ovarian tumors with high-dose megestrol acetate and had seven patients with complete response and four patients with a partial response. He suggested that the greatest benefit of hormonal therapy is the adjuvant effect on primary chemotherapy.

Based on the reported studies, it is apparent that future cooperative studies with large numbers of patients are needed to evaluate definitely the role of sex steroid hormone receptors in follow-up and treatment of patients with ovarian cancer.

At the present time, for ovarian carcinoma, assessment of sex steroid hormone receptors may be of some value in determining the probable primary site of adenocarcinomas of unknown origin, as well as providing a basis for rational development of new strategies in the management of ovarian carcinoma.

6.3. Endometrium

There is increasing evidence in the literature that response to hormonal therapy and prognosis in endometrial cancer are related to the steroid hormone receptor status of these endometrial cancers (Creasman et al., 1980, 1985; Ehrlich et al., 1981; Quinn et al., 1985; Kauppila et al., 1986). Results in patients treated for endometrial carcinoma are also affected by other clinical and histopathologic variables. Several investigators have reported on the association of ER and PgR status with several of these variables (Creasman et al., 1985; Kauppila et al., 1986; Liao et al., 1986). When hormone-receptor status has been correlated to clinical stage of endometrial cancer, no statistically significant trend has been observed with advancing stage (Creasman et al., 1985; Ehrlich et al., 1988). On the other hand, Kauppila (1984) observed a correlation between decreasing ER and PgR with advancing stage. Most studies have demonstrated higher sex steroid hormone receptor levels in well-differentiated tumors than in anaplastic tumors (Bennradd et al., 1980; Ehrlich et al., 1981; Creasman et al., 1985).

Negative association between receptor status, metastasis, and recurrence is reported by Creasman et al. (1985) and Ehrlich et al. (1988). No association among myometrial invasion, positive peritoneal cytology and retroperitoneal lymph node metastasis, and the receptor status of endometrial cancer has been observed (Kauppila et al., 1986; Liao et al., 1986; Ehrlich et al., 1988)

Several investigators have demonstrated a better prognosis for ER^+ and PgR^+ endometrial cancer than for cancers that lack these receptors (Beatson, 1896; Huggins and Bergenstal, 1952; Folca et al., 1961). Ehrlich et al. in 1988 reported a significant relationship only between PgR status and survival.

In the cumulative world literature, the response to progestin for PgR^+ endometrial cancer is 72% (Martin et al., 1979; Bennradd et al., 1980; Creasman et al., 1980), whereas the response rate for PgR^- endometrial cancer is 12% (Kauppila et al., 1982; Pollow et al., 1983a; Quinn et al., 1985; Ehrlich et al., 1988). These data strongly support the role of progesterone receptors in the management of advanced or recurrent endometrial cancer.

Special attention should be given to the methodology used for assaying hormone receptors in endometrial cancers, since endometrial stroma have considerable receptor activity. Biochemical hormone-receptor assays cannot distinguish between tumor tissue and a stromal component, whereas immunocytochemical assays tend to correct this deficiency. With the use of monoclonal immunostaining technique, divergent receptor localization in stroma and myometrium vs neoplastic epithelial components suggests that the biochemical assay of endometrial tumors may not reflect cancer-relevant receptor content (Budwit-Novanty et al., 1986).

6.4. Cervix

Estrogen and progesterone receptors have been detected in normal, premalignant lesions and neoplastic processes of the cervix (Soutter et al., 1981; Spona et al., 1986; Sadan et al., 1989). The number of cervical carcinomas that were positive for ER has varied from 13 to 71% (Martin and Hahnel, 1978; Soutter et al., 1981, 1984; Martin et al., 1982; Ford et al., 1983; Gao et al., 1983; Hunter et al., 1987; Sadan et al., 1989). The variation in the percentage of hormone-receptor-positive tumors is probably attributable to the difference in the methodology and in the criteria used to define the positivity and negativity of a tumor for hormone-receptor proteins.

Immunocytochemical hormone receptor analysis on cervical tissue has shown nuclear staining characteristic of positive hormone-receptor expression in squamous cells, endocervical glands, and stromal cells (Kupryjanczyk and Moller, 1988). No cyclic changes in ER expression in the uterine cervix has been observed. However, the presence of local inflammatory process strongly influences the ER content in cervical mucosa. This may suggest that synthesis of ER in cervical mucosa can be influenced by underlying stroma (Kupryjanczyk and Moller, 1988).

Reports in the literature regarding prognostic significance of hormone receptors in cervical cancer is limited and somewhat controversial. Hunter et al. in 1987 found no correlation between sex steroid hormone receptors and menopausal status, stage, cell type, or histological grade of cervical cancer. A weak correlation between the presence of PgR and length of survival was found, but there was no correlation between ER and survival. The authors concluded that measurement of hormone receptors has limited value in clinical management of cervical carcinoma. Meanwhile, in other studies, it is suggested that receptor status furnishes useful prognostic information (Martin et al., 1982; Gao et al., 1983; Potish et al., 1986). Gao et al. (1983) demonstrated longer survival for premenopausal patients who were PgR-positive. Martin and associates (1982) reported the association of longer survival in patients with positive ER expression in their cervical tumors. Potish et al. (1986) suggested that clinical stage and receptor level independently predict survival in patients with cervical cancer.

Although the independent prognostic value of receptors has been demonstrated, their therapeutic utility remains to be proved. Cervical cancer is generally refractory to hormonal therapy (Verga and Henriksen, 1964; Smith et al., 1967; Malkasian et al., 1977). Thus, the role of receptor-level measurement may be limited to select poor prognostic groups of patients for inclusion into more aggressive chemotherapy.

The question of whether it is safer to prescribe estrogen for contraception or replacement therapy to patients with premalignant and malignant uterine cervices was addressed in 1989 by Sadan et al., who measured the levels of ER and PgR in normal and abnormal uterine cervices. They found that the concentration of PgR was significantly higher in nonaffected cervices than in patients with preinvasive and invasive carcinoma of the cervix; however, the ER concentration did not differ between women with normal and abnormal uterine cervices. Thus, they concluded that estrogen-replacement therapy should be given when indicated to those who have lost their ovaries following surgery and/or radiotherapy for invasive carcinoma of the cervix.

6.5. Prostate

There are some suggestions that hormonal factors may be etiologically important in the development of prostate cancer. This observation is based on the androgen dependence of most prostate cancer, absence of prostate cancer in eunuchs, and induction of prostate cancer in Noble rats by the chronic administration of estrogen and androgen (Moore, 1936; Noble, 1977).

Prostatic cells are dependent on androgen to carry out their normal metabolic function. This occurs after conversion of androgen in the prostate to dihydrotestosterone (DHT) within the prostatic cell (Bruchovsky and Wilson, 1968). The major circulating androgen is testosterone, 90% of which is produced by the testes. Approximately 40% of testosterone is bound to albumin and 57% is bound to sex steroid-binding globulin. The remaining 3% of circulating testosterone remains unbound as the functionally active form of the hormone. Unbound testosterone enters by passive diffusion into the cytoplasm, where it is converted to DHT by the 5-α reductase enzymes. After conversion, DHT binds to an androgen receptor and is carried to the nucleus, where it binds to nuclear chromatin, resulting in initiation of transcription and formation of messenger RNA and subsequent synthesis of proteins that are important for the metabolic functions of the prostatic cells (Walsh, 1975; Ghanadian, 1982).

Testosterone production in the adult male is dependent on an intact hypothalamic pitutary–testicular axis (Walsh and Sirteri, 1975). Androgen withdrawal leads to marked atrophy of the prostatic epithelium. This is the basic rationale for endocrine manipulation of prostatic adenocarcinoma. Removal of androgen effects from prostatic cells may be achieved by removal of circulating androgen by orchiectomy, adrenalectomy, or hypophysectomy; by suppression by leuteinizing hormone, thereby reducing the testosterone secretion from the testis; and by inhibition of androgen effect.

Bilateral orchiectomy reduces circulating testosterone levels from approx 500 ng/100 mL to 50 ng/100 mL (Mackler et al., 1972; Shearer et al., 1973). This reduction in circulating androgen level has been associated with clinical remission in the majority of the patients treated (Walsh and Sirteri, 1975). Adrenalectomy and hypophysectomy have not been uniformly effective as primary treatment or as therapy for relapses after orchiectomy or hormone therapy, and the complications from these procedures should be weighed against the clinical benefit in a given patient (Mertes and Nicol, 1966; Walsh and Sirteri, 1975).

Estrogens suppress pitutary leutinizing-hormone secretion, reduce testosterone steroidogenesis in the testis, and influence the metabolism of prostatic cells (Pierepoint and Griffiths, 1970; Yanihara and Troen, 1972; Menon and Walsh, 1979). The most commonly used estrogen preparation is diethylstibestrol (DES). Daily administration of 1 mg of DES suppresses testosterone levels to the castrate range or near it, with no associated increased risk of cardiovasular complications or deaths (Beck et al., 1978).

Other hormone preparations, such as chloratrianisene, progestins, and gonadotropin-releasing hormone agonists and antagonists, also significantly supress plasma testosterone levels, but their superiority to DES is not well established yet (Beck et al., 1978; Geller et al., 1978; Baba et al., 1982; Corbin, 1982).

Two antiandrogens, cyproterone acetate and flutamide, have been evaluated in clinical studies. Therapeutically, these agents were found to be equally as effective as standard endocrine therapy in untreated patients with prostate cancer. However, no benefit was derived from the use of these antiandrogens in the treatment of estrogen-unresponsive patients (Tvetor et al., 1979; Narayana et al., 1981).

The antiestrogen tamoxifen has also been utilized in both previously untreated and androgen-independent prostate cancer patients. No significant response in either group of patients has been observed (Glick et al., 1980, 1982).

Overall, hormonal manipulation is effective in providing symptomatic relief for the patients with prostatic cancer. Most patients manifest some response to endocrine therapy; however, the response is clinically significant in only about 80% of the cases (Young and Kent, 1968). Orchiectomy and estrogen therapy seem to have equivalent therapeutic value, and there is little to be gained from using both modalities. Orchiectomy ensures the removal of the source of continuing testosterone production, eliminates the concern about patient compliance, and is associated with the least cardiovascular complications (Blachard et al., 1973; Young and Kent, 1968;

Murphy et al., 1983). Significant variability of survival in patients treated with endocrine therapy for prostate cancer is reported (Jordan et al., 1977; Reiner et al., 1979). This has prompted the development of biochemical assays to predict endocrine responsiveness in prostate cancer patients. Generally, in order for steroid hormones to effect target tissues, an intracellular receptor protein must be present. Several investigators have studied the relationship between androgen-receptor content of prostate cancer and response to endocrine therapy (De Voogt and Dingian, 1978; Mortelli et al., 1980; Trachtenberg and Walsh, 1982). These studies have yielded conflicting results. In a study conducted by Trachtenberg and Walsh (1982), no significant correlation between cytosol androgen receptor and patients' survival was noted. However, there was a remarkable relationship between nuclear androgen-receptor content and survival of patients with prostatic cancer.

Studies on ER and PgR in prostate cancer patients is also controversial. Although Young et al. (1979) reported a correlation between response to hormone therapy and ER content, other investigators found no such correlation (Wagner, 1978; Ekman and Snochowski, 1979).

7. Sex Steroid Hormone Receptors in Non-Sex Organ Malignancies

7.1. Central Nervous System

Sex steroid hormone receptors have been detected in various areas of the central nervous system, and the changes in receptor distribution and concentration during ontogeny has led to the hypothesis that brain tumors, at least in some stages of development, might contain hormone receptors and that some brain tumors might be hormonally dependent (McEwen et al., 1975, 1982).

Limited studies on sex steroid hormone receptors in intracranial tumors other than meningiomas have shown mixed results. In contrast to most authors, who have found no detectable amount or very low concentrations of hormone receptors (Markwalder et al.,

1983; Fujimoto et al., 1984), Brentani et al. (1985) and Staykovic and his associates (1990) found progesterone receptor and/or androgen receptors in concentrations between 10 and 20 fmol/mg of cytosalic proteins in some glioblastomas and oligodendrogliomas. These receptors were present in high concentration in a chordoma.

Hormonal dependency of meningioma is implied by a higher incidence of tumors in women than in men and by their accelerated growth during pregnancy (Poisson, 1984). Several investigators have detected PgR in a high percentage of menigioma specimens and have noted PgRs to be more common than ERs in these tumors (Lee, 1984b; Poisson, 1984; Lesch and Gross, 1987). To assess the functional significance of such hormone-receptor positivity in control of meningioma growth, a functional assay, the human tumor-stem-cell clonogenic assay (HTSCCA), was performed in 17 meningioma specimens. The HTSCCA revealed that only two (15%) of 13 specimens were sensitive to estradiol, whereas five (31%) of 16 specimens were sensitive to progesterone. No specimen that was negative for PgR was sensitive to progesterone by HTSCCA. These results suggest that progesterone additions or ablation may be a reasonable therapeutic approach for meningiomas (Grunbert et al., 1987). Androgen-receptor proteins are also found in meningiomas. However, when eight meningiomas were subject to in vitro growth studies in varying concentrations of dihydrotestosterone, no significant in vitro response was observed. It seems that androgens do not appear to play as important a role as progesterone or estrogen in meningioma growth in vitro (Olsen et al., 1988).

7.2. Malignant Melanomas

The better survival rate in women, the adverse effect of pregnancy, and the exacerbation of disseminated disease in menopause provide clinical evidence that malignant melanoma might be a sex-hormone-dependent tumor (Bodenham and Hale, 1972; Sadoff et al., 1973). The signficance of ER in malignant melanoma remains controversial. Many investigators have found some degree of ER expression in malignant melanoma by either biochemical assay or enzyme immunoassays (Ferno et al., 1987; Walker et al., 1987), but others have failed to show ER positivity using immunocytochemical techniques with a monoclonal antibody directed against the human ER protein (H222SPY). Flowers et al. (1987) suggested that the apparent estrogen-binding capacity of human melanoma tissues is the result of interactions other than those with ER. Nevertheless, in a study by Walker and his associates (1987), it was found that disease-free intervals in women with ER^+ lesions were significantly longer than those with ER^- tumors ($p < 0.05$). It was also demonstrated that ER status is a significant variable of survival, along with thickness level and nodal status. These observations suggest that ER may be a marker for a more biologically indolent melanoma. Furthermore, it has been observed that a malignant hamster melanoma cell line, HM–I, binds estrogens specifically and with high affinity, and that hamster melanoma cells positive for this binding protein respond to estrogen (Schleicher et al., 1987).

Nesbit et al. (1979) treated 26 patients with advanced malignant melanoma with tamoxifen and observed an overall response rate of 14%. Masied et al. (1981) also used tamoxifen in five patients with disseminated melanomas, and two patients experienced partial response of nodal and pulmonary lesions. However, Creagan et al. (1982) failed to show any response to tamoxifen therapy in 17 patients with advanced malignant melanoma.

7.3. Larynx and Lung

The presence of ER and PgR in some laryngeal-carcinoma cell lines prompted Urba and his associates (1990) to treat 12 patients with recurrent, advanced laryngeal carcinoma with tamoxifen; however, no clinical response was observed in any of the patients.

Estrogen and progesterone receptors have been detected in only a few cases of pulmonary lymphangioliomyomatosis (Colley et al., 1989). This is a rare disease characterized by conspicuous proliferation of pulmonary smooth-muscle cells around lymphatic and blood vessels and in the interstitium. Young women of child-bearing age are almost exclusively affected. Immunocytochemical hormone-receptor assays have shown strong PgR expression and weak ER expression in abnormal proliferating smooth-muscle cells of lung tissue of patients with this disease. Abnormal proliferation of smooth-muscle cells in pulmonary lymphangiomyomatosis is thought to be influenced by estrogen and progesterone receptors. This seems to be the basis for response to oophorectomy and hormone therapy in a few patients studied (Colley et al., 1989; Schiaffino et al., 1989). To the best of our knowledge, no evidence of hormone-receptor expression in normal lung tissue or neoplastic pulmonary processes has yet been reported. Immunocytochemical studies performed for tissue specificity of specific monoclonal antibodies for ER and PgR in lung tissues have reportedly been negative (Greene and Press, 1987).

7.4. Esophagus

The role of ER in the growth of human esophageal carcinoma is limited to a few studies in vitro. Using tumor tissue of an ER-positive but androgen-receptor-negative line of squamous cell carcinoma (ES–8), Utsumi et al. (1989) suggested that the inhibitory effect of estrogen on tumor line is mediated by ER. Matsuoka and associates (1990) developed an in vitro assay system for predicting the estradiol sensitivity of clinical cancer cells by measuring the effects of estradiol on the net DNA synthesis of primary culture cells. In this study, a case of ER^+ esophageal cancer showed a growth inhibition of primary carcinoma cells by estradiol treatment. These results may indicate tumor response to estradiol by using a rapid sensitivity test in vitro.

7.5. Stomach

Yokozaki and associates in 1988 demonstrated the presence of estrogen receptor in human gastric carcinomas by immunocytochemistry using a specific monoclonal antibody to hormone ER in 30 of 108 cases studied. They found no difference in the frequency of ER expression between female and male patients. Poorly differentiated tumors had higher incidence of ER expression. Patients with ER^+ tumors showed a much worse prognosis than those with ER^- gastric carcinomas.

In another study conducted by Wu et al. in 1990, the level of PgR, ER, and androgen receptors in the superficial part of gastric cancer from 16 patients with gastric adenocarcinoma was determined and compared with that of corresponding normal gastric mucosal tissues. Progesterone receptor was detected in high quantity in 100% of gastric tumors, whereas ER was expressed in only 50% of the cases studied. Androgen-receptor expression was noted only in two of 16 cases. There was no statistical difference between gastric cancers and normal gastric tissue in levels of sex steroid hormone receptors. Wu et al. concluded that gastric mucosa may be the target tissue for progesterone action. In addition, the absence of concordance between the levels of PgR and ER in gastric tumor tissue raises the possibility that the PgR in gastric adenocarcinomas is probably estrogen-independent.

In a randomized, controlled study, Harrison et al. (1989) assessed the therapeutic value of adjuvant tamoxifen therapy in 100 patients with gastric carcinoma. ER expression was demonstrated in 55.8% of the cases studied by the immunocytochemical method. However, tamoxifen therapy had no effect on the survival of patients with gastric carcinoma. Patients with ER^+ tumors had shorter survival times, which may suggest that ER status may be an independent prognostic factor in gastric carcinomas.

7.6. Pancreas and Liver

Sex steroid hormone receptor expression has been seen in hepatocellular carcinoma, normal adult pancreatic tissue, and adenocarcinoma of the pancreas (Corbishley et al., 1986; Erdstein et al., 1989; Nagasue et al., 1989).

7.7. Colon

In a study analyzing 12 primary colonic and 16 primary rectal carcinomas for sex steroid hormone receptors, positive expression of androgen and progesterone was seen. No evidence of ER expression was found (d'Lstria et al., 1986). However, Alford et al. (1979) demonstrated the presence of ER in normal colonic mucosa as well as in 25% of the large-bowel adenocarcinoma. Panettiere and Chen (1982) used tamoxifen in the treatment of 51 patients with advanced colorectal cancers. Only 8% of patients showed partial regression, but overall the survival of patients was similar to patients who did not respond. This probably indicates that tamoxifen is ineffective in management of colorectal cancer.

7.8. Hematopoietic System

Estrogen and progesterone receptors were studied in 23 patients with chronic lymphocytic leukemia. ER and PgR activity was found, respectively, in 52 and 26% of patients. No sigificant correlation was noted between ER/PgR status and other parameters, such as age, sex, stage, androgen and glucocorticoid receptors, and estradiol and progesterone levels. Administration of tomoxifen (30 mg/d for 3 mo) showed no objective response (Zaniboni et al., 1986).

7.9. Kidney

About half of renal-cell carcinomas have been shown to contain ER protein (Concolino et al., 1978). In reviewing the literature, Bloom (1973) reported that 15% of patients treated with progesterone therapy had objective response of their metastasis. However, a preliminary report of a prospective randomized study had shown no benefit with progesterone or testosterone therapy compared to a placebo (Dekernion and Berry, 1980).

7.10. Bone and Soft Tissue

There are factors suggesting that sex steroid hormones may have a favorable influence on the natural history of sarcoma (Cantin and McNeer, 1967; Nosanchuk et al., 1969). Some soft-tissue tumors had shown regression of growth when treated with testosterone or testolactone (Cole and Guiss, 1969; Waddell, 1975). The presence of steroid receptors for androgen, estrogen, and progesterone has been reported in different sarcomas (Ghaudhuri et al., 1980). This warrants further study on the therapeutic implication of hormonal therapy in the treatment of patients with bone and soft-tissue tumor.

References

Alford, J. C., H. M. Do, G. W. Geelhoed, N. T. Tsangaris, and M. E. Lippman (1979), *Cancer* **48,** 980–984.

Allred, D. C., M. A. Bustamante, C. O. Daniel, H. V. Caskill, and A. B. Cruz (1990), *Arch. Surg.* **125,** 107–113.

Anderson, J. N. (1984), in *Hormone Action,* (Goldgerger, R. F. and K. R. Yamamoto, eds.), vol. **3B,** Plenum, New York, pp. 169–212.

Anderson, J., S. M. Bentzen, and H. S. Poulsen (1988a), *Eur. J. Clin. Oncol.* **24,** 377–384.

Anderson, J., T. F. Orntoft, and H. S. Poulsen (1988b), *J. Histochem. Cytochem.* **12,** 1553–1560.

Anderson, J., T. Orntoft, and H. S. Poulsen (1986), *Cancer* **53,** 691–694.

Baba, S., G. Janestscheck, K. Pollow, K. Hahn, and G. H. Jacob (1982), *Br. J. Urol.* **54,** 393–398.

Bacus, S., J. L. Flowers, M. F. Press, and K. S. McCarty, Jr. (1988), *Am. J. Clin. Pathol.* **90,** 233–239.

Barnes, D. M., R. R. Millis, I. A. Fentimen, and R. D. Rubens (1989), *Lancet* **1,** 1126,1127.

Barnes, R. and S. Masood (1990), *Am. J. Clin. Pathol.* **94,** 533–537.

Beatson, G. T. (1896), *Lancet* **2,** 107.

Beck, P. H., J. W. McAninch, J. L. Goebal, and R. E. Stutzman (1978), *Urolology* **11,** 157.

Bennradd, T. J., L. G. Friberg, A. J. M. Koenders, and S. Kullander (1980), *Acta Obstet. Gynecol. Scand.* **59,** 155.

Berger, U., P. Wilson, P. A. McClelland, J. Davidson, and R. C. Coombes (1987), *Hum. Pathol.* **18,** 1263–1267.

Blachard, C. E., D. P. Byar, and W. P. Jordan, Jr. (1973), *Urology* **1,** 533–560.

Bloom, H. J. G. (1973), *Cancer* **32,** 1066–1071.

Bodenham, D. C. and B. Hale (1972), in *Endocrine Therapy in Malignant Disease,* (Stoll B., ed.), W. B Saunders, Philadelphia, pp. 377–383.

Brentani, M. M., M. T. P. Lopes, V. R. Martins, and J. P. P. Plese (1985), *Eur. J. Cancer Clin. Oncol.* **21,** 711–714.

Bruchovsky, N. and J. D. Wilson (1968), *Biol. Chem.* **243,** 2021.

Budwit-Novanty, D. A., K. S. McCarty, E. B. Cox, J. T. Soper, D. G. Mutch, W. J. Creasman, J. L. Flowers, and K. S. McCarty, Jr. (1986), *Cancer Res.* **46,** 5419.

Cantin, J. and G. P. McNeer (1967), *Surg. Gynecol. Obstet.* **125,** 1–5.

Chamness, G. C., W. D. Mercer, and W. L. McGuire (1980), *J. Histochem. Cytochem.* **28,** 792–798.

Charpin, C., M. P. Martin, B. DeVictor, M. N. Lavant, and M. C. Habib (1988), *Cancer Res.* **48,** 1578–1586.

Charpin, C., P. M. Martin, J. Jacquemier, M. N. Lavant, Pourrean, Schneider, N., and M. Toga (1986), *Cancer Res.* **46**(Suppl.), 4271S–4277S.

Chen, P., Z. Mei, X. Yao, and X. Meng (1989), *Cancer* **63,** 139–142.

Chevallier, B., G. Heintzmann, V. Mosseri, J. P. Dauce, P. Bastit, Y. Graic, P. Brunelle, J. P. Basuyan, M. Comoz, and B. Asselain (1988), *Cancer* **62,** 2517–2524.

Clark, G. M., W. L. McGuire, C. A. Hubray, O. H. Pearson, and J. S. Marshall (1983), *N. Engl. J. Med.* **309,** 1343–1347.

Clark, J. H., E. J. Peck, W. T. Schrader, and B. W. O'Malley (1976), *Methods Cancer Res.* **12,** 367–417.

Clark, J. H., J. W. Hardin, S. Upchurch, and H. Eriksson (1978), *J. Biol. Chem.* **253,** 7630–7634.

Cohen, O., G. Brugan, D. Seigneurin, and J. Demongeot (1988), *Cytometry* **9,** 579–587.

Cole, N. M. and L. W. Guiss (1969), *Arch. Surg.* **98,** 530–533.

Colley, M. H., E. Geppert, and W. A. Franklin (1989), *Am. J. Surg. Pathol.* **13**(9), 803–807.

Concolino, G., A. Marrachi, C. Conti, R. Tenaglia, F. Di Silveria, and U. Brace (1978), *Cancer Res.* **38,** 4340–4344.

Corbin, A. (1982), *Yale J. Biol. Med.* **55,** 27.

Corbishley, T. P., M. J. Logbal, M. L. Wilkinson, and R. Williams (1986), *Cancer* **57**(10), 1992–1995.

Creagan, E. T., J. N. Ingle, D. L. Ahmann, and S. J. Green (1982), *Cancer* **49,** 1353,1354.

Creasman, W. T., K. S. McCarty, Sr., T. F. Barton, and K. S. McCarty, Jr. (1980), *Obstet. Gynecol.* **55,** 363.

Creasman, W. T., R. A. Sasso, J. C. Weed, and K. S. McCarty, Jr. (1981), *Gynecol. Oncol.* **12,** 319–327.

Creasman, W. T., J. T. Soper, K. S. McCarty, Jr., K. S. McCarty, W. Hinshaw, and D. L. Clarke-Pearson (1985), *Am. J. Obstet. Gynecol.* **151,** 922.

Dekernion, J. B. and D. Berry (1980), *Cancer* **45,** 1947–1956.

DeSombre, E. R. and E. V. Jensen (1980), Cancer **46,** 2783–2788.

De Voogt, H. J. and P. Dingian (1978), *Urol. Res.* **6,** 151.

Dickson, R. B., A. Kasid, K. K. Huff, S. E. Bates, C. Knabbe, D. Bronzert, E. P. Gelmann, and M. E. Lippman (1987), *Proc. Natl. Acad. Sci. USA* **84,** 837–841.

d'Lstria, M, S. Fasano, F. Catuagro, F. Gaeta, L. Bucci, G. Benassai, F. Mazzeo, and G. Delrio (1986), *Dis. Colon Rectum* **29**(4), 263–265.

Dressler, L. G., L. C. Seamer, M. A. Owens, G. M. Clark, and W. L. McGuire (1988), *Cancer* **61,** 420–427.

Ehrlich, C. E., P. C. Young, and R. E. Cleary (1981), *Am. J. Obstet. Gynecol.* **141,** 539.

Ehrlich, C. E., P. C. M. Young, F. B. Stehman, G. P. Sutton, and W. M. Alford (1988), *Am. J. Obstet. Gynecol.* **158,** 796.
Ekman, P. and M. Snochowski (1979), *Eur. J. Cancer* **15,** 257.
Engelsman, E., J. P. Persiin, C. B. Korsten, and F. J. Cleton (1973), *Br. Med. J.* **2,** 750–752.
Erdstein, J., S. Wisebord, S. Y. Mishkin, and S. Mishkin (1989), *Hepatology* **9**(4), 621–624.
Ferno, M., A. Borg, C. Inguar, and P. E. Jonsson (1987), *Anticancer Res.* **7**(4B), 741–743.
Flowers, J. L., G. V. Burton, E. B. Cox, K. S. McCarty, Jr., G. A. Dent, K. R. Geisinger, and K. S. McCarty, Jr. (1986), *Ann. Surg.* **203,** 250–254.
Flowers, J. L., H. F. Seigler, K. S. McCarty, Sr., J. Konrath, and K. S. McCarty, Jr. (1987), *Arch. Dimatol.* **123**(6), 764,765.
Folca, P.J., R. F. Glascock, and W. T. Irving (1961), *Lancet* **ii,** 796.
Ford, L. C., J. S. Berek, L. O. Lagasse, N. F. Hacker, Y. L. Heins, and R. J. Delange (1983), *Gynecol. Oncol.* **15,** 27–31.
Fujimoto, M., E. Yoshino, K. Hirakawa, J. Fujimoto, and T. Tamaya (1984), *Clin. Neuropharmacol.* **7,** 357–362.
Galli, M. C., C. DeGiovanni, G. Nicoletti, S. Grilli, P. Nanni, G. Prodi, G. Gola, R. Rocchetta, and C. Orlandi (1981), *Cancer* **47,** 1297–1302.
Gao, Y. L., L. B. Twiggs, B. S. Leung, W. C. Y. Yu, R. A. Potish, T. Okagaki, L. L. Adcock, and K. A. Prem (1983), *Am. J. Obstet. Gynecol.* **140,** 299–306.
Gardner, D. G. and J. L. Wittliff (1973), *Biochemistry* **12,** 3090–3096.
Geisler, H. E. (1985), *Semin. Oncol.* **12** (1 Suppl.), 20–22.
Geller, J., J. Albert, and S. S. C. Yen (1978), *Urology* **12,** 537.
Ghanadian, R. (1982), in *Recent Advances in Urologic Cancer,* (Javadpour, N., ed.), Williams and Wilkins, Baltimore, p. 68.
Ghaudhuri, P. K., M. J. Walker, C. W. Beattie, and T. K. Das Gupta (1980), *Cancer Res.* **40,** 861–865.
Ghosh, L., B. C. Chosh, and T. K. Das Gupta (1978), *J. Surg. Oncol.* **10,** 221.
Glick, J. H., A. Wein, K. Padavic, W. Negendank, D. Harris, and H. Brodovsky (1980), *Cancer Treat. Rep.* **64,** 813.
Glick, J. H., A. Wein, K. Padavic, W. Negendank, D. Harris, and H. Brodevsky (1982), *Cancer* **49,** 1367.
Gorski, J., D. Toft, G. Shyamala, D. Smith, and A. Notides (1968), *Recent Prog. Horm. Res.* **24,** 45–80.
Greene, G. L. and E. V. Jensen (1982), *J. Steroid Biochem.* **16,** 353–359.
Greene, G. L. and M. F. Press (1987), in *Immunological Approaches to the Diagnosis and Therapy of Breast Cancer,* Plenum, New York, pp. 119–135.
Greene, G. L., L. E. Class, H. Fleming, E. R. DeSombre, and E. V. Jensen (1980), *Proc. Natl. Acad. Sci. USA* **77,** 5115–5119.

Greene, G. L., N. B. Sobel, and W. J. King, and E. V. Jensen (1984), *J. Steroid Biochem.* **20,** 51–56.
Gronroas, S. M., L. Kangas, D. Maenpa, R. Vanhavanta, A. Nieminen, and R. Johansson (1984), *Br. J. Obstet. Gynecol.* **91,** 427–478.
Grunbert, S. M., A. M. Daniels, H. Muensch, J. R. Daniels, L. Bernstein, V. Kortes, and M. H. Weiss (1987), *J. Neurosurg.* **66**(3), 405–408.
Hamilton, T. C., P. Davies, and K. Griffiths (1981), *J. Endocrinol.* **90,** 421–431.
Harding, M., S. Cowan, D. Hole, L. Cassidy, H. Kitchener, J. Davis, and R. Leake (1990), *Cancer* **1:65**(3), 486–491.
Harrison, J. D., D. L. Morris, I. O. Ellis, T. A. Jones, and I. Jackson (1989), *Cancer* **1:64**(5), 1007–1010.
Harwitz, K. B., W. L. McGuire, O. H. Pearson, and A. Segaloff (1975), *Science* **189,** 726, 727.
Henson, J. C., E. Longeval, W. H. Mattheiem, M. C. Deboel, R. J. Sylvester, and G. Leclercq (1977), *Cancer* **39,** 1971–1977.
Hill, S. M., S. Fuqua, G. C. Chamness, G. L. Greene, and W. L. McGuire (1989), *Cancer Res.* **49,** 145–148.
Holt, J. A., M. A. Lorincz, and V. D. Hospelhorn (1983), *J. Steroid Biochem.* **18,** 41–50.
Holt, J. A., C. R. Lyttle, M. A. Lorincz, S. D. Stern, M. F. Press, and A. L. Herbst (1981), *J. Natl. Cancer Inst.* **67,** 307–318.
Huggins, C. and C. V. Hodges (1941), *Cancer Res.* **1,** 293.
Huggins, C. and D. M. Bergenstal (1952), *Cancer Res.* **12,** 134–141.
Hunter, R. E., C. Longcope, and P. Keough (1987), *Cancer* **60,** 392–396.
Isola, J. J., M. J. Helle, and H. J. Helin (1990), *Am. J. Clin. Pathol.* **93,** 370–382.
Iversen, O. E., E. Skaarand, and E. Otaaker (1986), *Gynecol. Oncol.* **23,** 65–76.
Jacobs, S. R., W. L. Wolfson, L. Cheng, and K. J. Lewin (1983), *Cancer* **51,** 1621–1624.
Janssens, J. P., K. Pylser, J. Bekaert, J. Roelens, J. Stuyck, L. J. Dekeyser, J. M. Lauweryns, and W. DeLoekey (1985), *Cancer* **55,** 2600–2611.
Jensen, E.V. (1970), in (Griffiths, K. and E. G. Pierrepoint, eds.), Alpha Omega Alpha, Cardiff, p. 151.
Jensen, E. V., J. Greene, and E. R. DeSombre (1986), *Lab. Manage.* 25–42.
Jensen, E. V. (1968), *Proc. Natl. Acad. Sci. USA* **59,** 632–639.
Jordan, W. P., Jr., C. E. Blachard, and D. P. Byar (1977), *South. Med. J.* **70,** 1411.
Kasid, A. and M. E. Lippman (1987), *J. Steroid Biochem.* **27,** 465–470.
Kauppila, A. (1984), *Acta Obstet. Gynecol. Scand.* **63,** 441.
Kauppila, A., E. Kuyansuu, and R. Vihke (1982), *Cancer* **50,** 2157.
Kauppila, A., P. Vierikke, S. Kivinen, F. Stenback, and R. Vihko (1983), *Obstet. Gynecol.* **61,** 320–326.

Kauppila, A. J. I., H. E. Istolo, S. T. Kivinen, and R. K. Vitiko (1986), *Obstet. Gynecol.* **67,** 463.
King, W. J. and G. C. Greene (1984), *Nature* **307,** 747–754.
King, W. J., E. R. DeSombre, E. V. Jensen, and G. L. Greene (1985), *Cancer Res.* **37,** 4669–4671.
Kupryjanczyk, J. and P. Moller (1988), *Int. J. Gynecol. Pathol.* **7,** 75–85.
Kurzon, R. M. and L. A. Sternberger (1978), *J. Histochem. Cytochem.* **26,** 803.
Lautta, M. (1984), *Acta Obstet. Gynecol. Scand.* **63,** 497–503.
Lee, S. H. (1978), *Am. J. Clin. Pathol.* **70,** 197–203.
Lee, S. H. (1989), *Cancer* **64,** 1461–1466.
Lee, S. H. (1984), *J. Histochem. Cytochem.* **32,** 305–310.
Lee,Y. T. (1984), *J. Surg. Oncol.* **25**(4), 255–262.
Lesch, K. P. and S. Gross (1987), *J. Neurosurg.* **67**(2), 237–243.
Leung, B. S., W. S. Fletcher, T. D. Lindell, D. C. Wood, and W. W. Krippaechne (1973), *Arch. Surg.* **106,** 515–519.
Liao, B. S., L. B. Twiggs, B. S. Leung, W. C. Y. Yu, R. A. Potish, and K. A. Prem (1986), *Obstet. Gynecol.* **67,** 463.
Logeat, F., M. Vu Hai, A. Fournier, P. Legroin, and G. Buttin (1983), *Proc. Natl. Acad. Sci. USA* **90,** 6456–6459.
Lorincz, M. A., J. A. Holt, and G. L. Greene (1985), *J. Clin. Endocrinol. Metab.* **61,** 412–417.
Lozowski, M. S., Y. Mishriki, S. Chao, R. Grimson, P. Pai, M. A. Harris, and J. Lundy (1987), *Acta Cytol.* **31,** 557–562.
Luft, R., H. Olivecrona, and J. D. Ikkos (1958), in *Endocrine Aspects of Breast Cancer* (Currie, A. and R. Alastair, eds.), Livingstone of Glasgow, Edinburgh, pp. 77–35.
Lundy, J., M. Lozowski, D. Sadri, and Y. Mishriki (1990), *Arch. Surg.* **125,** 174–176.
Mackler, M. A., J. P. Liberti, M. J. V. Smith, W. W. Koontz, Jr., and G. R. Prout, Jr. (1972), *Invest. Urol.* **9,** 423.
Malkasian, G. D., D. G. Decker, and E. O. Jorgensen (1977), *Gynecol. Oncol.* **5,** 109–120.
Markwalder, T. M., D. T. Zava, and R. V. Markwalder (1983), (letter) *Surg. Neurol.* **20,** 163.
Martelli, A., M. Soli, E. Bercovich, G. Prodi, S. Grilli, C. DeGiovanni, and M. C. Gali (1980), *Urology* **16,** 245.
Martin, D. J. and R. Hahnel (1978), *Aust. NZ J. Obstet. Gynecol.* **18,** 55–59.
Martin, D. M., P. H. Rolland, M. Gammerre, H. Serment, and M. Toga (1979), *Int. J. Cancer* **23,** 321.
Martin, J. D., R. Hahnel, A. J. McCartney, and T.Woodings (1982), *N. Engl. J. Med.* **306,** 485.
Martin, P. M. and P. J. Sheridan (1982), *J. Steroid Biochem.* **16,** 215.

Masied, A., P. Bultrich, and J. Bittran (1981), *Cancer Treat. Rep.* **65,** 531,532.
Masood, S. (1988a), *Cancer Detect. Prev.* **12,** 283, 290.
Masood, S. (1988b), *Diagn. Cytopathol.* **4,** 42–47.
Masood, S. (1989), *Arch. Pathol. Lab. Med.* **113,** 26–30.
Masood, S. (1990a), *Acta Cytol.* **34,** 735 (abstract).
Masood, S. (1990b), *Acta Cytol.* **34,** 736 (abstract).
Masood, S. (1990c), *Am. J. Clin. Pathol.* **93(3),** 437 (Abstract).
Masood, S. (1991), *Am. J. Clin. Pathol.* **95,** 35–40.
Masood, S. and H. Johnson (1987), *Am. J. Clin. Pathol.* **87,** 30–36.
Masood, S., S. Dee, and J. D. Goldstein (1989a), *Am. J. Clin. Pathol.* **92,** 528.
Masood, S., J. Hertmann, R. C. Nuss, and G. J. Benrubi (1989b), *Gynecol. Oncol.* **34,** 57–60.
Masood, S., V. Lerch, and N. Rodenroth (1989c), *J. Histotechnol.* **12,** 265–269.
Masood, S., L. Lu, and N. Rodenroth (1990), *Mod. Pathol.* **3.6:** 724–728.
Mass, H., B. Engle, H. Hohmeister, F. Lehmann, and G. Trams (1972), *Am. J. Obstet. Gynecol.* **113,** 377–382.
Matsuoka, H., H. Ueo, K. Yano, Y. Kindo, K. Shivabe, T. Mitsudomi, and K. Sugimachi (1990), *Cancer Res.* **1:50**(7), 2113–2118.
McClelland, R. A., U. Berger, L. S. Miller, T. J. Powels, and R. C. Coombes (1986), *J. Clin. Oncol.* **4,** 1171–1176.
McEwen, B. S., A. Biegon, P. G. Davis, L. C. Krey, V. N. Luine, M. Y. McGinnis, C. M. Paden, B. Parsons, and T. C. Rainbow (1982), *Recent Prog. Horm. Res.* **38,** 41–92.
McEwen, B. S., C. J. Denef, J. L. Gerlach, and L. Plapinger (1975), *Steroid Hormones: Humoral Signals Which Alter Brain Cell Properties and Function,* MIT Press, Cambridge, MA, pp. 599–620.
McGuire, W. L., K. B. Horwitz, A. H. Pearson, and Segaloff, A. (1977), *Cancer* **39,** 2936–2974.
McGuire, W. L., P. P. Carbone, and E. P. Vollmer, eds. (1975), *Estrogen Receptors in Human Breast Cancer* Raven, New York, pp. 1–85.
Menon, M. and P. C. Walsh (1979), in *Prostate Cancer* (Murphy, B. P., ed.), PSG, Littleton, MA, pp. 175–200.
Mercer, W. D., M. E. Lippmen, T. M. Wahl, C. A. Carlson, D. A. Wahl, D. Lezette, and P. O. Teague (1980), *Cancer* **46,** 2859–2868.
Mertes, J. and C. S. Nicol (1966), *Annu. Rev. Physiol.* **28,** 57.
Meyer, J. S. and J. Y. Lee (1980), *Cancer Res.* **40,** 1890–1896.
Meyer, M. E., H. Gronemeyer, G. Turcotte, M. P. Bocqual, D. Tasset, and P. Chambon (1989), *Cell* **57,** 433–442.
Misrahi, M., M. Atger, L. d'Auriol, H. Loosfelt, C. Meriel, F. Fridlansky, A. Guiochon-Mantel, F. Galibert, and E. Milgrom (1987), *Biochem. Biophys. Res. Commun.* **143,** 740.
Moore, R. A. (1936), *Am. J. Pathol.* **12,** 599.

Mouridsen, H. T., J. Bayer, and N. Keiding (1987), *Cancer Res.* **47,** 6126–6133.

Murphy, G. P., S. Beckley, M. F. Brady, T. Ming Chu, J. B. deKernion, C. Dhabuwala, J. F. Gaeta, R. P. Gibbons, S. A. Loening, C. F. McKiel, D. G. McLeod, J. Edson Pontes, G. R. Pront, P. T. Scardino, J. U. Schlegel, J. D. Schmidt, W. W. Scott, N. HY. Slack, and M. S. Soloway (1983), *Cancer* **51,** 1264.

Nagasue, N., H. Kohno, Y. C. Chang, T. Hayashi, T. Nakamura, and H. Yukaya (1989), *Cancer* **63**(1), 1112–1116.

Narayana, A. S., S. A. Loening, and D. A. Culp (1981), *Br. J. Urol.* **53,** 152.

Nenci, I. (1978), *Cancer Res.* **38,** 4204.

Nenci, I., M. D. Becati, A. Diffanelli, and G. Lanza (1976), *J. Steroid Biochem.* **7,** 505.

Nesbit, R. A., R. L. Woods, M. H. M. Tattersall, R. M. Fox, J. F. Forbes, I. R. Mackay, and M. Goodyear (1979), *N. Engl. J. Med.* **301,** 1241, 1242.

Noble, R. L. (1977), *Cancer Res.* **37,** 1929.

Noleboom, W. D. and J. Gorski (1965), *Arch. Biochem. Biophys.* **11,** 559–568.

Nosanchuk, J. S., L. Weatherbee, and G. L. Brody (1969), *JAMA* **208,** 2439–2441.

Olsen, J. J., D. W. Bech, J. W. Maclendre, and P. Min-Loh (1988), *Cancer* **61**(5), 952–955.

Osborne, C. K. and W. L. McGuire (1984), *J. Clin. Oncol.* **2,** 1102–1109.

Oxley, D. K., G. T. Haven, J. L. Wittliff, and D. Gilbo (1982), *Arch. Surg.* **78,** 587–596.

Panettiere, F. J. and J. T. Chen (1982), *Asco Abst.* 94.

Pedersen, B. V. (1983), *Breast Cancer Res. Treat.* **3,** 103–110.

Perrot-Applanot, M., M. J. Groyer-Picard, P. F. Lorenzo, A. Jolivet, M. T. V. Hai, C. Pallud, F. Spyratos, and E. Milgrom (1987), *Cancer Res.* **47,** 2652–2661.

Pertschuk, L. P. (1976), *Res. Commun. Chrom. Pathol. Pharmacol.* **14,** 771.

Pertschuk, L. P., E. H. Tobin, D. J. Brigati, D. S. Kim, N. D. Bloom, E. Gaetjens, P. J. Berman, A. C. Carter, and G. A. Degenshein (1978), *Cancer* **41,** 907.

Pertschuk, L. P., E. H. Tobin, E. Gaetjens, A. C. Carter, G. A. Degenshein, N. D. Bloom, and D. J. Brigati (1980), *Cancer* **46,** 2896–2901.

Pertschuk, L. P., J. G. Feldman, K. B. Eisenberg, A. C. Carter, W. L. Thelmo, W. P. Cruz, S. M. Thorpe, I. J. Christensen, B. B. Rasmussen, and C. Rose (1988), *Cancer* **62,** 342–347.

Pertschuk, L. P., R. N. Eisenberg, and A. C. Carter (1987), *Lab. Invest.* **56,** 59A.

Pierepoint, C. G. and K. Griffiths (1970), *Steroids* **15,** 89.

Poisson, M. (1984), *Clin. Neuropharmacol.* **7,** 320–324.

Pollow, K., B. Manz, and J. H. Grill (1983a), in *Steroids and Endometrial Cancer* (Jasonni, V. M., ed.), Raven, New York, pp. 33–60.

Pollow, K., A. Schmidt-Matthiesen, and G. Hoffmann, et al. (1983b), *Int. J. Cancer* **31,** 603–608.

Potish, R. A., L. B. Twiggs, L. L. Adcock, K. A. Prem, J. E. Savage, and B. S. Leung (1986), *Cancer* **58,** 1709–1713.

Press, M. F., J. A. Holt, A. L. Heibst, and G. L. Greene (1985), *Lab. Invest.* **53,** 349–361.

Press, M. J. and G. L. Greene (1988) *Endocrinology* **122,** 1165–1175.

Quinn, M. A., M. Cauchi, and D. Fortune (1985), *Gynecol. Oncol.* **21,** 314.

Quinn, M. D. (1984), *Aust N. Z. J. Obstet. Gynecol.* **24,** 153–187.

Raam, S., N. Robert, C. A. Pappas, and H. Tamura (1988), *J. Natl. Cancer Inst.* **80,** 756–761.

Raam, S. R., R. Gelman, J. L. Cohner, A. Bacharach, A. J. Fishchinger, H. I. Jacobson, A. A. Keshgegian, S. J. Konopka, and J. L. Wittliff (1981), *Eur. J. Cancer* **17,** 643–649.

Reiner, W. G., W. W. Scott, J. C. Eggleston, and P. C. Welsh (1979), *J. Urol.* **122,** 183.

Richman, G. M., J. A. Holt, M. A. Lorincz, and A. L. Heibst (1985), *Obstet. Gynecol.* **65,** 257–263.

Rochefort, H., F. Capony, M. Garcia, and F. Vignon (1986), *Ann. NY Acad. Sci.* **464,** 190–201.

Rose, C. (1986), *Cancer Surv.* **5,** 505–525.

Runge, H. M., G. Teufel, J. Neulen, H. Geyer, and A. Pfleiderer (1986), *Cancer Chemother. Pharmacol.* **16,** 58–63.

Sadan, O., R. P. Frohlic, J. A. Driscoll, A. Apostoleris, N. Savaga, and H. Zakut (1989), *Gynecol. Oncol.* **34**(2) 159–163.

Sadoff, L., J. Winkley, and S. Tyson (1973), *Oncology* **27,** 244–257.

Sainsbury, J. R. C., J. R. Farndon, G. K. Needham, A. J. Malcolm, and A. L. Harris (1987), *Lancet* **I,** 1398–1402.

Savlov, E. D., J. L. Wittliff, R. Hilif, and T. C. Hall (1974), *Cancer* **33,** 303–339.

Schiaffino, E., E. Tavani, L. Dellafiore, and C. Schmid (1989), *Appl. Pathol.* **7**(4), 265–272.

Schleicher, R. L., M. H. Hitselberger, and C. W. Beattie (1987), *Cancer Res.* **47**(2), 453–459.

Schwartz, E. P., M. J. Merine, V. A. Livols, P. E. Schwartz, R. Lawrence, N. MacLusky, and A. Eisenfeld (1985), *Obstet. Gynecol.* **66,** 428–433.

Schwartz, P. E., V. A. Livols, N. Hildreth, N. J. MacLusky, F. N. Naftolin, and A. J. Eisenfeld (1982), *Obstet. Gynecol.* **59,** 229–238.

Shearer, R. J., W. F. Hendry, I. F. Sommerville, and J. D. Ferguson (1973), *Br. J. Urol.* **5,** 667.

Shintaku, P. and J. W. Said (1987), *Am. J. Clin. Pathol.* **87,** 161–167.
Sklarew, R. J. and L. P. Pertschuk (1987), *J. Histochem. Cytochem.* **25,** 1253–1259.
Sklarew, R. J., S. C. Bodmer, and L. P. Pertschuk (1990), *Cytometry* **11,** 359–378.
Slaman, D. J., G. M. Clark, S. T. Wong, W. J. Levin, A. Ullrich, and W. L. McGuire (1987), *Science* **235,** 177–182.
Slotman, B. J., R. Kuhnel, B. R. Rae, G. H. Dijkhuizen, J. de Graaff, and J. G. Stolk (1989), *Gynecol. Oncol.* **33**(1), 76–81.
Smith, J. P., F. Rutledge, B. C. Burns, Jr., and S. Soffar (1967), *Am J. Obstet. Gynecol.* **97,** 800–807.
Soutter, W. P., R. J. Pegararo, D. V. Green-Thompson, D. V. Naidoo, S. M. Joubert, and R. N. Philpott (1984), in *Cancer of the Uterine Cervix: Biochemical and Clinical Aspects* (McBrien, D. C. H. and T. F. Slater, eds.), Academic, London, vol. 1, p. 344.
Soutter, W. P., E. J. Pegoraro, D. V. Green-Thompson, D. V. Naidoo, S. M. Joubert, and R. H. Philpott (1981), *Br. J. Cancer* **44,** 154–159.
Spona, J., E. E. Gitsch, H. Kubista, H. Salzer, and B. Kohler (1986), *Cancer Res.* (Suppl.) **46,** 4310s–4312s.
Stoykovic, R. R., M. Jovancevic, D. J. Santel, N. Greevic, and S. Gamulin (1990), *Cancer* **65,** 1968–1970.
Straus, M. J., R. Moran, R. E. Mullor, and H. H. Wotiz (1982), *Oncology* **39,** 197–200.
Teufel, G., H., Geyer, G. deGregario, A. Fuchs, W. Kleine, and A. Pfleiderer (1983), *Geburtshilfe Frauenheilkd* **43,** 732–740.
Theillet, C., R. Lindereau, C. Escot, P. Hutzell, M. Brunet, J. Gest, J. Schlom, and R. Callahan (1986), *Cancer Res.* **46,** 4776–4781.
Thorpe, S. M. (1988), *Acta Oncologica* **27,** 1–19.
Trachtenberg, J. and P. C. Walsh (1982), *J. Urol.* **127,** 466.
Tvetor, K. J., A. Attramadol, R. Hannestad, and B. Otner (1979), *Scand. J. Urol. Nephrol.* **13,** 237.
Urba, S. G., T. E. Carey, V. Kudla-Hatch, G. T. Wolf, and A. A. Forastiere (1990), *Laryngoscope* **100**(1), 76–78.
Utsumi,Y., T. Nakamura, N. Nagasue, H. Kubota, and S. Morikawa (1989), *Cancer* **1:64**(1), 88–93.
Verga, A. and E. Henriksen (1964), *Obstet. Gynecol.* **23,** 51–62.
Vinko, R., H. Isotalo, A. Kauppila, and P. Vierikko (1983), *J. Steroid Biochem.* **19,** 827–832.
Waddell, W. R. (1975), *Ann. Surg.* **181,** 299–302.
Wagner, R. K. (1978), *Acta Endocrinol.* **88**(Suppl.) 3.
Walker, M. J, C. W. Beattie, M. K. Patel, S. M. Ronan, and T. K. Das Gupta (1987), *J. Clin. Oncol.* **5**(8), 1256–1261.

Walker, R. A., D. H. Cove, and A. Howell (1980), *Lancet* **1,** 171.

Walsh, P. C. (1975), *Urol. Clin. North Am.* **2,** 125.

Walsh, P. C. and P. K. Sirteri (1975), *J. Urol.* **114,** 254–256.

Walter, P., S. Green, G. Greene, A. Krust, J. M. Borrert, J. M. Jeltsch, A. Staub, E. Jensen, G. Scrag, and M. Waterfield (1985), *Proc. Natl. Acad. Sci. USA* **82,** 7889–7893.

Welshons, W. V., M. D. Liberman, and J. Grosk (1984) *Nature* **307,** 747–749.

Wiehle, R. D. and J. L. Wittliff (1983), *Fed. Proc.* **42,** 1877.

Wittliff, J. L. (1975), *Methods Cancer Res.* **11,** 293–354.

Wittliff, J. L. (1977), Presentation at the Southeastern Cancer Study Group, Atlanta, GA, October.

Wu, C. W., C. W. Chi, T. J. Chang, W. Y. Lui, and F. K. P'eng (1990), *Cancer* **15, 65**(6), 1396–1402.

Wurz H., E. Wassner, and P. Citoler, et al. (1983), *Tumor Diagn. Ther.* **4,** 15–20.

Yanihara, T. and P. Troen (1972), *J. Clin. Endocrinol. Metab.* **3,** 968.

Yokozaki, H., N. Takekura, A. Takaraski, and J. Tabuchi et al. (1988), *Virchows Arch.* **413**(4), 297–302.

Young, H. H. II, and J. R. Kent (1968), *J. Urol.* **99,** 788–792.

Young, J. D., Jr., M. S. Suresh, and N. Bashirelahi (1979), *Trans. Am. Assoc. Genitourin. Surg.* **71,** 23.

Zaniboni, A., D. DeLorenzo, E. Simoncini, P. Marpicati, F. Gorni, G. Marini, and G. Marianone (1986), *Acta Hematol.* **75**(2), 92–95.

Chapter 9

Tissue Polypeptide Antigen and Specific TPA

Peter Oehr, Manfred L. Lüthgens, and Qian Liu

1. Introduction

Tissue polypeptide antigen (TPA) was originally described by Björklund and Björklund (1957). It was isolated from the insoluble residues of pooled tumors. Horse antiserum against the protein recognized both soluble form of TPA in human sera and body fluids, and an insoluble form in human tissues. Originally TPA was thought to be a tumor marker and, more recently, a proliferation marker (Björklund, 1980). TPA levels are elevated in the sera of patients with carcinomas, including breast cancer and tumor of the gastrointestinal, urogenital, and respiratory tract (Menendez-Botet et al., 1978; Björklund, 1980; Lüthgens and Schlegel, 1980, 1983, 1985; Schlegel et al., 1981; Skryten et al., 1981; Oehr et al., 1981, 1982b, 1984a; Inoue et al., 1985; Panucci et al., 1985, 1986; Salvati et al., 1985; Mross et al., 1985; Liu et al., 1989). The correlation

From: *Serological Cancer Markers* Edited by Stewart Sell ©1992 The Humana Press, Totowa, NJ

between serological TPA levels and tumor progression has been studied for several years (Björklund, 1980; Lüthgens and Schlegel, 1980, 1985; Skryten et al., 1981; Inoue et al., 1985; Salvati et al., 1985). Generally there is an inverse relationship between TPA level and a favorable prognosis (Björklund, 1980; Lüthgens and Schlegel, 1980, 1985; Schlegel et al., 1981; Oehr et al., 1984a; Salvati et al., 1985; Bönnen et al., 1989). Serum and urinary TPA determinations show the highest sensitivity for early tumor detection in urinary bladder cancer. This is the case for transitional bladder cancer (Adolphs and Oehr, 1984, Oehr et al., 1984a; Costello et al., 1985; Carbin et al., 1989) as well as squamous cell cancer (El-Ahmady et al., 1989). There are isolated reports of elevated TPA levels in serum of patients with tumors other than carcinomas, e.g., in lymphoma (Inoue et al., 1985).

Elevated serological TPA levels have also been reported for several acute and chronic inflammatory conditions, e.g., cirrhosis of the liver and acute hepatitis (Björklund, 1980; Mross et al., 1985).

The use of anti-TPA antibodies or histochemical detection of micrometastases, for differential diagnosis of carcinosarcoma, and for staging of different cancer diseases has become an important new tool in pathology (Nathrath et al., 1984; Oehr and Vogel, 1984; Oehr et al., 1984b; Vogel et al., 1985).

Purified TPA is closely related to keratins (Lüning and Nilsson, 1983; Weber et al., 1984; Lüning al., 1985). Keratins are the intermediate filament (IF) protein characteristic of epithelial cells. The original demonstration of a relationship between TPA and human keratins 8, 18, and 19 was based on immunofluorescence and immunoblotting experiments. Rabbit polyclonal TPA antibody was shown to have reacted with keratins 8, 18, 19 expressing epithial cell lines and cells in human tissues. Conversely, antibodies to keratins 8, 18, and 19 reacted with a TPA B1 preparation, purified from pooled human carcinomas (Weber et al., 1984). These data explained earlier work where TPA was shown to be present in the cytoskeletal network of HeLa cells (Kirsch et al., 1983). The work of Kirsch and Weber also clarified why certain biochemical properties such as the high alfa-helix, the rod-like morphology, and partial amino acid sequence data were reminiscent of IF proteins (Lüning et al., 1980; Redelius et al., 1980; Lüning and Nilsson, 1983). Drahovsky et al. (1984) have demonstrated that TPA mAbs stained PtK-1 cells coincident with keratin and vimentin filaments in double labeling experiments. Ochi (1985) found positive immunoreactivity of TPA with poly- and monoclonal keratin antibodies, and reported that binding of ^{125}I-TPA to keratin antibodies could be displaced by unlabeled keratin. Moreover, alignment of short TPA sequences (Redelius et al., 1980; Lüning et al., 1985) with keratin sequences (Hanukoglu and Fuchs, 1982, 1983; Lüning and Nilsson, 1983; Lüning et al., 1985; Magin et al., 1986; Leube et al., 1986) revealed significant homology, particularly with bovine and human keratin 8, and with human keratins 6 and 14. Indeed, sequences in the coil 2 of human keratin 8 (Leube et al., 1986) are identical with the TPA CNBr C and E fragments (Redelius et al., 1980). These results suggest that TPA may not be a specific marker of cell proliferation, as originally suggested by Björklund (1980), but rather keratin-derived products released from certain cells.

TPS is called specific TPA by Björklund. It differs from TPA by applying an IRMA assay with the monoclonal antibody M3 instead of polyclonal antibodies as a tracer. According to Björklund, TPS has nothing to do with cytokeratins and is, in contrary to TPA, only related to cell proliferation. More recent findings, however, show that TPS and TPA antibodies bind to keratin 8 and 18 positive tissue as well as to keratin negative tissues (Oehr et al., 1991; Liu et al., 1991).

This, however, does not detract from the uefulness of TPA and TPS as diagnostic and prognostic markers in clinical oncology. The aim of this chapter is to give an overview of current knowledge on the nature of TPA and TPS in order to stimulate research on TPA, TPS, cytokeratins, and possibly other yet unknown molecules related to TPA. It should also demonstrate the utility of the antigens in experimental model systems, predicting their use as a tool for in vivo diagnosis and therapy of cancer in the present decade.

2. TPA and TPS in the 1990s

2.1. Biology

The nature of TPA and TPS is still the subject of considerable dispute. In general., TPA is found in a wide variety of simple and organized organisms (Björklund, 1980). It can be found in increasing concentrations of tumor tissue culture as well as in single cell suspensions of slime molds during the logarithmic growth phase and in the subsequent stationary phase when the cells are partially dying (Oehr et al., 1991).

Immunofluorescent staining of HeLa cell tissue culture shows disappearence of the cytoskeletal pattern at certain mitotic stages (metaphase, anaphase) and spotlike concentrations appear in the cell. Using double staining for TPA and cytokeratin 18 or for TPS and TPA, one can see that these spots appear analogous to each other (Oehr et al., 1991).

It should also be mentioned that TPA levels are elevated during pregnancy (Oehr et al., 1982a; Inaba et al., 1985, 1987). Inaba and coworkers reported that, in normal pregnancy, serum TPA levels were found to be increased according to the gestational weeks. The values became normal within 5 d after termination. They made the hypothesis that TPA was produced in the placental chorion, concentrated in the amniotic fluid and then partly passed into the maternal circulation. Therefore, Inaba proposed to call TPA an oncoplacental antigen (Inaba et al., 1985, 1987). Previously, it had been called a tumor-germinal-pregnancy associated antigen, because it also occurred in elevated concentrations in different pregnancy associated body fluids as well as in seminal fluid (Oehr et al., 1982b).

2.2. Relation of TPA and TPS to Keratin and Nonkeratin Epitopes

As explained in the introduction, TPA antibodies and the in vitro TPA test kit can detect keratin-related antigens. New experiments have shown that this is also the case for TPS determinations. The TPS IRMA from BEKI BARN applies the M3 antibody as a tracer. It quantitatively detects cytokeratin 8 with a sensitivity similar to that of the TPA IRMA assay from Sangtec Medical AB. In comparison to TPA, there is a more than tenfold increase sensitivity of the TPS assay for an epitope in purified cytokeratin 18; the results suggest that this TPA-binding epitope is highly repetitive (Oehr et al., 1991). Although TPA and TPS do not show exactly the same positivity in tumor tissues, it can be generally concluded that there is good homology between these two markers and cytokeratins 8 and 18. On the other hand, it was found that antibodies to both TPA and TPS also react positively with tissue sections in the nonlymphatic area of the spleen, where the cytokeratins should not be present (Liu et al., 1991). This was confirmed by the quantitative in vitro determination of TPA and TPS in spleen extract which showed that TPA and TPS were about 30 times more concentrated in the noncellular fraction (Oehr et al., 1991). This raises the possibility that both TPA and TPS react with epitopes that are also present in substances other than keratins. It leaves the resemblance between TPA, TPS, and keratins open for discussion.

2.3. Release of TPA and TPS

Wth respect to Björklund, TPA and TPS are proliferation markers. According to Björklund, TPA and TPS are released from the individual tumor cells in small blebs. New investigations with high resolution immunofluorescence, however, give evidence that this hypothesis might be owing to an artefact (Oehr et al., 1991). The findings of Osborn and Weber suggest that TPA might be unrelated to proliferation of tumor cells (Weber et al., 1984). This is confirmed by immunohistochemical investigations, which show that neither TPA nor TPS positivity correlate well with KI 67, a marker for dividing cells (Liu et al., 1991). Unfortunately, this proliferation marker question is still vigorously debated. The only striking piece of evidence that shows a clear relationship between cell division and TPA release is the fact that tumor cells in tissue culture treated with demecholcine, a reversible cell division inhibitor, do not continue to produce elevated TPA levels (Oehr et al., 1991). This finding does not necessarily mean that TPA is excreted from dividing cells but might indicate that TPA is released from tumor cells when they occasionally die during the mitotic cycle. In tissue culture, the highest TPA values were found after the growth curve of cells had changed from the logarithmic phase to the stationary phase, including a high rate of cell death.

There is histological proof that TPA release in vivo follows damage of TPA-positive tissue (Oehr et al., 1984b, 1986). This happens mainly at the borderline of necrotic areas when the tumor is growing and the blood flow to the tumor tissue is decreasing. An artificial example for such a case is the high TPA concentration increase in serum after surgical interruption of the blood flow to a liver metastasis. There are also data from experimental animal-tumor models as well as from sections of human cancer tissues that support the idea of TPA release from damaged TPA (TPS) positive tissue (Oehr et al., 1991).

Another interesting piece of evidence for the cell damage hypothesis is the human model of anaplastic thyroid cancer. This tumor is histologically TPA-negative. During its fast tumor growth the anaplastic TPA-free tumor tissue surrounds the TPA positive follicles, which then die as a result of lack of nutrient and mechanical pressure. As a consequence, free TPA can be histologically stained in the area of necrotic tumor-surrounded follicles. By the nature of this organ, these follicles are in close contact with blood vessels (endocrine), which would explain the availability of cell fragments to the circulation. Serum level of TPA also increases in these patients (Oehr, 1984b). The substances measured afterwards in serum or plasma seem to be degradation products of TPA or TPS. Since these products carry epitopes that are also found in keratins 8 and 18, it makes sense to perform keratin assays in addition to the assays of TPA and TPS. This could lead to a new family of tumor markers like the mucins or carcinoembryonal antigens. New keratin-like tumor markers could give valuable additional clinical information or increase of sensitivity when combined with established markers for cancer of the lung, breast, and other organs as has been recently shown by Liu and coworkers for TPS and NSE in lung cancer or TPS and mucin markers for cancer of the breast (Liu et al., 1989a,b).

On the basis of the actual data, TPA release is a result of both proliferation activity and loss of TPA from the dying cell or cancer tissue. Contrary to the observation of Björklund who proposes that TPA is released in blebs from the divided tumor cells at the end of the mitotic cycle, it seems that proliferation can lead to cell death causing release of TPA, TPS, or keratin-like degradation products. This interpretation can also explain why elevation of TPA and TPS is correlated with activity of tumor growth, as evidenced by clinical studies.

2.4. Clearance of TPA and TPS

Experiments with purified ^{125}I labeled TPA have been carried out with rats. Within 8 h, TPA was concentrated in the liver, passed through the bile duct system, and disappeared in the gastrointestinal tract. No accumulation of radioactivity was observed in the urogenital tract (Oehr, Björklund, and Gyries, unpublished data). However, TPA or TPS determination in urine show positive reactions. It is postulated that these results arise from either antigen degradation products which are filtered by the kidney, or TPA and TPS that are released from the urinary bladder, since elevated levels are mostly found in early stages of urinary bladder cancer and infection (Oehr et al., 1981; El-Ahmady et al., 1989). In addition, urinary bladder epithelium is one of the self-renewing tissues of the human body surface structures. Shedding of cells into the urine itself may also cause an increase of urinary TPA or TPS. Any irritation of the bladder mucosa might stimulate this process.

2.5. Experimental Results for In Vivo Diagnosis and Therapy

2.5.1. Advantage of the TPA and TPS Animal Tumor Systems

The utility of TPA and TPS for in vivo diagnosis and therapy has mainly been shown by experimental work with HeLa tumor-bearing rats. The advantage of this system is the great similarity of TPA antigen distribution in humans and rodents, as can be seen

Table 1
Degree of Staining in Various Organs of the Nude Rat, Humans, and an Experimental Tumor Cell System of Human Origin

Tissue	Rat	Human
Liver		
Hepatocytes	–	–
Bile ducts	+++	++
Pancreas		
Secratory acini	–	–
Duct epithelia	++	+
Lung		
Alveolar epithelia	–	+
Bronchial epithelia	+	+
Kidney		
Bowman's capsule	–	–
Henle's loop, thin segment	++	+
Collecting ducts	++	+
Urothelium of the renal pelvis	++	+
Intestine		
Goblet cells	+	+
Spleen		
Matrix	not done	+
Lymphocytes	–	–
Erythrocytes	–	–
Muscle		
Smooth	–	–
Striated	–	–
Connective tissue	–	–
HeLa cell carcinoma	+ to +++	+++[a]

[a] Tissue culture.

from Table 1. The disadvantages of the classical models using the nude mouse and CEA or other antigens was the lack of antigen in healthy normal tissue of the rodents. Scintigraphic studies of radioactivity accumulation in mice after infusion of anti-CEA showed high tumor uptake of radiolabeled antibody, but these results were

Table 2
In Vivo Background Reduction
by Blocking of Specific Epitopes in Organs

Tumor/organ	Group 1	Group 2	Group 3
Tumor/kidney	2.1	0.6	5.7
Tumor/spleen	2.3	0.6	9.3
Tumor/liver	2.7	0.5	7.3
Tumor/lung	1.9	0.8	4.1
Tumor/stomach	2.1	1.3	17.0
Tumor/intestine	6.0	2.1	12.8
Tumor/muscle	6.0	3.0	6.4

Tumor/organ index taken from tissue-radioactivity/min/g after intravenous application of labeled specific and/or nonspecific antibodies. Days refer to the day of animal sacrification after application of radiolabeled antibodies. Injection of specific nonlabeled anti-TPA antibodies was made 2 d prior to application of radiolabeled antibodies. Group 1: HeLa, RNU, $n = 3$, 125-I anti-TPA, day 5. Group 2: HeLa, RNU, $n = 3$, 125-I IgG, day 5. Group 3: HeLa, RNU, $n = 1$, anti-TPA, 125-I anti-TPA, day 5.

not applicable to humans, since CEA in tumor patients is found in the tumor as well as in healthy tissues. As a consequence, the radiolabel is accumulated in the healthy organs leading to high background radioactivity.

2.5.2. Biological In Vivo Background Reduction

The improved exerimental antigen model made it possible to develop a new technique to decrease the specific background binding of the antibodies to healthy tissue: preinjection of low concentrations (1:70,000 dilution) of a specific antibody two days prior to its radiolabeled counterpart (50 µg for a rat with 180 g) led to decreased accumulation of biological background radioactivity in the healthy tissue and thus to an improvement in the relation of tumor/tissue uptake ratio (Table 2). The reason for this improvement is presumably the blocking of specific TPA epitopes in normal tissue. This effect is also seen after multiple injections of radiolabeled antibodies into tumor-bearing rats; there is a significant increase of

Table 3
Effect of Multiple Injections of Radiolabeled M3-anti-TPS on the Uptake of Radioactivity in Tumor and Organs of Rats[a]

	Number of repeated antibody injections	
Tumor/organ	One (day 4)	Two (day 4 and 6)
Tumor/blood	0.3	2.7
Tumor/kidney	5.2	7.8
Tumor/spleen	5.8	17.5
Tumor/liver	4.3	23.7
Tumor/muscle	4.6	22.4

[a]Determinations were made 5 d after the last antibody injection.

radiolabeled uptake after repeated antibody injection (Table 3). Here again, the reason might be the blocking of specific epitopes in normal tissue followed by improved binding to the more abundant epitopes in the tumor after the second and third antibody injections. This effect could be important for diagnostic as well as therapeutic purposes.

2.5.3. Scintigraphic Imaging of TPA- and TPS-Positive Tumors

TPA as well as TPS antibodies have successfully been used for localization of tumors in animals as well as in humans. Since most of the antigen is in the cytoplasm of tumor tissue, the major tumor sites located by anti-TPA, anti-TPS, and anticytokeratin antibodies are the necrotic areas of the tumor tissue (Oehr, unpublished data; Sundström, 1990). This has been shown by autoradiographic staining after immunoscintigraphy (Oehr, unpublished data); it also occurs during increased uptake 14 d after tumor irradiation (Table 4), when irradiation damage of tumor tissue appears. In addition, the increased uptake could be caused by improved vascular permeability as a result of edema after irradiation.

Table 4
Increased Tumor Uptake of 3-Anti-TPA Antibodies in Rats After Irradiation[a]

	Tumor weight		
Tumor/organ	0.3 g	0.3 g[b]	0.2 g[c]
Tumor/liver	1.7	5.4	4.3
Tumor/lung	1.6	4.6	11.4
Tumor/kidney	1.2	3.2	2.8
Tumor/spleen	2.3	6.3	10.0
Tumor/intestine	7.6	19.0	71.4
Tumor/muscle	7.6	14.3	21.7

[a]Tumor and tissue were removed on day 5 after intravenous application of radiolabeled antibody.
[b]Irradiation 1 d after antibody injection.
[c]Irradiation 14 d prior to antibody injection.

2.5.4. Possible Antibody Guided Radiotherapy of Micrometastases

In animal experiments, M3-anti-TPS mAb was labeled with ^{131}I and injected intraperitoneally simultaneously with HeLa tumor cells (10 million per animal). Controls received the same number of HeLa cells simultaneously with either unlabeled M3-anti-TPS mAb or cadmium conjugated M3-anti-TPS mAb. The treatments were repeated on days 4 and 8. After 22 d, the animals were sacrificed and the tumor weights determined. The radioimmunotreated tumors had an average weight of 0.7 g, the antibody-treated tumors had an average weight of 11.8 g, and the cadmium M3-anti-TPS-treated tumors had an average weight of 9.0 g. Since single cells can be more easily reached by antibodies than solid tumors, the results show the potential of this approach to reduce the risk of survival of micrometastases after surgery.

References

Adolphs, H. D. and P. Oehr (1984), *Urol. Res.* **12,** 125.
Björklund, B. and V. Björklund (1957), *Int. Arch. Allergy* **10,** 153–184.
Björklund, B., B. Wiklund, B. Lüning, K. Andersson, E. Kallin, and V. Björklund (1980), *Tumor Diagnostik* **2,** 78–84.
Bönnen, U., P. Oehr, U. Bönnen, Q. Liu, and H. J. Biersack (1989), *Med. Nucl.* **1,** 355–365.
Carbin, B.-E., P. Ekman, P. Eneroth, and B. Nilson (1989), *Urol. Res.* **17,** 269–272.
Costello, C. B. and S. Kumar (1985), *J. Royal Soc. Med.* **78,** 207–210.
Drahovsky, D., S. Kaul, and H. P. Zimmerman (1984), *Protides of the Biological Fluids,* vol. 32, Pergamon , Oxford, New York, pp. 719–722.
El-Ahmady, O., S. Hamza, M. Aboul-Ela, A. B. Halim, and P. Oehr (1989), *Recent Results in Tumor Diagnosis and Therapy* (R. Klapdor, ed.), W. Zuckschwerdt Verlag, München, San Francisco, pp. S5230-S5236.
Hanukoglu, I. and E. Fuchs (1982), *Cell* **31,** 243–252.
Hanukoglu, I. and E. Fuchs (1983), *Cell* **33,** 915–924.
Inaba, N., I. Fukazawa, Y. Ota, A. Nito, M. Ijichi, T. Sato, and H. Takamizawa (1985), *Acta Obst. Gynaec. Jpn.* **37,** 2139–2140.
Inoue, M., Y. Inoue, D. Hirmatsu, and G. Ueda (1985), *Cancer* **55,** 2618-2623.
Kirsch, J., P. Oehr, and C. Winkler (1983) *Tumordiagn. u. Ther.* **4,** 222–224.
Leube, R. E., F. X. Bosch, V. Romano, R. Zimbelmann, H. Höfler, and W. W. Franke (1986), *Differentiation* **33,** 69–85.
Liu, W., P. Oehr, M. Meier, M. Altreuther, J. Pollok, B. Schultes, U. Kania, A. Müller, M. Frings, A. Hirner, and H. J. Biersack (1989b), *Recent Results in Tumor Diagnosis and Therapy* (R. Klapdor, ed.), W. Zuckschwerdt Verlag, München, San Francisco, pp. S5167–S5170.
Liu, W., P. Oehr, U. Loos, B. Schultes, M. Praum, and H. J. Biersack (1989a), *Recent Results in Tumor Diagnosis and Therapy* (R. Klapdor, ed.), W. Zuckschwerdt Verlag, München, San Fransisco, pp. 5267–5269.
Liu, Q., M. Nap, and P. Oehr (1991), *Tumordiagn. u. Ther.* submitted.
Lüning, B., B. Wiklund, P. Redelius, and B. Björklund (1980), *Biochem. Biophys. Acta* **634,** 90–101.
Lüning, B., U. Nilsson, Lüning, M., and G. Thuresson (1985) *Protides of the Biological Fluids,* vol. 32, (H. Peeters, ed.), Pergamon, Oxford, New York, pp. 717-718.
Lüthgens, M. and G. Schlegel (1980), *Tumor Diagn.* **2,** 63–77.
Lüthgens, M. and G. Schlegel (1983), *Cancer Detect. Prevent.* **6,** 51-59.
Lüthgens, M. and G. Schlegel (1985), *Tumordiagn. u. Ther.* **6,** 1–7.
Margin, T. M., J. L. Jorcano, and W. W. Franjkke (1986), *Differentiation* **30,** 254–264.

Menendez-Botet, C. J., H. F. Oettgen, C. M. Pinsky, and M. K. Schwarz (1987), *Clin. Chem.* **24,** 868–872.

Mross, K. B., D. I. Wolfrum, and H. Rauchrecker (1985), *Oncology* **42,** 288–295.

Nathrath, W. B. J., P. Heidenkummer, H. Arnholdt, R. Bassermann, U. Löhrs, W. Permanetter, K. Remberger, and B. Wiebecke (1984), *Protides of the Biological Fluids,* vol. 31 (H. Peeters, ed.), Pergamon, Oxford, pp. 437–440.

Nathrath, W. B. J., P. Heidenkummer, V. Björklund, and B. Björklund (1985), *J. Histochem. Cytochem.* **33,** 99-109.

Ochi, Y., Y. Ura, M. Hamazu, M. Ishida, Y. Kajita, and Y. Nakajima (1985), *Clinica Chimica Acta* **15,** 157–167.

Oehr, P., G. Derigs, and R. Altmann (1981), *Tumor Diagn.* **2,** 283-290.

Oehr, P., O. Bellmann, and D. Hamann (1982a), *Clin. Biochem.* **15,** 13–16.

Oehr, P., L. Fischer, W. Kerjes, U. Kunath, H. J. Biersack, U. Sipeer, and C. Winkler (1982b), *Tumordiagn. Ther.* **3,** 195-198.

Oehr, P. and J. Vogel (1984), in *Protides of the Biological Fluids,* vol. 31 (H. Peeters, ed.), Pergamon, Oxford, pp. 727-730.

Oehr, P., L. Fischer, W. Kerjes, H. D. Adolphs, H. J. Biersack, and C. Winkler (1984a), *Campact News in Nucl. Med.* **15,** 152–154.

Oehr, P., J. Vogel, A. Lichius, B. Selbach, H.-J. Biersack, C. Winkler, and P. Gedigk (1984b), *Tumordiagn. Ther.* **5,** 129–138.

Oehr, P., J. Vogel, and M. Kramer (1986), *Arztl. Lab.* **32,** 166-172.

Oehr, P., Q. Liu, M. Nap, B. Schultes, M. Lechmann, Y. Ota, and H. Y. Jin (1991), *Tumordiagn. Ther.* submitted.

Panucci, A., C. Fabris, C. Del Favero, D. Basso, L. Marichioro, A. Piccoli, A. Burlina, and R. Naccarato (1985), *Br. J. Cancer* **52,** 801-807.

Panucci, A., C. Fabris, G. Del Favero, D. Basso, F. Di Mario, L. Marchioro, A. Piccoli, M. Lise, A. Burlina, and R. Naccarato (1986), *J. Clin. Pathol.* **39,** 75–77.

Rasmuson, T., G. R. Björk, L. Damber, S. E. Holm, L. Jacobsson, A. Jeppsson, B. Littbrand, T. Stigbrand, and G. Westman (1983), *Recent Results Cancer Res.* **84,** 331–343.

Redelius, P., B. Lüning, and B. Björklund (1980), *Acta Chem. Scand. B* **34,** 265–273.

Salvati, F., A. R. Cruciani, F. Flore, G. De Angelis, F. Pigorini, A. Antilli, F. Pau, R. Munno, and A. Cipri (1985), *Cancer Detect. Prvent.* **8,** 111–114.

Schlegel, G., M. Lüthgens, G. Eklund, and B. Björklund (1981), *Tumordiagn. Ther.* **2,** 6–11.

Skryten, A., B. Unsgaard, B. Björklund, and G. Eklund (1981), *Tumordiagn. Ther.* **3,** 117–120.

Sundström, B., B. Johansson, S. O. Hietala, and T. Stigbrand (1990), *Tumor Biol.* **11,** 158–166.

Vogel, J. and P. Oehr (1985), in *Protides of the Biological Fluids,* vol. 32 (H. Peeters, ed.), Pergamon, Oxford, pp. 743–746.

Weber, K. and G. Geisler (1984), *Cancer Cells 1. the Transformed Phenotype.* Cold Spring Harbor Laboratory, Cold Spring Harbor, NY, pp. 153–159.

Weber, K., M. Osborn, R. Moll, B. Wiklund, and B. Lüning (1984), *EMBO J.* **3,** 2707–2714.

Chapter 10

Tumor-Associated Carbohydrate Markers

Chemical and Physical Basis and Cell Biological Implications

Sen-itiroh Hakomori

1. Tumor-Associated Antigens: How Specific Should They Be?

Aberrant glycosylation associated with oncogenic transformation in experimental as well as human cancers was originally indicated by the change of glycolipid profile in virally transformed cells in vitro in 1968, 1969 (Hakomori and Murakami, 1968; Mora et al., 1969), and by the accumulation of fucose- and GlcNAc-containing glycolipids in human cancer in 1964 (Hakomori and Jeanloz); these glycolipids were identified later as Le^x, Le^a, and Le^b, regardless of host Lewis blood group status (Hakomori and Andrews, 1970; Yang and Hakomori, 1971). The first unequivocal evidence that glycolipids were tumor-associated antigens (TAAs) was provided in 1977 by the observed accumulation of asialo-GM2 (Gg3) in KiMSV sar-

From: *Serological Cancer Markers* Edited by Stewart Sell ©1992 The Humana Press, Totowa, NJ

coma in Balb/c mice and by the fact that rabbit anti-Gg3 antibodies specifically stained KiMSV sarcoma cells grown in vivo, but did not stain a variety of other Balb/c cells and tissues (Rosenfelder et al., 1977), except a few cells in spleen and testis (Hakomori et al., 1980). The concept that TAAs are often carbohydrates evolved only after successful application of the monoclonal antibody (MAb) approach in analysis of TAAs expressed in human cancers. During the past decade, studies with specific MAbs have shown that many TAAs are carbohydrates, particularly bound to lipids (glycosphingolipids; GSLs) (*see,* for reviews, Hakomori and Kannagi, 1983; Hakomori, 1985). The general concept for the immunochemical basis of TAAs is summarized in Table 1.

Strictly speaking, on a chemical basis, there are no "tumor-specific" structures. Some carbohydrate structures to which anti-tumor antibody responses are directed are also found in normal tissues. However, since a number of mouse and human MAbs capable of recognizing carbohydrate TAAs can be established even after syngeneic immunization (Ito et al., 1984; Taniguchi and Wakabayashi, 1984) and autoantibody response to such antigens can be observed (Singhal et al., 1987), one has to assume that these "nonspecific structures" could be present at the tumor-cell surface, organized in such a way that they are recognized by the host immune cell as "foreign." An analogy can be found in the immune response of patients with syphilis. It is well known that "specific antibodies" called Wasserman antibodies, detected in sera of patients with syphilis, were widely used for the diagnosis of syphilis by Wasserman reaction or its modification. The antigen was originally isolated from syphiloma of fetal liver and was considered to be specific for *Treponema pallidum.* The antigen, however, was subsequently found to be a normal cellular component identified as diphosphatidylglycerol (cardiolipin) (Davis et al., 1967). The lipid antigen is cryptic in normal cells and tissues; our current knowledge indicates that cardiolipin is present only in mitochondrial membrane, and absent at the cell surface. However, the antigen could be "surface-exposed" in syphilitic lesions, causing an immune response.

Table 1
Immunochemical Basis of Tumor Specificity

A. There are no "tumor-specific" structures characterized on a chemical basis.
B. However, MAbs defining human TAAs have been established after immunization of mice with tumor cells or tumor cell membranes, and antibody-secreting hybridomas have been selected on the basis of preferential selectivity with tumor cells (or tissues) over normal cells.
C. "Tumor-associated" structures defined by these MAbs are:
   1. Relatively novel structures expressed highly at the tumor cell surface. The same structures are absent in progenitor cells, but can be found in other normal tissues. Examples: GD3 in melanoma; di- or trimeric Le^x; sialosyl dimeric Le^x; sialosyl Le^a in gastrointestinal cancer.
   2. Highly restricted structures immunologically detectable only in tumor cells. Examples: incompatible A, Tn, and sialosyl Tn in various cancers.
   3. Common structures abundant in normal cells or tissues, but with a very high concentration in tumors. Antibodies can recognize this high density or a specific conformation induced by high density. Examples: GM3 in melanoma; Le^x in gastrointestinal cancer. It is the antibody, not the antigen structure, that defines tumor specificity.

2. Conflicting Data on Carbohydrate TAAs

There has been long-standing controversy on the specificity of TAAs, based on differences in immunobiological, immunochemical, and chemical data. Existence of TAAs was first suggested by the observed resistance to tumor inoculation following syngeneic immunization of mice with killed tumor cells (irradiated or treated with cytostatic reagents). The antigen was therefore termed "tumor-associated transplantation antigen" (TSTA) in classic tumor immunology. However, TSTA has not been clearly demonstrable in spontaneous tumors (including various human cancers), and the biochemical properties of TSTA are still unknown, since host immune response to TSTA is mainly a cellular, rather than an antibody, response. The majority of TSTA may be polypeptide antigens (recognized by T-cell receptors) rather than carbohydrate antigens (which elicit antibody response mainly through T-cell-independent pathways).* Rabbit polyclonal antibodies directed to chemically well-defined glycolipid TAAs were the first clue, on a chemical basis, to the actual existence of TAAs (Rosenfelder et al., 1977). Following extensive application of the MAb approach in detection of TAAs through selection of hybridoma antibodies, which react with tumors but not with normal tissues, a large number of carbohydrate TAAs have been identified (*see,* for reviews, Hakomori, 1985, 1989). Although many TAAs are undetectable in normal cells and tissues by immunostaining with their MAb probes, they are detectable by chemical analysis or a MAb blotting test following extraction from normal cells and tissues. Only a few TAAs have been characterized as novel structures restricted mainly to tumors.

---

*The carbohydrate antigen Le^x is strongly immunogenic in inducing antibody-producing response, and anti-Le^x antibodies are present even in sera of athymic *nu/nu* mice (Umeda et al., 1986). Immunization of mice with Le^x-containing cells did not produce T-cell response, and antibody responses directed to various glycolipids can be produced by direct stimulation in vitro of B-cells by lipopolysaccharide alone (Handa et al., unpublished). Polysaccharides are classified as type 2 antigens and are generally considered not to require the action of antigen-specific T-cells in order to stimulate responses (e.g., Paul, 1989, and references cited therein). These facts suggest that anticarbohydrate antibody response, in general, is T-cell-independent. Some carbohydrate antigens, however, may cause T-cell responses. GM3 present in high density at the melanoma cell surface may cause suppressor T as well as cytotoxic T-cell responses, depending on conditions. Cytotoxic T-cell response is produced by liposomes containing *N*-glycolyl GM3 at high density. These responses are not restricted by major histocompatibility antigens (*see* Taniguchi et al., 1989; Harada et al., 1989). T hapten (Galβ1 →3GalNAc) linked to BSA may cause cytotoxic T-cell response, as determined by a delayed hypersensitivity test (Henningsson et al., 1987) and by T-cell proliferative response in vitro (Singhal et al., 1991). These interesting observations obviously require extensive follow-up studies.

Nevertheless, a nonnovel common structure highly expressed in tumors may be recognized by the host immune system as a TAA. A good example is GM3 ganglioside in melanoma cells, defined by MAb M2590 (Taniguchi and Wakabayashi, 1984; Hirabayashi et al., 1985), which was established after syngeneic C57/BL mice were immunized extensively with B16 melanoma (*see* Section 5).

Since carbohydrate antigens are easily detectable by biochemical procedures after extraction of cells or tissues, the chemical quantity of antigens present in tissues can be compared with their MAb-based immunohistological staining patterns or biodistribution pattern in vivo based on infusion of radiolabeled MAb. Interestingly, distribution patterns derived from these three approaches are quite inconsistent. For example, when terataocarcinoma expressing Le^x was inoculated in syngeneic mice and studied with ^{125}I-labeled anti-Le^x MAb (anti-SSEA-1), only tumor cells showed a major accumulation of antibody. Accumulation of labeled antibody in kidney was minimal, even though kidney sections showed strong immunofluorescence with labeled antibody, and Le^x glycolipid was detected in significant quantity in kidney (Ballou et al., 1984, 1986). Biodistribution of ^{125}I-labeled anti-GM3 MAb DH2 in mice bearing B16 melanoma also showed high accumulation in tumor cells, whereas binding to various other tissues was minimal, regardless of the chemical quantity of GM3 present (Dohi et al., 1988).

3. Chemical and Structural Basis of Carbohydrate TAAs

Many TAAs have been identified as carbohydrates bound to lipid (glycolipid) or to protein (glycoprotein) (Fig. 1). Some epitopes are expressed in both glycolipids and glycoproteins (e.g., lactoseries structures); others are expressed exclusively in glycolipids (e.g., ganglioseries and globoseries structures) (Fig. 1, items 1 and 2). Some structures are associated exclusively with mucin-type glycoproteins, e.g, T, Tn, and sialosyl Tn (Fig. 1, item 3). A novel tumor-associated antigenicity was recently found, i.e., a peptide epitope is maintained by a single *O*-linked glycosylation, as shown by MAb

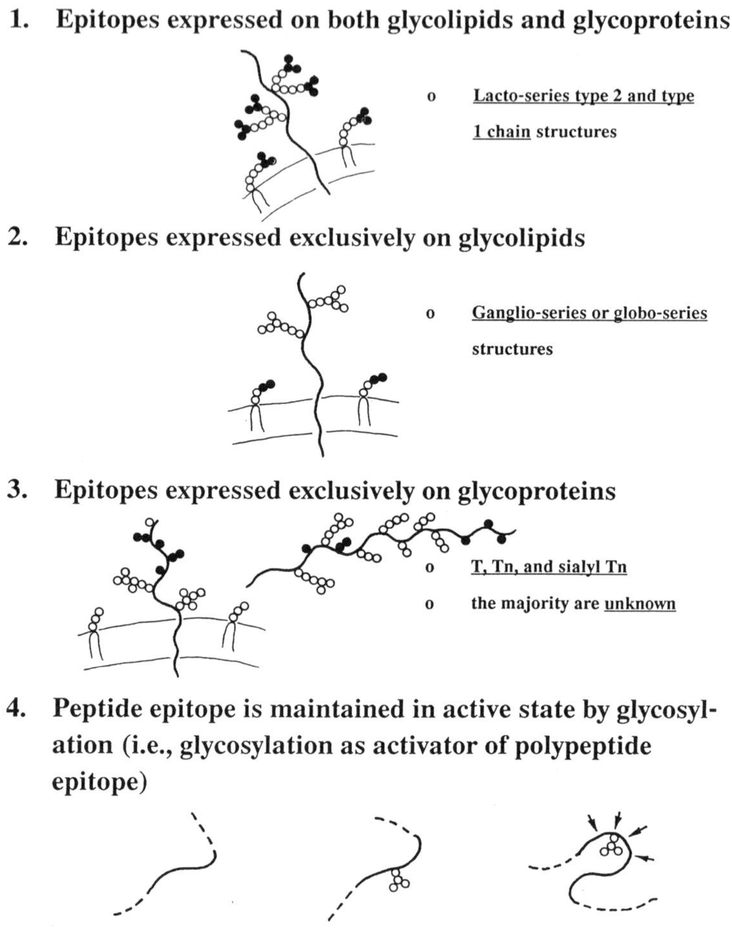

Fig. 1. Expression mode of carbohydrate TAAs. Four different types of epitopes are illustrated. Epitopes of type 3 are carried mainly by high-mol-wt mucin-type glycoproteins. An example of type 4 is oncofetal epitope associated with fibronectin, as discussed in the text.

FDC6, which is directed not to α-GalNAc or any carbohydrate chain, but to a hexapeptide, VTHPGY, with a specific conformation (Matsuura et al., 1988) (Fig. 1, item 4; Table 2, item G).

Carbohydrate TAAs can be formed by three basic processes, as shown (with examples) in Table 3, i.e., incomplete synthesis,

Table 2
Directions of Aberrant Glycosylation

A. Changes in ganglioseries structure
   1. Accumulation of GM3, GD2, GM2, GD3, and so on, in melanoma, neuroblastoma, and the like: LacCer →GM3 →GD3→GD2→ GD1b GT1b
   2. Accumulation of Fuc-GM1 in small-cell lung carcinoma: GM1 →Fuc-GM1

B. Changes in globoseries structure
   1. Accumulation of Gb3 in Burkitt's lymphoma, esophageal cancer: LacCer →Gb3→Gb4
   2. Neosynthesis of extended globoseries, e.g., globo-H: Gb4→ Gal-Gb4→ Fuc-Gal-Gb4

C. Changes in lactoseries type 1 chain
   1. Enhanced synthesis of 2→3 sialosyl Le^a, 2→3/2→6 sialosyl Le^a, Le^a, Le^b, 2→3 sialosyl Lc_4; coexpression of Le^a and Le^b

D. Changes in lactoseries type 2 chain
   1. Enhanced chain elongation without branching
      a. nLc_4, nLc_6, nLc_8, and so on
      b. Le^x, Le^y, dimeric Le^x, trimeric Le^x, sialosyl Le^x, sialosyl dimeric Le^x, and so on

E. Synthesis of incompatible blood-group antigens (*see* Table 4)

F. Mucin glycoprotein
   1. T, Tn, sialosyl Tn

G. Oncofetal fibronectin, defined by MAb FDC6
   1. —Val—Thr—His—Pro—Gly—Tyr— no activity
   2. —Val—Thr—His—Pro—Gly—Tyr— strong activity

```
                |
                O
                |
             GalNAc
```

Polypeptide conformation is converted to antigenically active by GalNAc addition.

Table 3
Basic Changes in Glycolipids
Associated with Oncogenic Transformation

A. Incomplete synthesis with or without accumulation of precursor structures
   1. Gb3 in Burkitt's lymphoma
   2. GD2 and GD3 in melanoma, neuroblastoma, and T-cell leukemia
   3. Gg3 in Hodgkin's lymphoma, and mouse lymphoma and sarcoma
   4. Tn antigen expressed in various cancers

B. Enhanced synthesis of neostructures
   1. Dimeric or trimeric Le^x, trifucosyl Le^y, sialosyl Le^x, and sialosyl Le^a in various adenocarcinomas (gastrointestinal, pulmobronchial, genitourinary)

C. Organizational changes of carbohydrates in membranes
   1. Occur in all types of tumors
   2. High exposure as a result of loss of crypticity, which is influenced by:
      a. Adjacent glycoconjugates that interact with glycolipids
      b. Density of glycolipids
      c. Ceramide composition (short-chain fatty acid > long-chain fatty acid > α-OH fatty acid)

neosynthesis, and organizational changes. TAAs resulting from incomplete synthesis are relatively novel structures in normal tissues, representing precursors of more complex carbohydrates, and are greatly accumulated in tumor cells as a result of either blocked synthesis of the more complex structure or enhanced synthesis of the precursor (Table 3, item A). The most remarkable example of the occurrence of TAAs as a result of incomplete synthesis is that of Tn antigen expressed in various human cancers. Tn expression is obviously caused by blocked synthesis of *O*-linked mucin-type carbohydrate chain in which α-GalNAc is located at the innermost residue directly linked to Ser or Thr. The residue is exposed and

Table 4
Changes of Histoblood Antigens in Human Cancer

A. Deletion of A and B determinants (Masamune et al., 1952; Davidsohn et al., 1966) and associated accumulation and disorganization of precursor (H and *N*-acetyllactosamine) (Dabelsteen et al., 1983).
B. Expression of incompatible A antigen in O or B tumor:
   1. Identification as Tn antigen (Hirohashi et al., 1985);
   2. Real A antigen expression (ALe^b, ALe^d) (Clausen et al., 1986);
   3. Other structures (Forssman, fucoseless A) are of minor importance.
C. Expression of incompatible PP_1P^k antigen in small p tumor (Levine et al., 1951; Kannagi et al., 1982; Hattori et al., 1987).
D. Change of carrier isotype in A tumor (Dabelsteen et al., 1988). Type 2 and type 3 chain A are absent in normal adult colonic mucosa, but are expressed in tumors.

displays strong immunogenicity. Many of the accumulated lactoseries antigens with novel structures are assumed to be products of neosynthesis (Table 3, item B).

Organizational changes of carbohydrate antigens in membranes, observed in essentially all types of experimental and human cancer, are caused by a demasking effect by deletion of adjacent glycoconjugates (Urdal and Hakomori, 1983; Wiels et al., 1984) , or by a high density of carbohydrates, which may cause changes of organization and conformation of individual carbohydrates (Nores et al., 1987). In glycolipid antigens, ceramide composition greatly influences the exposure of carbohydrate chains, and hence their immunogenicity and antigenicity (Yoshino et al., 1982; Kannagi et al., 1983b; Symington et al., 1984) (Table 3, item C).

The general direction of aberrant glycosylation found in each type of carbohydrate chain is indicated in Table 2. Enhanced synthesis of precursor structure coupled with blocked synthesis of complex structure in ganglio- and globoseries glycolipids has been

Table 5
Tn and Sialyl-Tn Structures:
Antigens Expressed Exclusively in Glycoproteins

Structure	Name	MAbs
1. GalNAcα1→*O*-Ser/Thr (polypeptide)	Tn	NCC-Lu35 and -81 (Hirohashi et al., 1985) Cu-1 (Takahashi et al.,1988)
2. GalNAcα1→*O*-Ser/Thr (polypeptide) 6 ↑ NeuAcα2	sialosyl Tn	TKH1 and -2 (Kjeldsen et al., 1988); MLS102 (Kurosaka et al., 1988)

clearly observed and results in accumulation of precursors for ganglio- and globostructures, such as Gb3, GD2, GD3, and Gg3. In contrast, "neosynthesis" often occurs in lactoseries type 1 and type 2 chains, as well as in blood-group A, Lewis, and P determinants, resulting in the synthesis of "incompatible blood-group antigens." The chemical nature of incompatible A antigens has been studied extensively; it is currently believed that the majority are crossreacting Tn (Hirohashi et al., 1985) and 10–20% are real A antigen, particularly type 1 chain (Clausen et al., 1986; Metoki et al., 1989). Changes of blood-group antigens in human cancer are summarized in Table 4.

The most well-characterized carbohydrate antigens found in mucin-type glycoproteins are Tn (GlcNAcα1→*O*-Ser/Thr) and sialosyl Tn (NeuAcα2→6GalNAcα1→*O*-Ser/Thr) (*see* Table 5). T antigen, often referred to as Galβ1→3GalNAcα1→*O*-Ser/Thr, the core structure of *O*-linked carbohydrate chains, may not be accurately described as tumor-associated, because MAbs directed to Gal β1→3GalNAcα1→R did not react with tumors, whereas MAbs directed to Galβ1→3GalNAcβ1→R showed clear specificity to a variety of human cancers (Ørntoft et al., unpublished data).

Carbohydrate TAAs can be classified into three groups, i.e., epitopes expressed on (1) both glycolipids and glycoproteins, (2) glycolipids only, and (3) glycoproteins only. The first group corresponds essentially to lactoseries structure, and is found most abundantly in the most common human cancers, such as lung, gastrointestinal, breast, colorectal, liver, and pancreatic cancer. The structure has a common backbone consisting of Galβ1→3GlcNAcβ1→3Gal (type 1) or Galβ1→4GlcNAcβ1→3Gal (type 2) (*see,* for reviews, Hakomori and Kannagi, 1983; Hakomori, 1985). The novel type 2 chain structures, and their defining MAbs established in this laboratory, are listed in Table 6. All these structures are characterized by unbranched linear type 2 chains with internal fucosylation as the backbone (Table 6, structures 1, 2, and 5); terminal fucosylation (structure 3) or sialylation (structure 4) is also found in some cases. Of particular interest in this structural series is the expression of real A antigen (type 1 chain A, i.e., ALe^b and ALe^d) in tumors of individuals of blood-group O or B (Clausen et al., 1986; Metoki et al., 1989). The structures (not shown in the table) are defined by combinations of MAbs capable of distinguishing various A antigens carried by different carbohydrate chains (Clausen et al., 1985a,b; Abe et al., 1984). Aberrant expression of blood-group antigens in human cancer is summarized in Table 4.

The second group of epitopes, expressed exclusively on glycolipids, has been found mainly on ganglio- or globoseries structures (Hakomori and Kannagi, 1983; Hakomori, 1985). These antigens (shown in Table 7, pp. 220,221) are abundantly expressed in specific types of human cancer, such as melanoma, Burkitt's lymphoma, neuroblastoma, and small cell lung carcinoma, but not in common human cancers. The antibody MBr1 was originally established as being directed to human breast carcinoma. The antigen was identified as "globo-H": fucosylgalactosylgloboside (IV^3Fucα1→2 GalGb4). However, it also crossreacts with ganglio-H and mucin-type H, which have the common structure Fucα1→2Galβ1 →3 GalNAc. Since the major antigen in breast cancer has been found to be mucin-type glycoprotein, the real antigen could be mucin-type H.

Table 6
Lactoseries Structures: Antigens Expressed in Both Glycoproteins and Glycolipids

	Structure	Name	MAbs
1.	Galβ1→4GlcNAcβ1→3Galβ1→4GlcNAcβ1→3Galβ1→4Glcβ1→1Cer 3 3 ↑ ↑ Fucα1 Fucα1	Difucosyl y_2 (dimeric Le^x)	FH4 (Hakomori et al., 1984; Fukushi et al., 1984a)
2.	Galβ1→4GlcNAcβ1→3Galβ1→4GlcNAcβ1→3Galβ1→4GlcNAcβ1→3Galβ1→4Glcβ1→1Cer 3 3 3 ↑ ↑ ↑ Fucα1 Fucα1 Fucα1	Trimeric Le^x	FH5 (Hakomori et al., 1984; Fukushi et al., 1984a)
3.	Galβ1→4GlcNAcβ1→3Galβ1→4GlcNAcβ1→3Galβ1→4Glcβ1→1Cer 2 3 3 ↑ ↑ ↑ Fucα1 Fucα1 Fucα1	Trifucosyl Le^y	AH6, KH1 (Abe et al., 1983; Nudelman et al., 1986)
4.	Galβ1→4GlcNAcβ1→3Galβ1→4GlcNAcβ1→3Galβ1→4Glcβ1→1Cer 3 3 3 ↑ ↑ ↑ NeuAcα2 Fucα1 Fucα1	Sialosyl difucosyl Le^x	FH6 (Fukushi et al., 1984b)
5.	Galβ1→4GlcNAcβ1→3- Galβ1→4GlcNAcβ1→3Galβ1→4GlcNAcβ1→3Galβ1→4GlcNAcβ1→3Galβ1→4Glcβ1→1Cer 3 ↑ Fucα1		ACFH18 (Nudelman et al., 1988)

The third group of epitopes, expressed exclusively in glycoproteins, has been recently identified as Tn (Hirohashi et al., 1985) and sialosyl Tn (Kjeldsen et al., 1988; Kurosaka et al., 1988), the precursors of *O*-linked carbohydrate chains. Tn and sialosyl Tn can be regarded as blood-group antigens, since a genetically-defined rare population expresses these antigens highly in blood cells and tissues (Kjeldsen et al., 1989). These structures and their defining antibodies are shown in Table 5.

In addition to these three groups, a new type of tumor-associated epitope has been found recently in "oncofetal fibronectin" (Matsuura and Hakomori, 1985). The epitope is a pentapeptide sequence (VTHPGY) whose conformation is maintained in an active state by glycosylation, i.e., *O*-glycosylation at "T" of the above sequence converts an inactive pentapeptide into an active form, whereas the carbohydrate has no epitope (Matsuura et al., 1988) (Fig. 1; Table 2, item G).

4. Enzymatic Basis of Aberrant Glycosylation

The enzymatic basis of most of these carbohydrate changes, with a few exceptions, has not been investigated. However, three basic changes in glycolipids associated with oncogenic transformation can be considered, as shown in Table 4. They are: (1) incomplete synthesis with or without accumulation of precursor glycolipid; (2) enhanced synthesis of neoglycolipid essentially absent in progenitor cells; and (3) organizational changes in cell membrane, observed in essentially all tumors.

An important enzymatic basis for the accumulation of lactoseries type 2 chain glycolipid (Table 6) in colon cancer is the enhancement of β1→3GlcNAc transferase, rather than any other glycosyltransferase (Holmes et al., 1987). Thus, unbranched core structure, to which sialosyl or fucosyl substitution could occur, accumulated greatly. There was no indication in colon cancer of enhanced sialosyl- or fucosyltransferase (Holmes et al., 1987). However, this conclusion was based on restricted determination conditions. There are indications that sialosyl- or fucosyltransferases are also enhanced (unpublished observations). In normal human epi-

Table 7
Globo- or Ganglioseries Structures: Antigens Expressed Exclusively in Glycolipids

	Structure	Source/ Name	MAbs
Globoseries			
1.	Galα1→4Galβ1→4Glcβ1→1Cer	Burkitt's lymphoma	Anti-BLA (Nudelman et al., 1983)
2.	Fucα1→2Galβ1→3GlcNAcβ1→3Galα1→4Galβ1→4Glcβ1→1Cer	Breast cancer (globo-H antigen)	MBr1 (Bremer et al., 1984)
3.	Fucα1→2Galβ1→3GlcNAcβ1→3Galα1→4Galβ1→4Glcβ1→1Cer (Gal 3 ↑ GalNAcα1)	Colorectal cancer (globo-A antigen and type 3 chain A)	HH5 (Clausen et al., 1986)
4.	GalNAcα1→3GlcNAcβ1→3Galα1→4Galβ1→4Glcβ1→1Cer	Gastric/lung cancer (Forssman antigen)	(Hakomori et al., 1981)

Ganglioseries			
5.	NeuAcα2→3Galβ1→4GlcCer	Human/mouse melanoma (GM3 ganglioside or lactone)	M2590 (Taniguchi and Wakabayashi, 1984; Hirabayashi et al., 1985) DH2 (Dohi et al., 1988)
6.	NeuAcα2→8NeuAcα2→3Galβ1→4GlcCer	Human melanoma (GD3 ganglioside)	4.2 (Nudelman et al., 1982)
7.	NeuAcα2→8NeuAcα2→3Galβ1→4GlcCer 4 ↑ GalNAcβ1	Neuroblastoma, melanoma (GD2 ganglioside)	(Cahan et al., 1982)
8.	Fucα1→2Galβ1→3GlcNAcβ1→4Galβ1→4GlcCer 3 ↑ NeuAcα2	Small-cell lung carcinoma (fucosyl GM1)	(Nilsson et al., 1984)

thelia, the majority of type 2 chains are branched, possibly through β1→6GlcNAc transferase (Koenderman et al., 1987), leading to synthesis of an I-type structure that is subsequently converted to branched H and branched blood-group-A and -B antigens. Some of these I antigens are partially sialylated to result in G8 or G9 gangliosides (Watanabe et al., 1978, 1979; Kannagi et al., 1983a). Tumor tissues of epithelial origin (the most common type of human cancer) are characterized by: (1) blocked synthesis of the β1→6GlcNAc branch in type 2 chain; (2) enhanced synthesis of unbranched type 2 chain (representing I antigen); (3) subsequent 2→3 or 2→6 sialylation, resulting in 2→3 or 2→6 terminally sialylated gangliosides; or (4) α1→3 fucosylation at the subterminal internal residue. Occurrence of process (3) followed by process (4) results in sialosylfucosyl structures. The basic difference in the glycosylation process for lactoseries structures is illustrated in Fig. 2.

5. Organizational and Physical Basis of Tumor Specificity

All glycolipid antigens may share a common physical structure organized in the lipid bilayer. Recent analysis of the conformational structure of GSL antigens indicates that the axis of ceramide is perpendicular to the axis of the carbohydrate chain (Kaizu et al., 1986; Hakomori, 1986). Furthermore, hydrophobic structures, such as the *N*-acetyl group of GalNAc or GlcNAc, are oriented toward the upper surface of the carbohydrate chain, whereas hydrophilic groups are more abundant on the lower surface, which faces the polar surface of the lipid bilayer. Thus, epitopes carried by GSLs could constitute the hydrophobic area on the surface of carbohydrate chains laid on the lipid bilayer (Fig. 3, item 3 [*see* p. 226]). This property is not limited to glycolipid TAAs, but is common to all types of glycolipid antigens. However, highly immunogenic TAAs are the rigid structures formed by GalNAc or GlcNAc with fucosyl or sialosyl substitution, which prevent free rotation and enhance rigidity of the carbohydrate chain (Fig. 3, item 1). These structures show high rigidity as a result of steric hindrance (conformations based on hard-sphere exanomeric [HSEA] calculation), and form large hydrophobic areas surrounded by hydrophilic areas (Fig. 3, item 2), providing the antibody-binding sites.

Anomalous conformations specific to tumors may also be formed by common structures, such as GM3 or Le^x, when they are organized in high density at the surface membrane. A good example is MAb M2590, which was selected on the basis of negative reactivity with nonmelanoma cells and tissues and exclusive positive reactivity with melanoma. Surprisingly, this MAb was found to be directed to GM3, a very common ganglioside present in various normal tissues. Subsequent studies, however, indicate that M2590 does not react with GM3 at low density, indicating that it is capable of recognizing GM3 at densities above a certain threshold value (Nores et al., 1987). In addition, cytotoxic T-cell response in vitro was shown to be induced by GM3 liposome present at high density, but not low density (Taniguchi et al., 1989; Harada et al., 1989). This example clearly indicates that tumor specificity cannot be defined by primary chemical structure, but rather is defined purely by host immune response, i.e., by the ability to recognize density and yet ill-defined tertiary structure (organization) of carbohydrate antigen present at the tumor cell surface. The same antigen at the surface of normal cells has different organization and density, and is not recognized as tumor antigen by the host immune system. Similar density-dependent recognition has been described for anti-Le^x MAb (Hakomori et al., 1981) and for the cytotoxic effect activated by anti-GD3 MAb directed to melanoma (Welt et al., 1987). Obviously, if the TAA is a unique structure highly expressed in tumors, it will be the most appropriate tumor marker,

---

Fig. 2 *(see following pages)*. Synthetic pathways for branched polylactosamine (PLA) structures (**A**), found predominantly in normal adult tissues, and unbranched PLA structures (**B**), found mainly in fetal and cancer tissues. A variety of unbranched PLAs could be synthesized by chain elongation of lactosamine through enhanced activity of $\beta1 \rightarrow 3$GlcNAc transferase (and relative suppression of $\beta1 \rightarrow 6$GlcNAc transferase), leading to various unbranched type 2 chain structures that are subsequently $2 \rightarrow 3$ sialylated, $2 \rightarrow 6$ sialylated, or $2 \rightarrow 3$ fucosylated to yield a number of TAA epitopes.

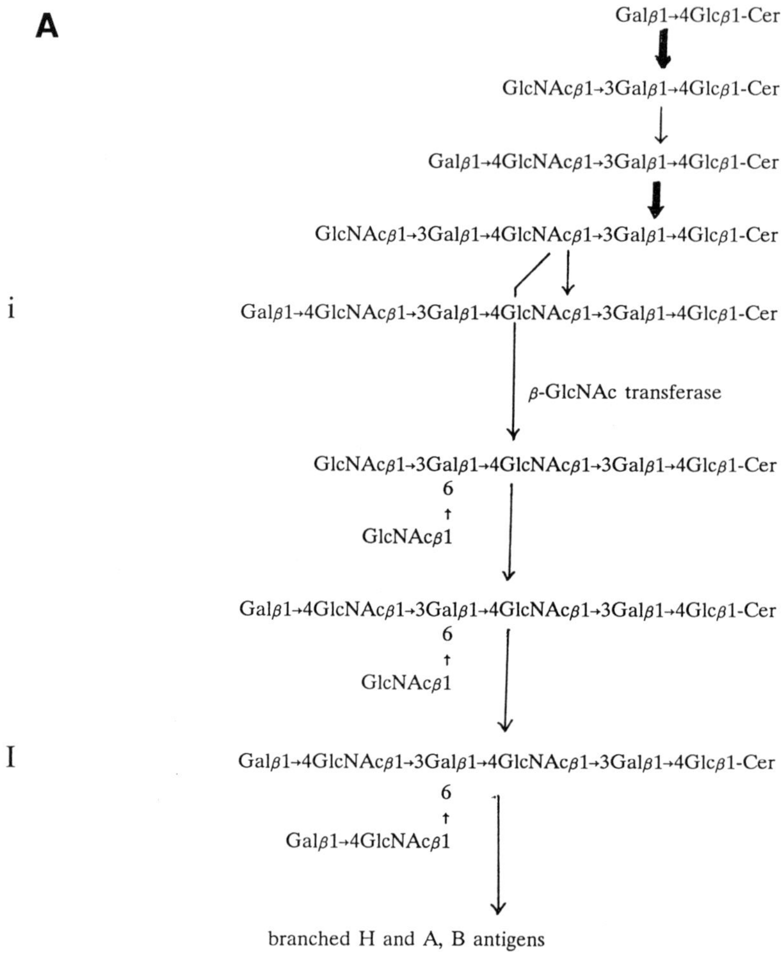
A
Galβ1→4Glcβ1-Cer
GlcNAcβ1→3Galβ1→4Glcβ1-Cer
Galβ1→4GlcNAcβ1→3Galβ1→4Glcβ1-Cer
GlcNAcβ1→3Galβ1→4GlcNAcβ1→3Galβ1→4Glcβ1-Cer
i
Galβ1→4GlcNAcβ1→3Galβ1→4GlcNAcβ1→3Galβ1→4Glcβ1-Cer
β-GlcNAc transferase
GlcNAcβ1→3Galβ1→4GlcNAcβ1→3Galβ1→4Glcβ1-Cer
6
GlcNAcβ1
Galβ1→4GlcNAcβ1→3Galβ1→4GlcNAcβ1→3Galβ1→4Glcβ1-Cer
6
GlcNAcβ1
I
Galβ1→4GlcNAcβ1→3Galβ1→4GlcNAcβ1→3Galβ1→4Glcβ1-Cer
6
Galβ1→4GlcNAcβ1
branched H and A, B antigens

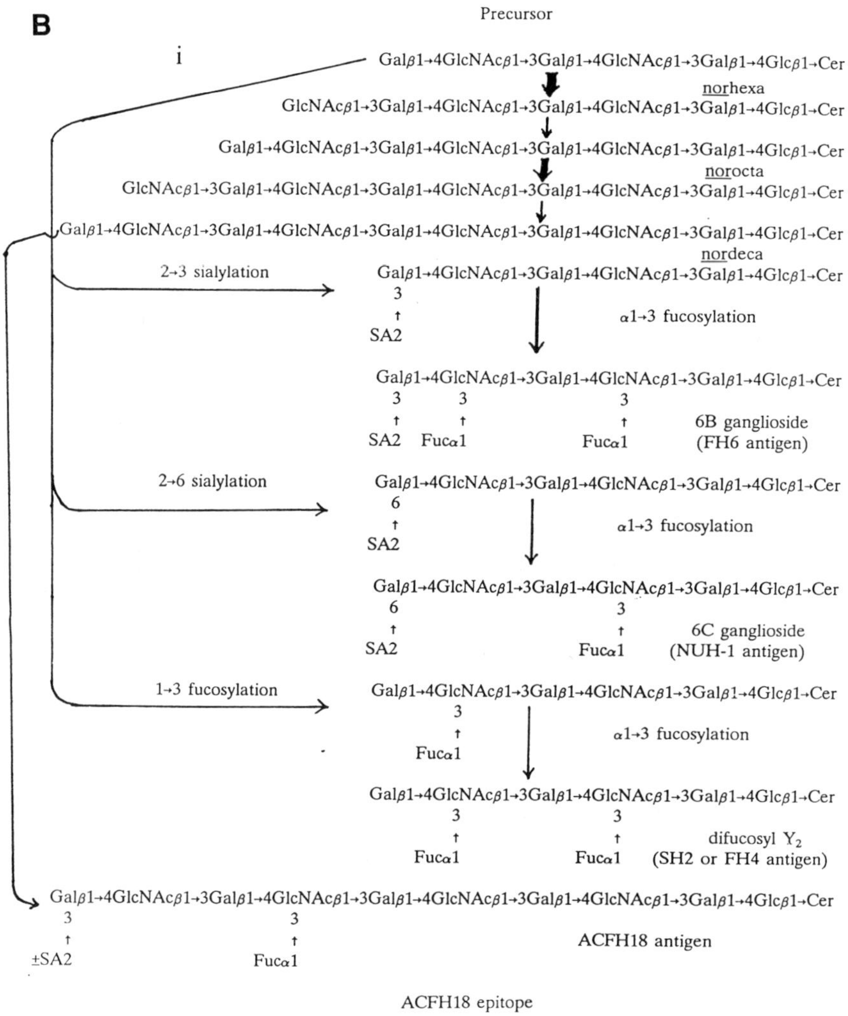
B
Precursor
i
Galβ1→4GlcNAcβ1→3Galβ1→4GlcNAcβ1→3Galβ1→4Glcβ1→Cer
norhexa
GlcNAcβ1→3Galβ1→4GlcNAcβ1→3Galβ1→4GlcNAcβ1→3Galβ1→4Glcβ1→Cer
Galβ1→4GlcNAcβ1→3Galβ1→4GlcNAcβ1→3Galβ1→4GlcNAcβ1→3Galβ1→4Glcβ1→Cer
norocta
GlcNAcβ1→3Galβ1→4GlcNAcβ1→3Galβ1→4GlcNAcβ1→3Galβ1→4GlcNAcβ1→3Galβ1→4Glcβ1→Cer
Galβ1→4GlcNAcβ1→3Galβ1→4GlcNAcβ1→3Galβ1→4GlcNAcβ1→3Galβ1→4GlcNAcβ1→3Galβ1→4Glcβ1→Cer
nordeca
2→3 sialylation
SA2
α1→3 fucosylation
SA2 Fucα1 Fucα1
6B ganglioside
(FH6 antigen)
2→6 sialylation
6C ganglioside
(NUH-1 antigen)
1→3 fucosylation
difucosyl Y_2
(SH2 or FH4 antigen)
±SA2 Fucα1
ACFH18 antigen
ACFH18 epitope

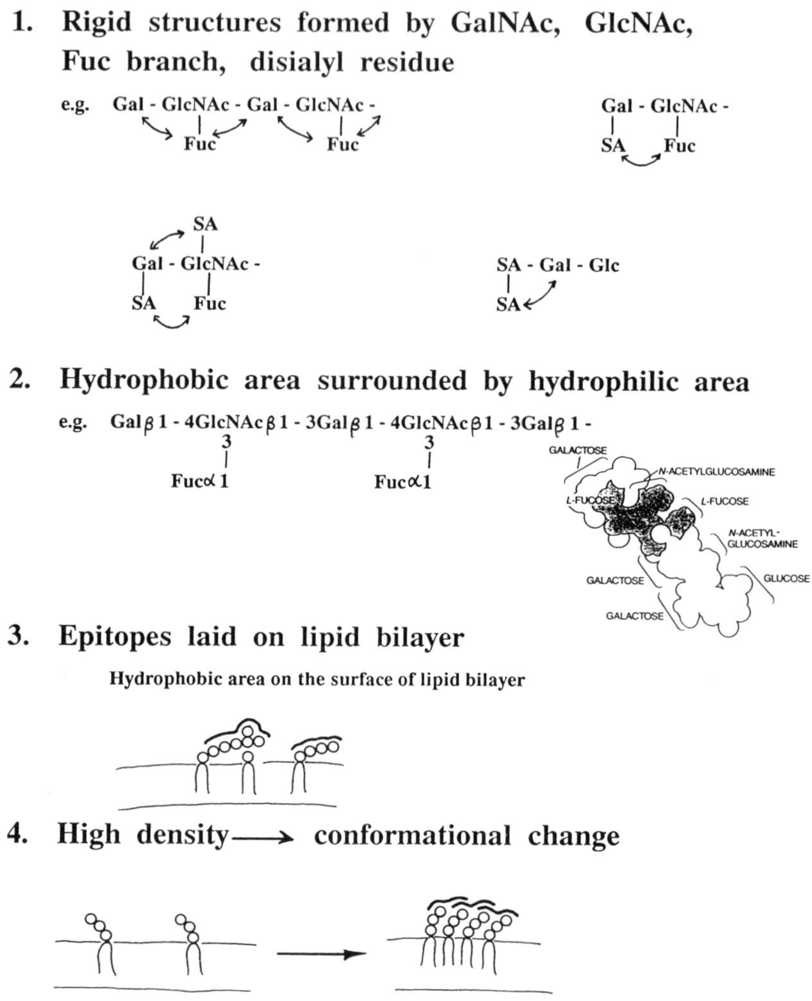

Fig. 3. Physical structural factors affecting tumor specificity and immunogenicity of carbohydrate TAAS. Factor 1: Rigid structure formed by branched sugar residues that restrict free rotation, e.g., Fuc and Gal residues of Le^x; adjacent linked sialyl and Fuc residues in type 1 or type 2 lactosamine structure. Factor 2: Large hydrophobic area surrounded by a hydrophilic area, providing a site for preferential binding of antibody. The illustration shows a minimum–energy conformational model of dimeric Le^x structure, with the exposed hydrophobic area at the top surface of the carbohydrate chain indicated by shading. Factor 3: Prefer-

i.e., target, for antibody-mediated drug delivery or immunotherapy. The tumor-associated specificity of Tn and sialosyl Tn antigens, highly expressed in a variety of human cancers, provides one such example (Hirohashi et al., 1985; Takahashi et al., 1988; Kjeldsen et al., 1988). On the other hand, even highly novel structures detectable in tumors, if their quantity and cell-surface density are low, may not be appropriate tumor markers; e.g., Forssman antigen expressed in a variety of human cancers (Hakomori et al., 1977; Taniguchi et al., 1981).

6. Cell Biological Significance of Aberrant Glycosylation in Tumors

A large number of structural changes resulting from aberrant expression of glycosyltransferases and hydrolases have been observed, but the exact details of changes in glycosyltransferases and their organization (which obviously provide the basis of aberrant glycosylation expressed in essentially all tumor cells) are not known.

Aberrant glycosylation in some virus-transformed cells has been correlated to oncogene activation. The level of GM3 has been shown to be closely correlated to expression of *src* gene in chick embryonic fibroblasts transformed with *src* oncogene (Hakomori et al., 1977). NIH 3T3 cells transfected and transformed by *ras*-K oncogene were characterized by synthesis of gangliotriaosylceramide (Tsuchiya and Hakomori, 1983). However, the majority of glycosylation changes cannot be correlated to oncogene expression, or vice versa. It is important to emphasize that essentially all experimental tumors in human as well as animal systems have been characterized by aberrant glycosylation, but that the majority do not express oncogenes. The highest incidence of oncogene expression, even by combination of polymerase chain reaction, is <40%.

---

ential orientation of carbohydrate chain on the lipid bilayer. In this model, the epitope is stabilized by fixation of carbohydrate chains on the hydrophilic heads of lipid molecules, and hydrophobic areas are exposed on top of the chains. Factor 4: A given glycolipid structure assumes a different conformation when packed at high density in the lipid bilayer.

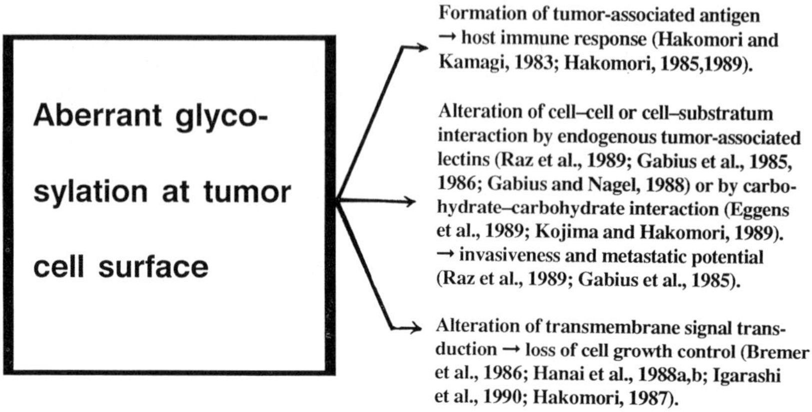

Fig. 4. Cell biological significance of aberrant glycosylation at the tumor-cell surface. Three possible consequences are briefly described, and references listed.

How can we explain aberrant glycosylation in the context of tumor cell biology? Is aberrant glycosylation an essential mechanism for maintenance of uncontrolled cell growth, metastatic potential, invasiveness, and the like? We have very few data relating to this fundamental question. Since certain oligosaccharides, particularly in multivalent form, strongly inhibit cell–cell adhesion, and certain sugar sequences are regarded as important recognition signals (Fenderson et al., 1984), carbohydrate-recognition mechanisms are of primary importance for understanding invasiveness and metastatic potential of tumors. On the other hand, gangliosides and their catabolites have been shown to affect transmembrane signal transduction through growth-factor-dependent receptor kinases, C kinases, and other protein kinases (Bremer et al., 1986; Hanai et al., 1988a,b; Igarashi et al., 1989, 1990). Major alteration of ganglioside metabolism may be implicated as being closely related to the failure of tumor cells to exert self-control of growth, although the possible mechanism for this is completely unknown. These possibilities are briefly summarized in Fig. 4.

Acknowledgment

The author's own work cited in this article has been supported by NIH Outstanding Investigator Grant CA42505 and by funds from The Biomembrane Institute.

References

Abe, K., S. B. Levery, and S. Hakomori (1984), *J. Immunol.* **132,** 1951–1954.
Abe, K., J. M. McKibbin, and S. Hakomori (1983), *J. Biol. Chem.* **258,** 11793–11797.
Ballou, B., R. Jaffe, R. J. Taylor, D. Solter, and T. R. Hakala (1984), *J. Immunol.* **132,** 2111–2116.
Ballou, B., J. M. Reiland, G. Levine, R. J. Taylor, W.-C. Shen, H. J.-P. Ryser, D. Solter, and T. R. Hakala (1986), *J. Surg. Oncol.* **31,** 1–12.
Bremer, E.G., S. B. Levery, S. Sonnino, R. Ghidoni, S. Canevari, R. Kannagi, and S. Hakomori (1984), *J. Biol. Chem.* **259,** 14773–14777.
Bremer, E., J. Schlessinger, and S. Hakomori (1986), *J. Biol. Chem.* **261,** 2434–2440.
Cahan, L. D., R. Irie, R. Singh, A. Cassidenti, and J. C. Paulson (1982), *Proc. Natl. Acad. Sci. USA* **79,** 7629-7633.
Clausen, H., S. Hakomori, N. Graem, and E. Dabelsteen (1986), *J. Immunol.* **136,** 326–330.
Clausen, H., S. B. Levery, J. M. McKibbin, and S. Hakomori (1985a), *Biochemistry* **24,** 3578–3586.
Clausen, H., S. B. Levery, E. Nudelman, M. Baldwin, and S. Hakomori, (1986), *Biochemistry* **25,** 7075–7085.
Clausen, H., J. M. McKibbin, and S. Hakomori (1985b), *Biochemistry* **24,** 6190–6194.
Dabelsteen, E., N. Graem, H. Clausen, and S. Hakomori (1988), *Cancer Res.* **48,** 181–187.
Dabelsteen, E., P. Vedtofte, S. Hakomori, and W. W. Young, Jr. (1983), *Cancer Res.* **43,** 1451–1454.
Davidsohn, I., S. Kovarik, and C. L. Lee (1966), *Arch. Pathol.* **81,** 381–390.
Davis, B. D., R. Dulbecco, H. Eisen, H. S. Ginsberg, and W. B. Wood (1967), in *Microbiology*, Harper & Row, New York, pp. 880–896.
Dohi, T., G. Nores, and S. Hakomori (1988), *Cancer Res.* **48,** 5680–5685.
Eggens, I., B. A. Fenderson, T. Toyokuni, B. Dean, M. R. Stroud, and S. Hakomori (1989), *J. Biol. Chem.* **264,** 9476–9484.
Fenderson, B. A., U. Zehavi, and S. Hakomori (1984), *J. Exp. Med.* **160,** 1591–1596.
Fukushi, Y., S. Hakomori, E. Nudelman, and N. Cochran (1984a), *J. Biol. Chem.* **259,** 4681-4685.

Fukushi, Y., E. Nudelman, S. B. Levery, H. Rauvala, and S. Hakomori (1984b), *J. Biol. Chem.* **259,** 10511–10517.
Gabius, H.-J. and G. A. Nagel (1988), in *Lectins and Glycoconjugates in Oncology,* Springer-Verlag, Berlin.
Gabius, H.-J., R. Engelhardt, and F. Cramer (1986), *Anticancer Res.* **6,** 573–578.
Gabius, H.-J., R. Engelhardt, F. Cramer, R. Batge, and G. A. Nagel (1985), *Cancer Res.* **45,** 253–257.
Hakomori, S. (1985), *Cancer Res.* **45,** 2405–2414.
Hakomori, S. (1986), *Sci. Am.* **254,** 44–53.
Hakomori, S. (1987), in *Oncogenes and Growth Factors* (Bradshaw, R. A. and S. Prentis, eds.), Elsevier Science, Amsterdam, pp. 218–226.
Hakomori, S. (1989), *Adv. Cancer Res.* **52,** 257–331.
Hakomori, S. and H. Andrews (1970), *Biochim. Biophys. Acta* **202,** 225–228.
Hakomori, S. and R.W. Jeanloz (1964), *J. Biol. Chem.* **239,** 3606,3607.
Hakomori, S. and R. Kannagi (1983), *J. Natl. Cancer Inst.* **71,** 231–251.
Hakomori, S. and W. T. Murakami (1968), *Proc. Natl. Acad. Sci. USA* **59,** 254–261.
Hakomori, S., S. M. Wang, and W. W. Young, Jr. (1977a), *Proc. Natl. Acad. Sci. USA* **74,** 3023–3027.
Hakomori, S., J. A. Wyke, and P. K. Vogt (1977b), *Virology* **76,** 485–493.
Hakomori, S., E. Nudelman, S. B. Levery, and R. Kannagi (1984), *J. Biol. Chem.* **259,** 4672–4680.
Hakomori, S., E. Nudelman, S. B. Levery, D. Solter, and B. B. Knowles (1981), *Biochem. Biophys. Res. Commun.* **100,** 1578–1586.
Hakomori, S., W. W. Young, Jr., L. M. Patt, T. Yoshino, L. Halfpap, and C. A. Lingwood (1980), in *Structure and Function of Gangliosides* (Svennerholm, L., H. Dreyfus, and P.-F. Urban, eds.), Plenum, New York, pp. 247–261.
Hanai, N., T. Dohi, G. A. Nores, and S. Hakomori (1988a), *J. Biol. Chem.* **263,** 6296–6301.
Hanai, N., G. A. Nores, C. MacLeod, C.-R. Torres-Mendez, and S. Hakomori (1988b), *J. Biol. Chem.* **263,** 10915–10921.
Handa, K., Y. Kato, and S. Hakomori (1991), unpublished.
Harada, Y., M. Sakatsume, G. A. Nores, S. Hakomori, and M. Taniguchi (1989), *Jpn. J. Cancer Res.* **80,** 988–992.
Hattori, H., K. Uemura, H. Ogata, T. Katsuyama, T. Taketomi, and J. N. Kanfer (1987), *Cancer Res.* **47,** 1968–1972.
Henningsson, C. M. et al. (1987), *Cancer Immunol. Immunother.* **25,** 231–241.
Hirabayashi, Y., A. Hanaoka, M. Matsumoto, T. Matsubara, M. Tagawa, S. Wakabayashi, and M. Taniguchi (1985), *J. Biol. Chem.* **260,** 13328–13333.
Hirohashi, S., H. Clausen, T. Yamada, Y. Shimosato, and S. Hakomori (1985), *Proc. Natl. Acad. Sci. USA* **82,** 7039–7043.

Holmes, E. H., S. Hakomori, and G. K. Ostrander (1987), *J. Biol. Chem.* **262,** 15649–15658.

Igarashi, Y., S. Hakomori, T. Toyokuni, B. Dean, S. Fujita, M. Sugimoto, T. Ogawa, K. El-Ghendy, and E. Racker (1989), *Biochemistry* **28,** 6796–6800.

Igarashi, Y., K. Kitamura, T. Toyokuni, B. Dean, B. A. Fenderson, T. Ogawa, and S. Hakomori (1990), *J. Biol. Chem.* **265,** 5385–5389.

Ito, M., E. Suzuki, M. Naiki, F. Sendo, and S. Arai (1984), *Int. J. Cancer* **34,** 689–697.

Kaizu, T., S. B. Levery, E. Nudelman, R. E. Stenkamp, and S. Hakomori (1986), *J. Biol. Chem.* **261,** 11254–11258.

Kannagi, R., D. Roelcke, K. A. Peterson, Y. Okada, S. B. Levery, and S. Hakomori (1983a), *Carbohydr. Res.* **120,** 143–157.

Kannagi, R., R. Stroup, N. A. Cochran, D. L. Urdal, W.W. Young, Jr., and S. Hakomori (1983b), *Cancer Res.* **43,** 4997–5005.

Kannagi, R., P. Levine, K. Watanabe, and S. Hakomori (1982), *Cancer Res.* **42,** 5249–5254.

Kjeldsen, T., H. Clausen, S. Hirohashi, T. Ogawa, H. Iijima, and S. Hakomori (1988), *Cancer Res.* **48,** 2214–2220.

Kjeldsen, T., S. Hakomori, G. F. Springer, P. Desai, T. Harris, and H. Clausen (1989), *Vox Sang.* **57,** 81–87.

Koenderman, A. H., P. L. Koppen, and D. H. van den Eijnden (1987), *Eur. J. Biochem.* **166,** 199–208.

Kojima, N. and S. Hakomori (1989), *J. Biol. Chem.* **264,** 20159–20162.

Kurosaka, A., H. Kitagawa, S. Fukui, Y. Numata, H. Nakada, I. Funakoshi, T. Kawasaki, T. Ogawa, H. Iijima, and I. Yamashina (1988), *J. Biol. Chem.* **263,** 8724–8726.

Levine, P., O. B. Bobbit, R. K. Waller, and A. Kuhmichel (1951), *Proc. Soc. Exp. Biol. Med.* **77,** 403–405.

Masamune, H., Z. Yosizawa, K. Oh-Uti, J. Matsuda, and A. Masukawa (1952) *Tohoku J. Exp. Med.* **56,** 37–42.

Matsuura, H. and S. Hakomori (1985), *Proc. Natl. Acad. Sci. USA* **82,** 6517–6521.

Matsuura, H., K. Takio, K. Titani, T. Greene, S. B. Levery, M. E. K. Salyan, and S. Hakomori (1988), *J. Biol. Chem.* **263,** 3314–3322.

Metoki, R., K. Kakudo, Y. Tsuji, N. Teng, H. Clausen, and S. Hakomori (1989), *J. Natl. Cancer Inst.* **81,** 1151–1157.

Mora, P. T., R. O. Brady, R. M. Bradley, and V. W. McFarland (1969), *Proc. Natl. Acad. Sci. USA* **63,** 1290–1296.

Nilsson, O., J.-E. Mansson, T. Brezicka, J. Holmgren, L. Lindholm, S. Sorenson, F. Yngvason, and L. Svennerholm (1984), *Glycoconjugate J.* **1,** 43–49.

Nores, G. A., T. Dohi, M. Taniguchi, and S. Hakomori (1987), *J. Immunol.* **139,** 3171–3176.

Nudelman, E., S. B. Levery, T. Kaizu, and S. Hakomori (1986), *J. Biol. Chem.* **261,** 11247–11253.

Nudelman, E. D., S. B. Levery, M. R. Stroud, M. E. K. Salyan, K. Abe, and S. Hakomori (1988), *J. Biol. Chem.* **263,** 13942–13951.

Nudelman, E., R. Kannagi, S. Hakomori, M. Parsons, M. Lipinski, J. Wiels, M. Fellous, and T. Tursz (1983), *Science* **220,** 509–511.

Nudelman, E., S. Hakomori, R. Kannagl, S. B. Levery, M.-Y. Yeh, K.-E. Hellstrom, and I. Hellstrom (1982), *J. Biol. Chem.* **257,** 12752-12756.

Ørntoft, T. F., N. Harving T. Kjeldsen, S. Hakomori, G. F. Springer, and H. Clausen, unpublished data.

Paul, W. E. (1989) *Fundamental Immunology,* Raven, NY, pp. 52, 53.

Raz, A., G. Pazerini, and P. Carmi (1989), *Cancer Res.* **49,** 3489–3493.

Rosenfelder, G., W. W. Young, Jr., and S. Hakomori (1977), *Cancer Res.* **37,** 1333–1339.

Singhal, A. K., M. C. Singhal, E. Nudelman, S. Hakomori, J. P. Balint, C. K. Grant, and H. W. Snyder, Jr. (1987), *Cancer Res.* **47,** 5566–5571.

Singhal, A., M. Fohn, and S. Hakomori (1991), *Cancer Res.* **51,** 1406–1411.

Symington, F.W., I. D. Bernstein, and S. Hakomori (1984), *J. Biol. Chem.* **259,** 6008–6012.

Takahashi, H. K., R. Metoki, and S. Hakomori (1988), *Cancer Res.* **48,** 4361–4367.

Taniguchi, M., M. Sakatsume, Y. Harada, G. A. Nores, and S. Hakomori (1989), in *Immune System and Cancer* (Hamaoka, T., ed.), Jpn. Sci. Soc., Tokyo, pp. 247–254.

Taniguchi, N., N. Yokosawa, M. Narita, T. Mitsuyama, and A. Makita (1981), *J. Natl. Cancer Inst.* **67,** 577–583.

Taniguchi, M. and S. Wakabayashi (1984), *Jpn. J. Cancer Res.* **75,** 418–426.

Tsuchiya, S. and S. Hakomori (1983), *EMBO J.* **2,** 2323–2326.

Umeda M., I. Diego, and D. M. Marcus (1986), *J. Immunol.* **137,** 3264–3269.

Urdal, D. L. and S. Hakomori (1983), *J. Biol. Chem.* **258,** 6869–6874.

Watanabe, K., M. Powell, and S. Hakomori (1978), *J. Biol. Chem.* **253,** 8962–8967.

Watanabe, K., M. E. Powell, and S. Hakomori (1979), *J. Biol. Chem.* **254,** 8223–8229.

Welt, S. W., E. A. Carswell, C.-W. Vogel, H. F. Oettgen, and L. J. Old (1987), *Clin. Immunol. Immunopathol.* **45,** 214–229.

Wiels, J., E. H. Holmes, N. Cochran, T. Tursz, and S. Hakomori (1984), *J. Biol. Chem.* **259,** 14783–14787.

Yang, H.-J. and S. Hakomori (1971), *J. Biol. Chem.* **246,** 1192–1200.

Yoshino, T., K. Watanabe, and S. Hakomori (1982), *Biochemistry* **21,** 928–934.

Chapter 11

Glycoamines: Structural–Functional Characterization of a New Class of Human Tumor Markers

Gennadi V. Glinsky

1. Introduction

Glycoamines (aminoglycoconjugates) represent a previously unknown class of endogenous biopolymers that circulate in mammalian blood plasma. The characterization of glycoamines as a new class of potential humoral tumor markers is of great interest, since the level of the free form of glycoamines is known to be elevated in blood plasma from animals and humans with a wide range of malignant neoplasms and leukoses (Glinsky, 1988a,b, 1989). It is important that at least in some forms of human malignant tumor the level of glycoamines is already increased at the early stages of the disease.

Structural–functional analysis of aminoglycoconjugates implies a structural–functional resemblance between glycoamines and linear polyamines (Glinsky, 1987, 1988a,b). Direct biological action of glycoamines may be attributed not only to the presence in them of free amino groups, but also to the active group of glyco-

From: *Serological Cancer Markers* Edited by Stewart Sell ©1992 The Humana Press, Totowa, NJ

amine amino acid radical and the keto groups of carbohydrates. In the last case, the mechanism of glycoamine action may be similar to the mechanism of the action of carbohydrate aldehydes. A reaction of this type may probably determine the covalent incorporation of glycoamines into proteins. But the hypothesis that seems the most intriguing for us is that glycoamines present a humoral "molecular imprint" of the carbohydrate epitopes of carbohydrate-containing antigens. A number of important biological functions of glycoamines may be determined by the carbohydrate part of the molecule. This paper presents some of the data on the structure, biology, and biochemistry of glycoamines. These data characterize glycoamines as polyfunctional substances that may reveal their biological activity at different levels of organization: from the molecular and subcellular to the organism level.

2. Structural Generalization

The chemical structure of glycoamines represents carbohydrate–amino acid conjugates that contain from 5 to 23 amino acids and from 1 to 17 carbohydrate residues. Amino acids in glycoamines are joined to the carbohydrate core part of the molecule via the ester bonds. The structure of over 53 aminoglycoconjugates isolated from the blood plasma of rodents and humans has been investigated (Glinsky, 1989).

We can now present two structural models of aminoglycoconjugates purified from blood plasma of oncology patients (Glinsky et al., 1990). These models are based on the data of the amino acid and carbohydrate composition, protein sequence, infrared spectroscopy, structural investigation of the carbohydrate core of the molecule, and intermediate products obtained after mild acidic and alkaline hydrolyses. In accordance with the first model, the amino acids are joined to the core carbohydrate components via ester bonds and separate amino acid–carbohydrate blocks are joined in the molecule through the glucose aldehydes by way of the formation of Schiff bases and Amadori products (Fig. 1). The structure of the

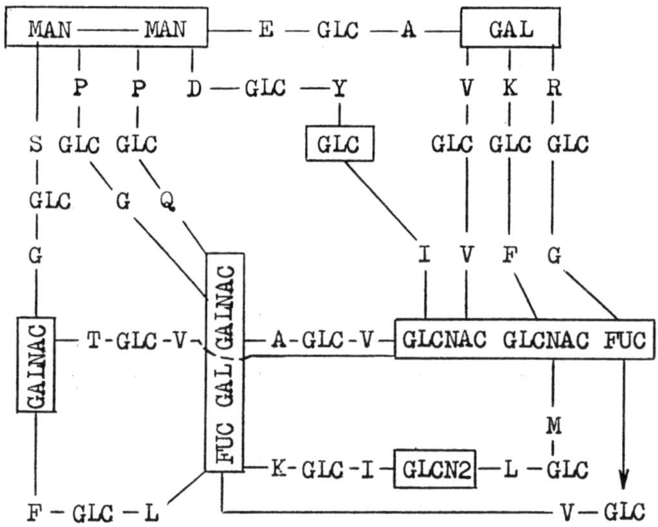

Fig. 1. Structure of the type-1 glycoamine.

second type of glycoamine differs to a certain extent from this model. According to structural analysis, the carbohydrate blocks are joined via the amino acid "bridges" with the formation of ester bonds, Schiff bases, and Amadori products. The monosaccharide components form the peripheral part of the molecule and their reducing ends are available for the interaction with 7-amino-4-methylcoumarin (AMC) in the reaction of reducing amination. The reducing ends of disaccharides and trisaccharides are blocked and become available for the interaction with AMC in the reaction of reducing amination after lithium borohydride hydrolysis, which probably destroys bonds that are more stable than Schiff bases, the Amadori product type bonds (Fig. 2). Thus, the structural analysis of glycoamines reveals that the amino acids and carbohydrates are linked by labile bonds. At least some of these bonds (Schiff bases and Amadori products) may be formed nonenzymatically. Further investigations showed that glycoamines are able to incorporate monomeric carbohydrates and amino acids by a nonenzymatic mecha-

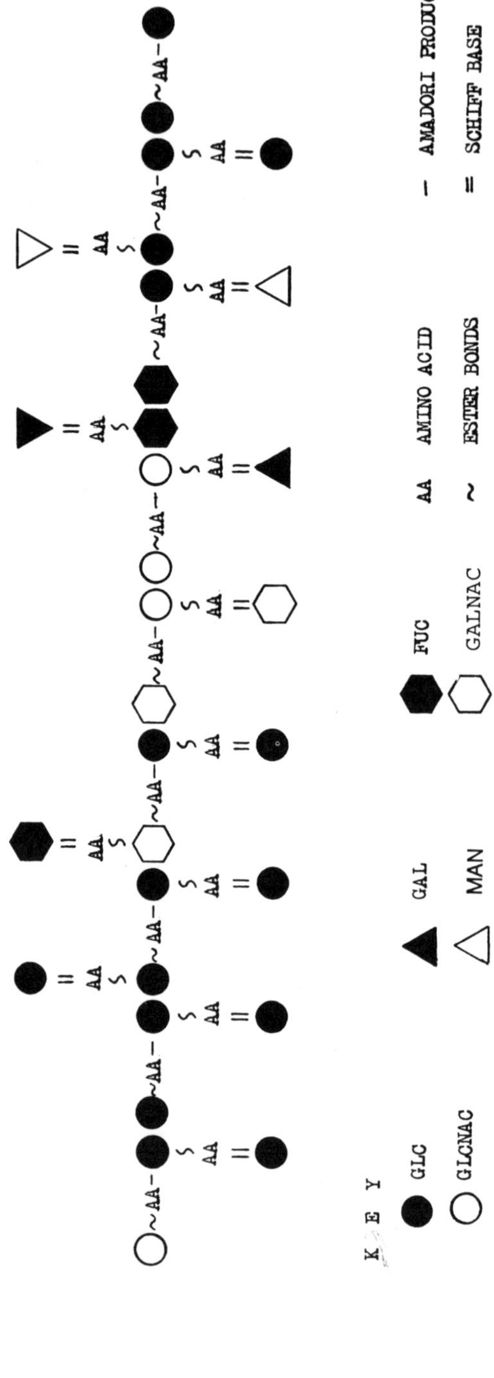

Fig. 2. Structure of the type-2 glycoamine.

nism (Glinsky and Linetsky, 1990). In the case of carbohydrates, the reaction involves the formation of Schiff bases, Amadori products, and fluorescent advanced nonenzymatic glycation products (Glinsky and Linetsky, 1990). In the case of amino acids, the reaction of nonenzymatic incorporation involves the formation of Schiff bases, subsequent spontaneous hydrolysis of Schiff bases accompanied by intramolecular rearrangement, with the formation of an ester bond between the amino acid carboxyl and carbohydrate hydroxyl and "secondary" blocking of the amino acid L-amino group as a result of the interaction with the aldehyde or keto group.

The results of investigations on the structure and biogenesis of glycoamines reveal a unique capacity of these compounds for nonenzymatic modification of the peripheral part of the molecule by way of incorporation of new amino acid and carbohydrate units. The analysis of the interrelation structure–function with the use of chemical, biochemical, spectroscopic, and biological methods indicates that amino acids and carbohydrates are the main structural–functional determinants of glycoamines. Thus, the structural studies on natural glycoamines and their synthetic analogs, along with the identification of the structural–functional determinants of aminoglycoconjugates, provide the chemical basis for the hypothesis on humoral molecular "imprints." Investigations of the biological properties of glycoamines reveal the carbohydrate component as their key structural–functional determinant. One of the main reactions of the biogenesis of glycoamines is the nonenzymatic interaction between the carbohydrate aldehydes and L-amino groups of amino acids (Glinsky and Linetsky, 1990).

3. Glycoamine-Dependent Mechanism of the Modification of In Vitro Formation of Multicellular Spheroids by Tumor Cells: Similarities of the In Vivo Malignant Growth

One of the characteristic features of the growth of malignant tumors cultivated in vitro is their ability to form three-dimensional spheroid-like structures—the multicellular spheroids (Mueller-Kleiser, 1987; Sutherland, 1988). The similar (according to biochemical, immunocytochemical, morphological, and cytological criteria) spheroid-like formations are detected in rodent and human malignant tumors in vivo. Therefore the multicellular spheroids are considered a cytofunctional analog of the avascular stage of in vivo tumor development (Sutherland, 1988). Under our experimental conditions, about 90 of the spheroids formed by tumor cells are in suspension and about 10% are attached to the substrate. The fraction of blood serum from tumor bearers with a mol wt over 100 kDa stimulates spheroid formation, increasing the number of spheroids in suspension twofold (Fig. 3). Glycoamines inhibit the tumor spheroid formation by over 95%, bringing about dramatic changes in adhesion properties of tumor cells and the disaggregation of multicellular spheroids. What is the mechanism of this phenomenon? One possible mechanism is the one we have discussed in detail previously (Glinsky, 1989). At that time we had available data on the biochemical synergism of glycoamines and linear polyamines as potential antiadhesion factors that favor the dissemination of tumor cells (Glinsky, 1989). Primary amine-dependent restraint on the activity of protease inhibitors may play an important role in this effect. The molecular scenario of the events may be following (Fig. 4).

Glycoamine-dependent restraint on the inhibitory activity of α-2-macroglobulin favors the thrombin-mediated activation of plasma transglutaminase and activates the proteolysis. Under the conditions of hyperpolyaminemia, the activated transglutaminase incorporates polyamines into proteins, preventing in this way the ε(γ-glutamyl) lysine protein–protein crosslinks required for cell adhesion and the formation of cell contacts. Simultaneously, the ε-lysine amino groups in proteins are liberated for the ubiquitination (intracellular proteins) and/or the nonenzymatic glycation. This leads in turn to the activation of proteolysis, the disturbances in protein functions, and finally to the invasion of tumor cells. The enhanced nonenzymatic glycation associated with the transglutaminase-dependent incorporation of polyamines into proteins may provide an

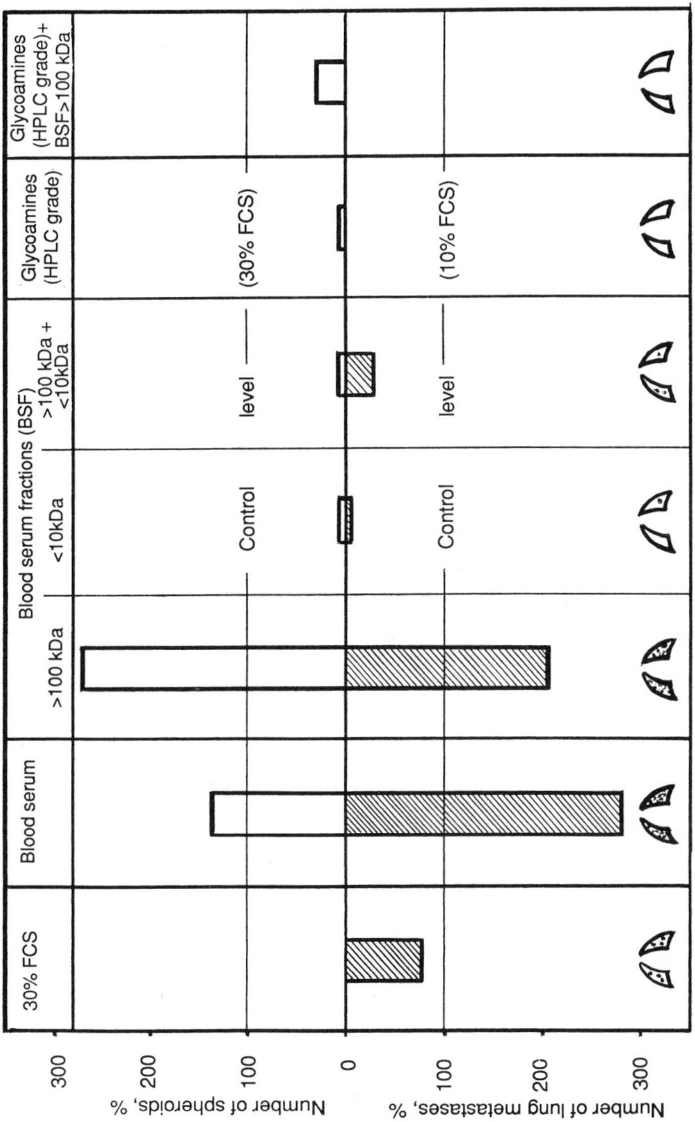

Fig. 3. Effects of glycoamines and fractions of blood serum on the spheroid formation in vitro and metastatic spreading in vivo.

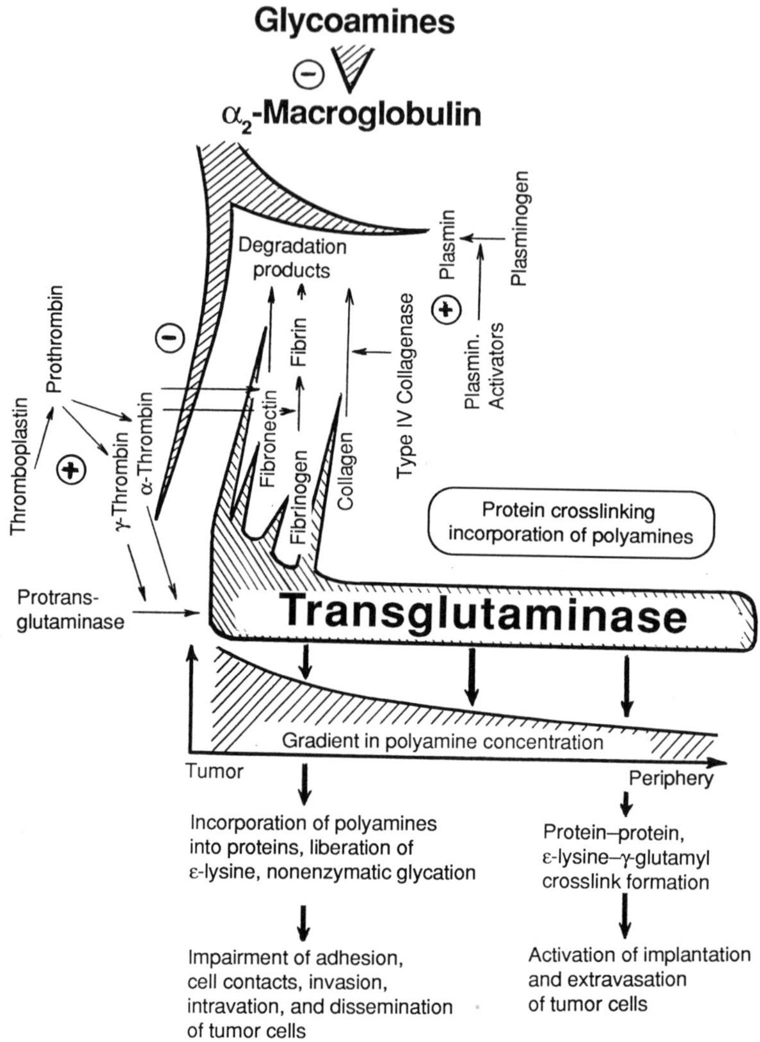

Fig. 4. "Cooperative" mechanism of the antiadhesive action of glycoamines and polyamines.

important factor that alters the sensitivity of tumor stroma to the proteolysis. Under decreased concentration of polyamines in the circulatory channel and in sites distant from the tumor tissues of host organism, the activated transglutaminase catalyzes the formation of ε(γ-glutamyl) lysine protein–protein crosslinks and sets of the implantation mechanism.

This pathway may be called a "cooperative" mechanism of the action of glycoamines when they function together with polyamines. Further in vivo and in vitro investigations on glycoamines have revealed a suppression of immunological response to tumor antigens. Thus, it is possible that glycoamines may be a humoral factor contributing to tumor-associated immunosuppression. The stimulation of spheroid formation in suspensions induced by serum proved to be caused by immunoglobulins and is probably associated with reactions of the antigen–antibody type. The fraction of blood serum with a mol wt below 10 kDa and glycoamines also inhibit the in vitro reassociation of lymphocyte–macrophage aggregates isolated from the spleen of tumor-bearing animals. These data, in conjunction with the analysis of glycoamine structure, enabled us to formulate the hypothesis of a monovalent mechanism of antiadhesive and immunosuppressive action of aminoglycoconjugates (Fig. 5).

Malignant transformation-associated aberrant glycosylation of cell-membrane glycomacromolecules of tumor cells alters their antigenic and adhesive properties. These alterations provide a trigger or specific T- and B-cellular immunological reactions. Aberrant glycosylation also leads to the modification of homo- and heterotypical cell adhesion and cell–cell contacts, since the oligosaccharide part of glycomacromolecules is known to play the key role in these processes. The carbohydrate epitopes of glycomacromolecular antigens are represented mainly by mono-, di-, and trisaccharides, as was shown by recent investigations. Tumor and serum glycosidases remove from the cell-membrane glycomacromolecules of tumor cells the mono-, di-, and trisaccharides, which are incorporated into glycoamine molecules by nonenzymatic mechanism. In this way specific humoral molecular "imprints" of the carbohydrate epitopes of glycomacromolecular antigens of tumor cell membranes are formed. These compounds may cause specific blocking of the antitumor immunological reactions and a modification of adhesive properties of tumor cells. In this way the monovalent

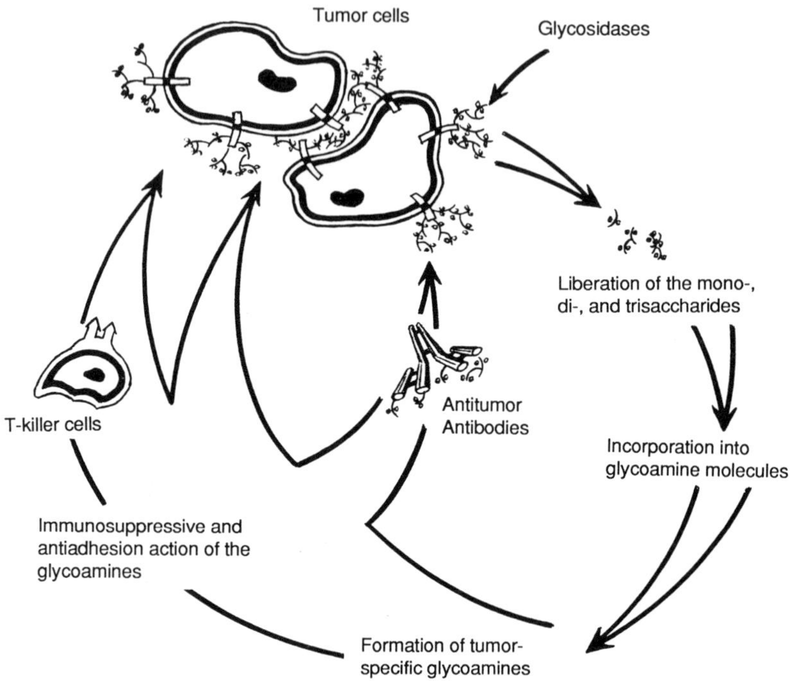

Fig. 5. "Monovalent" mechanism of the antiadhesive and immunosuppressive action of glycoamines.

mechanism of the antiadhesive and immunosuppressive action of glycoamines may be realized.

Of great importance is the phenomenon of complete correspondence between the effect of blood-serum fractions on spheroid formation in vitro and their effect on metastatic spreading in vivo after intravenous inoculation of tumor cells. The fraction of blood serum with a mol wt over 100 kDa increases the number of tumor-cell colonies in the lungs over twofold, whereas the fractions with a mol wt below 10 kDa considerably inhibit the formation of lung metastases and remove the stimulation of metastasizing by the high-mol-wt fraction of blood serum (Fig. 3).

4. The Biology of Glycoamines: Several Physiological and Pathophysiological Aspects

Amino acids and carbohydrates were identified as the main structural–functional determinants of the glycoamines. The functional identification of carbohydrate determinants was performed in the hemagglutination inhibition test, in the peptide–protein binding assay, in the lectin chromatography, and in the test of the inhibition of aggregate formation by tumor cells.

The suggested hypothesis of humoral molecular "imprints" that explains our experimental data is evidently only one of the numerous possible pathophysiological applications to cancer of the putative function of glycoamines as a circulatory form of the carbohydrate epitopes of glycomacromolecular antigens and endogenous ligands of mammalian lectins (Table 1). For example, of great interest is the study of aminoglycoconjugates as a transport form of carbohydrates and amino acids in view of the possibility of monomolecular transport of energetic and plastic substrates from the extracellular medium into the cell. It may well be that this process occurs in mammals with the participation of lectinlike cell-membrane proteins. Another example concerns the nonenzymatic covalent incorporation of glycoamines into proteins and, possibly, into other macromolecules. This reaction would alter the antigenic properties of macromolecules, permitting the development of autoimmune reactions. On the other hand, covalent incorporation of glycoamines into proteins may lead to an enhancement in their affinity for polyanions (proteoglycans, nucleic acids, cytoskeletal proteins) and to the molecular transcompartmentalization of the modified macromolecules (Fig. 6). Structural–functional resemblance between glycoamines and polyamines suggests that increased concentrations of the latter may cause the dissociation of the complex polyanion–glycoamine–modified protein by a competitive mechanism. Since cell proliferation significantly increases the levels of polyamines and glycoamines, this mechanism

Table 1
Postulated Biological Functions of Glycoamines (Aminoglycoconjugates)

Level	Postulated function
Organism	Modification of the action of the neuroendocrine system by altering peptide–protein binding in organism body fluids and the transport of regulatory biomolecules through biological barriers (blood–brain barrier, hematoparenchymatous barrier).
Organism	Alterations in half-lives of regulatory biomolecules caused by modifications of their extracellular catabolism (altered binding and availability of ligands for proteolytic degradation, disturbed function of protease inhibitors) and by alterations in the excretion and efficiency of the uptake of glycoamine-modified molecules by the tissue from blood.
Organism	Regulation of the reactions of nonenzymatic glycation of protein and control of the level of glucose aldehyde in blood.
Organism	Involvement in humoral mechanisms of the maintenance of immunity.
Tissue and cellular	Amplification and intratissue reprogramming of mitogenic and/or hormonal signal through the activation of serum growth factors and protein-bound hormones.
Tissue and cellular	Alterations in cell adhesion properties and structural–functional characteristics of the extracellular matrix glycoproteins.
Tissue and cellular	Modification of ligand–receptor interactions and the properties of membrane glycoproteins.
Intracellular	Monomolecular transport of energetic (hexoses) and plastic (amino acids) molecules—possibly also ions, metal, and the like. Role of the interaction of glycoamines and linear polyamines.

(continued)

Table 1 *(continued)*

Level	Postulated function
Intracellular	Intracellular transcompartmentalization of regulatory macromolecules. "Transport" and "sorting" of macromolecules, reprogramming of the genome, and control of translation by way of postponing the affinity of glycoamine-modified macromolecules for polyanion sites (the system proteins, nucleic acids, and proteins–cytoskeleton, protein–protein binding). Role of structural–functional resemblance between glycoamines and linear polyamines.
Intracellular	Modification of intracellular catabolism and processing of macromolecules (PEST- and ubiquitin-dependent proteolysis, splicing). Role of cytoskeleton, protein–protein binding, and linear polyamine.
Intracellular	Involvement of the enole form of glycoamines in free-radical reactions.

may provide a regulator of molecular transcompartmentalization during mitogenesis.

Because of their ability to circulate in free and protein-bound forms, the glycoamines may determine directed cell migration. If the composition of free and protein-bound glycoamines includes the carbohydrate epitopes involved in cell recognition and formation of cell–cell contacts, then glycoamines may determine both the "negative chemotaxis" and "positive haptotaxis," and control cell migration.

5. Glycoamines as One of the Key Humoral Factors of Cancer Pathogenesis

In conclusion, an attempt will be made to put forward a hypothesis on the role of glycoamines as a factor of dissemination of

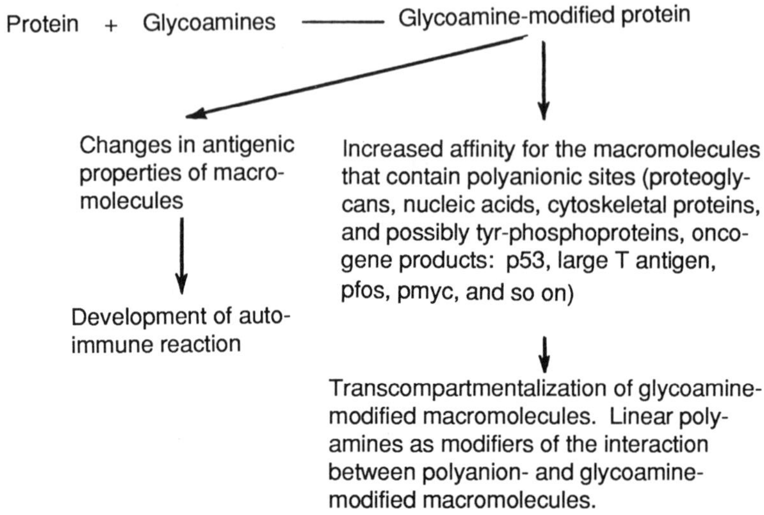

Fig. 6. Consequences of the covalent modification of proteins by glycoamines.

tumor cells in malignant growth. In Fig. 7 the results of experiments on the effect of combined administration of glycoamines and spermidine on the metastatic spreading of Lewis carcinoma under the ablation of primary tumor are represented. Administration of glycoamines and spermidine stimulated lung metastases threefold, mainly because of the increase in the number of metastases. We have shown that the effect of stimulation of metastatic spreading is exhibited under the condition that the administration of glycoamines and spermidine starts in the presence of primary tumor. The effect disappears when the administration starts one day after the ablation of primary tumor. Thus, the glycoamine- and spermidine-dependent stimulation of metastatic spreading is associated with the activation of tumor-cell dissemination from the primary focus.

How does the glycoamine-dependent mechanism of the dissemination of tumor cells operate? In vivo development of tumor at the avascular stage is characterized by the formation of multicellular spheroids and by the elevated levels of polyamines and

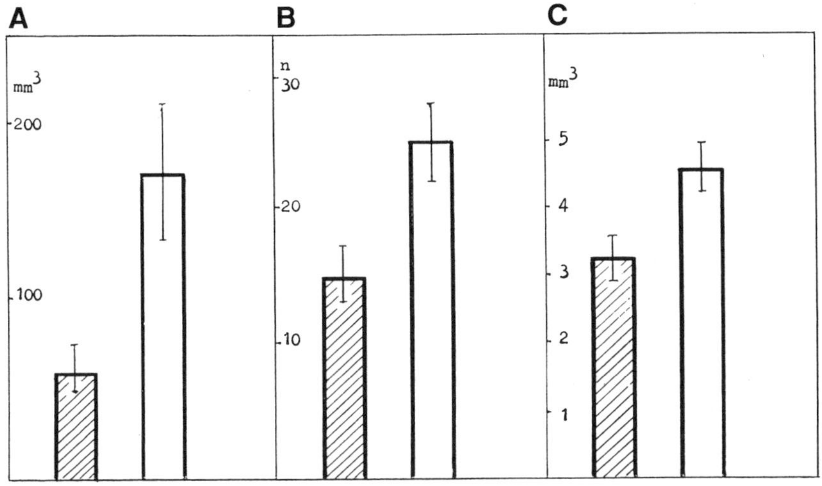

Fig. 7. Effect of combined administration of glycoamines and spermidine (▨, control; □, glycosamines + spermidine) on the metastatic spreading: **A,** metastases volume; **B,** number of metastases; **C,** average volume of one metastasis.

glycoamines in the tumor zone. These levels increase simultaneously with the growth of the mass of tumor cells (Fig. 8). The development of necrosis in the central zone of tumor spheroid with the release of hydrolytic enzymes brings about dramatic activation of catabolic reactions. The vascularization rapidly activates tumor growth, leading to a rapid increase in the concentration of polyamines and tumor-specific glycoamines in the tumor zone and to the formation of a sharp concentration gradient of polyamines and glycoamines among the tumor, normal tissues, and hemo- and lymphocirculatory channels. The "cooperative" and "monovalent" antiadhesion action of glycoamines causes the disaggregation, dissociation, and release of tumor cells from the multicellular spheroids into the zone of primary tumor. The presence of specific antibodies against tumor-cell glycomacromolecules in the extracellular fluid, lymph, and blood favors the translocation and spreading of tumor cells against the concentration gradient of polyamines and glycoamines. The presence of antitumor antibodies in the hemo-

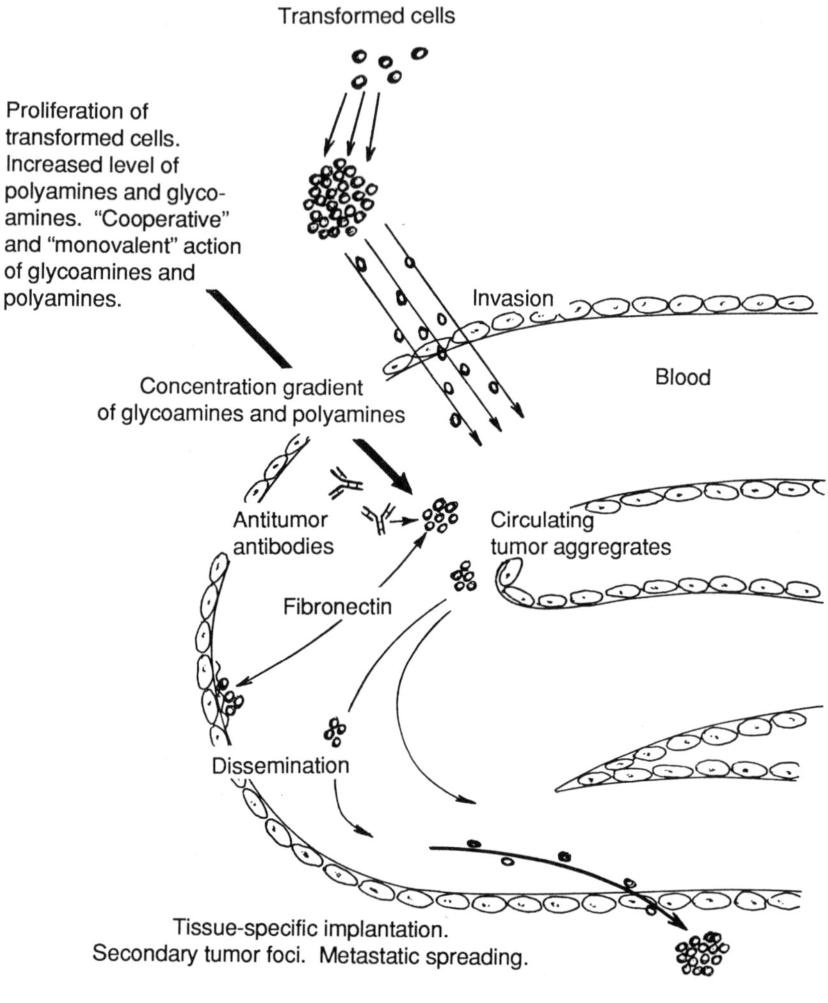

Fig. 8. Glycoamine-dependent mechanism of the dissemination of tumor cells.

and lymphocirculatory channels favors the formation of tumor aggregates and the dissemination of tumor cells (Fig. 8).

The represented views are based on the development of our previously suggested idea on the monomolecular, humorally mediated mechanism of the formation of biological properties of malignant tumors (Glinsky, 1989). The mechanism enables the revelation of causal–consequential relations among the most important attributes of malignancy: relative autonomy of growth; the disturbances in cell adhesion and cell–cell contacts; and the abilities for invasion, dissemination, implantation, metastatic spreading of tumor cells, and systemic disturbances in the metabolism. The autonomy of growth is a fundamental, basic property of neoplastic transformation. Proliferaton-associated excessive accumulation of primary amines (mono-, di-, and polyamines) and aminoglycoconjugates in the extracellular medium and biological fluids of tumor host would inevitably lead to the formation of the classical range of malignancy attributes. From Table 2, it is clear that the development of many, if not all, attributes of in vivo malignancy that characterize the progressive course of tumoral disease may be related to the biological action of glycoamines. It is also clear that the glycoamine conception concludes the key role of aberrant glycosylation in the pathogenesis of cancer. Do not the new facts in our knowledge about cancer as a disease today enable us to return to the old understanding of this disease as a polyetiological and monopathogenetic pathological process? In addition, these new facts enable us to understand cancer as a unique pathological process for every individual, requiring the development of individual means of therapy.

6. Conclusion: Aberrant Glycosylation, Glycoamines, and Immunoselective Mechanism of Tumor Progression

The process of cell adhesion consists of multiple steps, and the last model of such a multistep process was proposed by S. Hakomori and coworkers in 1989 (Eggest et al., 1989). The initial step is specific recognition between two cells in which multivalent carbohydrate–carbohydrate interactions mediated by bivalent cations may play a major role. Initial cell recognition through carbohydrate–carbohydrate interaction is followed by nonspecific adhesion, primarily mediated by Ca^{2+}-sensitive adhesion molecules

Table 2
Role of Glycoamines in the Formation of In Vivo Malignant Behavior of Tumor Cells

Biological properties of malignant tumors	Glycoamine-dependent mechanism of formation	Consequences for the interaction between tumor and organism in tumoral disease
1. Autonomous proliferation	Decreased binding in blood plasma of positive peptide growth factors and increased binding of negative growth factors.	Involvement of host growth factors in the in vivo growth of tumor and metastases.
2. Invasion	Blocking of the function of protease inhibitors (2-macroglobulin). Altered antigenic properties of host macromolecules.	Involvement of host proteases and immune system in the invasive growth of tumors.
3. Modification of adhesion. Dissemination of tumor cells from the primary focus, implantation.	Alpha-2 macroglobulin-dependent thrombin-mediated activation of plasma transglutaminase. Activation of the incorporation of primary amines into proteins and/or formation of specific protein–protein crosslinks. Carbohydrate epitope-dependent modification of the	Involvement of host blood-coagulation system and immune system (antibodies) in the modification of adhesive properties and dissemination and implantation of tumor cells.

	recognition function of the extracellular matrix glycoproteins and cell-membrane glycoproteins.	
4. Immunodepression	Carbohydrate epitope-dependent inhibition of the antibody- and cell-mediated immunological reactions.	Development of tumor-associated specific immunosuppression. Accumulation in the body of low-affinity antigen–antibody complexes, damage of renal function.
5. Systemic disturbances in the metabolism.	Modification of the blood plasma binding of neuropeptides and hormones, changes in the transport of peptide bioregulators through the blood–brain barrier, hematoparenchymatous barrier, and renal barrier. Altered half-lives of peptides and altered peptide–receptor interactions.	Formation of pathological biochemical axes: tumor–brain, tumor–liver, tumor–neuroendocrine system, and the like.

or sugar-binding proteins, or by pericellular adhesive meshwork proteins consisting of fibronectin, laminin, and their receptor systems (integrin). The third step of cell adhesion is the establishment of intercellular junctions, e.g., " gap junctions," in which a cell–cell communication channel is opened through a specific structural protein.

Of great importance is the fact that tumor cells retain to a great extent their ability to reveal initial stages of cell adhesion: at the same time cancer is characterized by profound disturbances in the subsequent stages of cell adhesion occurring with the involvement of extracellular matrix proteins and completing with the formation of specific "gap junctions."

Cell adhesion is processed mainly through recognition between similar types of cells. Thus, the "sorting-out" behavior of homotypic cell populations plays a major role in morphogenesis and organogenesis. Specific interaction between identical or similar carbohydrate chains highly expressed in the same type of cells may provide a better explanation for sorting out than the interaction of relatively nonspecific adhesive molecules (Eggest et al., 1989). We suggested that the recognition between identical types of cells that provides the basis for sorting one homotypic population out of a heterotypic assemblage of cells plays a major role in the metastatic spreading of tumor cells. This mechanism provides a basis for the formation of multicellular aggregates by tumor cells in the circulatory channel of tumor host and their subsequent arrest in blood vessel of target organs.

Since the glycoamines are able to block the cell adhesion process at various—both specific and nonspecific—stages, they can evidently be used as a new instrument in the pathogenetic antimetastatic cancer therapy. In this context of unquestionable theoretical and practical interest would be the elucidation of molecular determinants responsible for homotypic selection of tumor cells during tumor progression and structural identification of glycoamines and other serum factors involved in this process.

Two important conclusions can be drawn from the experiments on the investigation of the effect of glycoamines and fractions of blood serum on the cell aggregation in vitro and on metastasizing. First, the formation of oncoaggregates and reassociation of immunoaggregates occurs with the involvement of common or similar structural determinant, probably of carbohydrate nature. Second, the humoral (serum) constituents (glycoamines and high-mol-wt factors of blood serum) that are able to recognize these structural determinants are present not only in the cancer serum, but also (to a lesser extent) in the normal blood serum. Such structural determinants participating in the homotypic aggregation of histogenetically different types of cells may be, in particular, the carbohydrate determinants of the blood-group antigen (BGA) related glycoantigens, since normal blood serum contains anticarbohydrate antibodies (including those against BGA-related glycoepitopes), and preliminary data indicate the involvement of BGA-related glycoepitopes in the inhibition of hemagglutination by glycoamine.

At present most of the clinically used humoral tumor markers are glycomacromolecules (CEA, mucins, CA 19-9, C 15-3, CA 26); many of them contain the BGA-related glycoepitopes (Lewis family, T, Tn, I) (Magnani et al., 1982, 1983; Dube, 1987; Yamashita et al., 1987; Linsley et al., 1988) and reveal immunosuppressive properties (Hakim et al., 1984; Hakim, 1984). Blood serum from most healthy individual contains natural anticarbohydrate antibodies, including those against the BGA-related glycoepitopes (anti-A, B, H, O, I, and Lewis family; anti-Tn-antibodies; antiasialo GM_2 [Gal Nac β 1-4β Galβ 1-4 Glc-Cer]) (Lloyd, 1989). Blood serum from oncology patients reveals a decrease in the titers of anti-T, anti-Tn, anti-I, and anti-Forssman anticarbohydrate antibodies (Young et al., 1979; Springer, 1984; Dube, 1987). Finally, the most characteristic manifestation of aberrant glycosylation of cancer cells is neosynthesis (or ectopic synthesis), the synthesis of incompatible antigens and incomplete synthesis (with or without the accumulation of precursors) of the BGA-related glycoepitopes (Hakomori, 1984, 1989). BGA-related glycoepitopes are directly involved in the homotypic (tumor cells, embryonal cells) and heterotypic (tumor cells–normal cells) formation of cellular aggregates (e.g., Lewis X antigen, H antigen, polylactosamine sequences, and T- and Tn-antigen), which was demonstrated in different experimental systems (Springer et al., 1983; Springer, 1984; Fenderson et al., 1987, 1990; Glinsky, 1988a; Lindenberg et al., 1988).

It is very important that the characteristic presence of cancer BGA-related alterations in the tissue glycosylation pattern are detected in benign (premalignant) tumors with high risk of malignant transformation, in primary malignant tumors, and in metastases (Abe et al., 1986; Itzkowitz et al., 1986a,b, 1989; Kim et al., 1986; Hakomori, 1989), i.e., they were demonstrated as typical alterations in different stage of tumor progression. Lymphoid cell (lymphocytes, granulocytes, monocytes) are Lewis family glycoepitope-positive and contain T-antigen (Lloyd, 1988; Clausen and Hakomori, 1989; Stein et al., 1989) (demasked after treatment with neuraminidase). Based on these facts, we have suggested that the processes of thymic education and antigen presentation are accompanied by certain changes in the glycosylation pattern of the cellular membranes. These changes include the presentation of the BGA-related glycoepitopes—in particular, of their cryptic forms. A number of experimental data are now available that confirm this suggestion for antigen presentation. Effective antigen presentation occurs in cells expressing an increased number of histocompatibility antigens with decreased sialylation level (Booy et al., 1989). The cells infected with AIDS virus or cytomegalovirus start to express a high level of LeY and LeX glycoepitopes, respectively (Adachi et al., 1988; Andrews et al., 1989). This relatively nonspecific mechanism of the presentation of BGA-related glycoepitopes may be involved in the process of homotypic sorting of the cells at subsequent stages of formation of immune response. In view of this, natural anticarbohydrate antibodies may fulfill a double function: to accomplish the complement-dependent lysis of cells containing high-density BGA-related glycoepitopes (e.g., in the thymic education it may lead to negative selection of T-cells whose major histocompatibility complexes have a high affinity for their own presented antigens) and to favor the homotypic selection of cells revealing a medium or low density level of the BGA-related glycoepitopes. Similar mechanisms may be realized for tumor cells, but these interactions should also involve humoral glycomacromolecules that contain BGA-related glycoepitopes. It seems very intriguing to suggest that a similar mechanism is involved in the development of tumor progression and determines both its direction and the selection of metastasizing cell in cancer. Indirect confirmation of this idea is provided by two groups of facts: the preservation at all stages of tumor progression (from premalignant benign tumors with high risk of malignant transformation to metastatic foci) of the characteristic of primary malignant tumor alterations in the glycosylation pattern of BGA-related glycoepitopes of cellular membranes (Abe et al., 1986; Itzkowitz et al., 1986a, b, 1989; Kim et al., 1986; Hakomori, 1989) and the accumulation during tumor progression of tumor cells with a low density level of histocompatibility antigens on the cellular membrane (Tanaka et al., 1988).

Aberrant glycosylation of cell-membrane macromolecules is one of the universal phenotypic attributes of malignant tumors. A rather limited number of molecular probes based on monoclonal anticarbohydrate antibodies now enables the detection of over 90% of the most widespread human forms of cancer (Hakomori, 1988, 1989), whereas the use of most informative kits of molecular probes for oncogene detection enables the detection of no more than 21–30% of human cancer (Barbacid, 1986; Bos et al., 1987). It can be assumed that the conception of the oncogene that has significantly contributed to the understanding of molecular mechanisms of the control of cell proliferation and the autonomyzation of tumor-cell proliferation is, on the whole, of rather limited importance for the elucidation of mechanisms of the formation of other major biological properties of malignant cells. The concept of aberrant glycosylation undoubtedly is of more universal importance for the understanding of molecular mechanisms of the malignant behavior of transformed cells in vivo not only in the aspect of a classical approach to the knowledge of cellular and biological mechanisms of the formation of invasive and implantation properties, cell-adhesion disturbances, and the like, but also for the elucidation of mechanisms of distant or systemic action of a malignant tumor on the homeostasis of host organism. A number of theoretical and experimental preconditions implies that a malignant tumor is able to alter the glycosylation pattern of glycomacromolecules in the extracellular medium—in particular, in blood serum. At least partly, these alterations may be characterized as the formation of humoral molecular imprints of glycomacromolecular antigens expressed on the membranes of tumor cells. One of the mechanisms of this process is evidently the "throwing down" of glycomacromolecules from the membrane of tumor cells (Sakamoto et al., 1989). In view of the wide molecular range of biomolecules (from low-mol-wt glycoamines to high-mol-wt glycoproteins and multimolecular complexes) involved in these alterations and of the key role of the involved determinants in the development and maintenance of homeostasis, one can suggest that this mechanism is responsible for various distant (systemic) metabolic and biochemical effects of malignant tumors on the organs and tissues of the host organism. This stage of the biochemical generalization of cancer evidently may be characterized as the early or first phase of the morphological generalization of the pathological process that is typical of cancer—metastasis development.

When considering the causes of aberrant glycosylation of the glycomacromolecules of tumor-cell membranes, one usually mentions the alterations in the glycosyltransferase activity (e.g., the activation of glycosyltransferase V) and, more seldom, the elevation in the glycosidase activity. In view of the important role of the primary structure of the protein carrier of carbohydrates in the determination of glycosylation specificity, it can be suggested that alterations in the expression of such glycocarrier molecules (e.g., ectopic in site and/or time expression) are also one of the causes of the changes in the glycosylation pattern of the membranes of tumor cells. In functional and biological aspects, the alterations in the glycosylation of glycomacromolecules of tumor-cell membranes can be related to the changes that reflect the autonomyzation and enhancement of cell division and also to the changes associated with blocking the realization of the development and differentiation program. The alterations associated with the autonomyztion of cell division of transformed cells may be both the consequence of enhanced cell proliferation (since the entry of cells into mitotic cycle is accompanied by certain changes in the glycosylation of cellular membranes, and in tumor tissue the fraction of dividing cells is many orders of magnitude higher than that in the normal tissue) and the causal and/or supporting factors of the autonomous proliferation (e.g., the characteristic of transformation decrease in the level of GM_3-glycolipids of cellular membranes facilitates the dimerization of the EGF-receptor molecules [Igarashi, personal communication]). However, in the biological aspects it seems to us most important that a part of the alterations in the glycosylation of glycomacromolecules of cellular membranes of tumor cells is associated with the antigen-presentation function—a universal common biological function of all nucleus-containing cells of higher mammals and humans. In addition to the elevated (or even unchanged, but in combination with the increase in cell multiplication) genomic and mutation mutability of tumor cells, the antigen-presentation function and subsequent change in cellular surface with a definite type of the modification of the glycosylation pattern of cellular membrane glycoepitopes may provide the key cause of the phenotypic mutability and divergence of tumor cells. These phenotypic alterations evidently may provide the immunoselective basis for tumor progression with a rather strict determination in tumoral disease of the selection direction, the latter largely depending on the predisposition of immunoselective factors of the host organism. Thus, the progression of tumor and the formation of complete malignant phenotype, including the metastatic ability, may be represented as the consequence of a monopathogenetic immunoselective process with the following stages:

1. The autonomyzation of the proliferation of tumor cells;
2. Genomic and mutation mutability, and alterations in the primary structure of proteins;
3. Aberrant glycosylation of membrane glycomacromolecules and phenotypic divergence of tumor cells;

4. The formation of extracellular humoral "molecular imprints" of the glycoepitopes of glycomacromolecular antigens of cellular membranes of the tumor;
5. The immunoselection of tumor-cell clones with a low or medium density of membrane glycoepitopes with the involvement of the competition for common structural determinants of the immunocompetent cells and humoral factors (anticarbohydrate antibodies, soluble glycomacromolecules, and glycoamines); and
6. The formation of mechanisms of immunoresistance and homotypic association of tumor cells.

It seems very promising to consider as the key role the function in these processes of natural anticarbohydrate antibodies and BGA-related glycoepitopes.

Note added in proof: The results of a recently published investigation (Hansen et al., 1990) strongly support our hypothesis concerning the involvement of the BGA-related glycoepitopes in the immune cells cooperation. The most intriguing conclusion is that CD4 receptor recognizes certain BGA-related glycoepitopes (LeY, A1, Sialyl Tn). Thus, the lymphocytes have on their surfaces the certain glycoepitopes and corresponding binding (recognition) proteins (structures). All that they are needed for cells association in appropriate conditions.

References

Abe, K., S.-I. Hakomori, and S. Ohshiba (1986), *Cancer Res.* **46,** 2639–2644.

Adachi, M., N. Hayami, N. Kashiwagi, T. Mizuta, Y. Ohta, M. J. Gill, D. S. Matheson, T. Tamaoki, C. Shiozawa, and S.-I. Hakomori (1988), *J. Exp. Med.* **167,** 323–331.

Andrews, P. W., E. Gonozol, B. A. Fenderson, E. H. Holmes, G. O'Malley, S.-I. Hakomori, and S. Plotkin (1989), *J. Exp. Med.* **169,** 1347–1360.

Barbacid, M. (1986), *Carcinogenesis* **7,** 1037–1042.

Booy, C. J. P., L. J. Needjes, J. Boes, H. L. Ploegh, and C. J. M. Melief (1989), *Eur. J. Immunol.* **19,** 537–542.

Bos, J. L., E. R. Fearon, S. R. Hamilton, M. Verlaan-de Vries, J. H. van Boom, A. J. van der Eb, and B. Vogelstein (1987), *Nature* **327,** 293–297.

Clausen, H. and S.-I. Hakomori (1989), *Vox Sang.* **56,** 1–20.

Dube, V. E. (1987), *Cancer Metastasis Rev.* **6,** 541–567.

Eggest, I., B. Fenderson, T. Toyokuni, B. Dean, M. Stroud, and S.-I. Hakomori (1989), *J. Biol. Chem.* **264,** 9476–9484.

Fenderson, B. A., E. M. Eddy, and S.-I. Hakomori (1990), *Rev. Articles* **12,** 173–176.

Fenderson, B. A., P. W. Andrews, E. Nudelman, H. Clausen, and S.-I. Hakomori (1987), *Dev. Biol.* **122,** 21–27.

Glinsky, G. V. (1987), *J. Tumor Marker Oncol.* **1,** 249–294.

Glinsky, G. V. (1988a), *Proc. Acad. Sci. Ukr. SSR.* B series. **4,** 43–49 (Russ.).

Glinsky, G. V. (1988b), *Proc. Acad. Sci. Ukr. SSR.* B series. **3,** 69–72 (Russ.).

Glinsky, G. V. (1989), *J. Tumor Marker Oncol.* **4,** 193–221.

Glinsky, G. V. and M. D. Linetsky (1990), *J. Tumor Marker Oncol.* **5,** 137–160.

Glinsky, G. V., M. D. Linetsky, V. V. Liventsov, N. I. Surmito, A. B. Ivanova, M. V. Sidorenko, and V. B. Vinnitsky (1990), *J. Tumor Marker Oncol.* **5,** 119–136.

Hakim, A. A. (1984), *Neoplasma* **31,** 385–397.

Hakim, A. A., C. M. Siraki, and C. E. Joseph (1984), *Fed. Proc.* **43,** 1714.

Hakomori, S.-I. (1984), *Annu. Rev. Immunol.* **2,** 103–126.

Hakomori, S.-I. (1988), in *Altered Glycosylation in Tumor Cells,* Liss, New York, pp. 207–212.

Hakomori, S.-I. (1989), *Adv. Cancer Res.* **52,** 257–331.

Hansen, J.-E., H. Clausen, C. Nielsen, et al. (1990), *J. Virology* **64,** 2833–2840.

Igarashi, Y. (personal communication).

Itzkowitz, S. R., M. Yuan, L. D. Ferrell, A. Palekar, and Y. S. Kim (1986), *Cancer Res.* **46,** 5976–5984.

Itzkowitz, S. H., M. Yuan, C. K. Montgomery, T. Kjeldsen, H. K. Takahashi, W. L. Bigbee, and Y. S. Kim (1989), *Cancer Res.* **49,** 197–204.

Itzkowitz, S. H., M. Yuan, Y. Gukushi, A. Palekar, P. C. Phelps, A. M. Shamsuddin, B. F. Trump, S.-I. Hakomori, and Y. S. Kim (1986), *Cancer Res.* **46,** 2627–2632.

Kim, Y. S., M. Yuan, S. H. Itzkowitz, Q. Sun, T. Kaizu, A. Palekar, B. F. Trump, and S.-I. Hakomori (1986), *Cancer Res.* **46,** 5985–5992.

Lindenberg, S., K. Sundberg, S. J. Kimber, and A. Lundblad (1988), *J. Reprod. Fert.* **83,** 149–158.

Linsley, P. S., J. P. Brown, J. L. Magnani, and D. Horn (1988), *Cancer Res.* **48,** 2138–2148.

Lloyd, K. O. (1988), in *Altered Glycosylation in Tumor Cells,* Liss, New York, pp. 235–243.

Lloyd, K. O. and L. J. Old (1989), *Cancer Res.* **49,** 3445–3451.

Magnani, J., Z. Steplewski, H. Koprowski, and V. Ginsburg (1983), *Cancer Res.* **43,** 5489–5492.

Magnani, J., B. Nilsson, M. Brockhaus, J. D. Zop, Z. Steplewski, H. Koprowski, and V. Grinsburg (1982), *J. Biol. Chem.* **257,** 14365–14369.
Mueller-Klieser, W. (1987), *J. Cancer Res. Clin. Oncol.* **113,** 101–122.
Sakamoto, J., T. Watanabe, T. Tokumaru, H. Takagi, H. Nakazato, and K. O. Lloyd (1989), *Cancer Res.* **49,** 745–752.
Springer, G. F. (1984), *Science* **224,** 1198–1206.
Springer, G. F., R. Cheinsong-Popov, V. Schirrmacher, P. R. Desoi, and H. Tegtmeyer (1983), *J. Biol. Chem.* **258,** 5702–5706.
Stein, R., S. Chen, W. Grossman, and D. M. Goldenberg (1989), *Cancer Res.* **49,** 32–37.
Sutherland, R. M. (1988), *Science* **240,** 177–184.
Tanaka, K., T. Yoshioka, C. Bieberich, and G. Jay (1988), *Annu. Rev. Immunol.* **6,** 359–380.
Yamashita, K., K. Totani, M. Kuroki, Y. Matsuoka, I. Ueda, and A. Kobata (1987), *Cancer Res.* **47,** 3451–3459.
Young, W. W., S.-I. Hakomori, and P. Levine (1979), *J. Immunol.* **123,** 92–96.

Chapter 12

CA 15-3 Assay for the Detection of Episialin

A Serum Marker for Breast Cancer

John Hilkens

1. Introduction

Monoclonal antibody (MAb) technology has facilitated the development of several new assays to determine the levels of tumor-associated antigens in serum. Such markers are commonly used for the management of disease in cancer patients. For breast cancer, several assays have been developed based on MAbs against a sialomucin called episialin. These assays appear to be useful tools for monitoring breast cancer, since they show a higher sensitivity than the commonly used CEA assay.

Numerous MAbs have been raised against mucins on carcinoma cells. It has been shown, by competition assays, immunoprecipitation, peptide mapping, and so forth, that many of these MAbs are directed against an epithelial sialomucin that we now call episialin (Price et al., 1986; Abe and Kufe, 1987; Burchell et al., 1989; Xing et al., 1989; Hilkens et al., 1989). For a number of other

From: *Serological Cancer Markers* Edited by Stewart Sell ©1992 The Humana Press, Totowa, NJ

MAbs the evidence that they are directed against episialin is based only on reported characteristics of their antigens; i.e., highly polymorphic mucins with a high molecular weight and a basically similar tissue distribution. Table 1 shows an incomplete list of MAbs directed against this molecule. We have shown that some of these MAbs detect different glycoforms of episialin; i.e., the same protein backbone carrying different carbohydrate structures (Hilkens et al., 1989).

Episialin is a major sialylated glycoprotein present at the cell surface of most types of carcinoma cells. In normal tissues, the molecule is, with a few exceptions, present only at the apical side of exocrine cells, and is not in direct contact with the circulation. As determined with MAbs, the expression of the molecule in carcinoma cells is increased relative to that in the corresponding normal epithelial cells. For example, we have found that normal intestinal epithelium is rarely stained with various MAbs against episialin, but more than 90% of colorectal tumors are reactive with these MAbs (Zotter et al., 1987). Episialin is a membrane-bound glycoprotein, but it is released from the cell and appears in the serum of breast cancer patients.

Several of the MAbs against episialin have been used to develop serum assays, which are also listed in Table 1. One of these assays is the CA 15-3 test (centocor), a "sandwich" assay using MAb 115D8, developed in our group (Hilkens et al., 1984a), and MAb DF3, raised by Kufe and colleagues (Kufe et al., 1984). Both MAbs were initially employed in separate assays (the MAM-6 assay, Hilkens et al., 1984b,1986,1987; and the DF3 assay, Hayes et al., 1985), but have been combined in the CA 15-3 assay, in which they act as catcher and tracer, respectively.

In this chapter I will first briefly review some of the applications and limitations of these tests, with emphasis on the CA 15-3 assay, which is presently most widely used, and then discuss some of the recently obtained knowledge about the molecular structure of episialin, which has important implications for the usefulness and interpretation of the assay results. Finally, I will discuss the existence of various glycoforms of episialin, which explains the

Table 1
Monoclonal Anitbodies to Episialin and Episialin Detection Assays

MAb	Antigen designation	Assay designation	References
HMFG-1,2	HMFG/PEM	HMFG	Taylor-Papadimitriou et al., 1981; Burchell et al., 1984
SM3	PEM		Burchell et al., 1987
Ca1,2	Ca		Ashall et al., 1982; Bramwell et al., 1983
Mc5	NPGP		Ceriani et al., 1983
F36/22	DCA		Papsidero et al., 1983; Papsidero and Johnson, 1986
115D8	MAM-6	CA15-3, MAM-6	Hilkens et al., 1984a,b, 1986, 1987
DUPAN-2[a]	DUPAN-2		Metzgar et al., 1984; Lan et al., 1987
NCRC-11	NCRC-11	NCRC-11	Ellis et al., 1984; Price et al., 1986, 1987
E29	EMA		Cordell et al., 1985; Heyderman et al., 1985
OM-1	SGA		DeKretser et al., 1985,1986
DF3		DF3, CA 15-3	Kufe et el., 1984; Hayes et al., 1985, 1986
M26, M29	CAM	CA M26, CA M29	Linsley et al., 1988a
b12		MCA	Bieglmayer et al., 1988, 1989
3E1.2		MSA	Stacker et al., 1985, 1988
BC4E549[a]	CA 549		Bray et al., 1987

[a]Only indirect evidence that this MAb is directed against episialin.

variations in results obtained with various assays based on different MAbs against episialin.

2. Clinical Application of the CA 15-3 Assay

2.1. Circulating Episialin

In a large study using more than 1000 control sera of apparently healthy individuals, the normal level of the CA 15-3 assay was established (Hayes et al., 1986). Only 1.3% of the control sera showed an episialin level over 30 U/mL. Using this cutoff level, approx 70% of breast cancer patients with advanced metastatic disease have a positive result. About 30% of the patients with advanced disease never show elevated episialin levels in the circulation, although almost 100% of the breast carcinoma specimens are positive with MAbs 115D8 and DF3. Therefore, a much higher percentage of the patients with advanced stages of breast cancer was expected to have elevated levels of circulating episialin. The discrepancy in correlation between the immunohistological data and the serum-assay results could be attributable to the heterogeneous expression of episialin combined with the difficulty in quantitavely estimating the expression of the antigen by immunohistochemical methods. Alternatively, circulating episialin levels may depend on the differentiation of the tumor; differentiated tumors may release the antigen into pseudoductal structures, where the molecule is trapped. Also, the site of the metastases affects the serum level of episialin (Hayes et al., 1986; Colomer et al., 1989a).

Circulating episialin levels do not correlate to age or menopausal status (Schmidt-Rhode et al., 1987; Colomer et al., 1989c). Neither does smoking affect the levels of episialin, as determined with the CA 15-3 assay (Tobias et al., 1985). Also, the levels in patients with benign diseases of the breast do not differ significantly from those in healthy individuals (Hayes et al., 1986; Bonfrer, 1986; Kallioniemi et al., 1988; Colomer et al., 1989c). Elevated episialin levels, as determined with the CA 15-3 assay, were found in sera of some patients with hepatic (cirrhosis, hepatitis) and renal diseases. The level of episialin increases only slightly during pregnancy when determined with the CA 15-3 assay (Touitou et al., 1989), but a relatively larger increase was observed when determined with the MAM-6 or MCA assays (Hilkens et al., 1986; Bieglmayer et al., 1989).

Elevated levels of episialin have also been observed in sera of patients with other carcinomas, but the levels in these patients are usually lower and less frequently above the normal reference level. Among the exceptions are patients with ovarian cancer and adenocarcinomas of the lung, who have elevated levels of episialin in the circulation at high frequency (Schmidt-Rhode et al., 1987; Colomer et al., 1989b and Scambia et al., 1988, using the CA 15-3 assay; and Hilkens et al., 1986 and Koldowsky et al., 1986, using the MAM-6 assay). Increased levels of episialin are even detected in a low percentage of the sera of patients with certain nonepithelial cancers, such as leukemias, hepatomas, and sarcomas (Hayes et al., 1985; Hilkens et al., 1986).

Episialin levels in the circulation, as determined with the CA 15-3, MCA, or MAM-6 assay, are elevated in a higher percentage of breast cancer patients than CEA levels (Hayes et al., 1986; Hilkens et al., 1987; Bieglmayer et al., 1989; Colomer et al., 1989a).

2.2. Early Detection of Primary Breast Cancer

High episialin levels are present almost exclusively in patients with advanced breast cancer. Only a low percentage of patients with primary tumors (with or without locoregional metastases, but with no evidence of distant metastases) have elevated episialin levels in the circulation, as determined with the CA 15-3 test (Hayes et al., 1986; Pons-Anicet et al., 1987, 1988; Kallioniemi et al., 1988). Although the episialin levels in these patients are almost always below the cutoff level, the levels correlate to the size of the tumor (Pons-Anicet et al., 1987). The latter result suggests that episialin is also released by relatively small primary tumors. However, a low background level of episialin is always present in the circulation. The level varies in each individual and masks the contribution of episialin released by a small tumor burden. Therefore, even with more sensitive assays, the episialin level attributable to primary breast cancer will usually not exceed the cutoff levels determined in normal controls. Moreover, as discussed above, circulating episialin levels are also elevated in a number of benign diseases. In conclusion, the assays for episialin developed thus far are not suitable for early detection of primary breast cancer. An exception could be the MSA assay using MAb 3E1.2, which has been reported to be elevated in 70% of patients with early breast carcinoma (Stacker et al., 1988). However, this result is disputed and has not yet been confirmed.

2.3. Monitoring Breast Cancer

The levels of episialin in breast cancer patients, as detected with the CA 15-3 assay, correlates to changes in metastatic tumor burden, and the assay has been found useful in monitoring the clinical course of the disease (Pons-Anicet et al., 1987; Schmidt-Rhode et al., 1987; in Tondini et al., 1988; Colomer et al., 1989a; Van Dalen, 1989). If only patients with elevated antigen levels are considered, the response to or failure of therapy is indicated correctly in approx 90% of the cases in a retrospective study (Schmidt-Rhode et al., 1987). Recently, Kerin et al. (1989) obtained similar results in a prospective study. A rapid increase in episialin levels during therapy should be considered carefully, because "spiking" may occur, which could be mistaken for evidence of disease progression (Hayes et al., 1988a).

Several studies have shown that the CA 15-3 assay is not only more sensitive than the CEA assay, but also correlates more accurately to the extent of the disease (Pons-Anicet et al., 1987; Tondini et al., 1988; Colomer et al., 1989c). The difference in sensitivity has been proven most elegantly by Van Dalen et al. (1986) using receiver operating characteristics (ROC) curves (*see also* Swets, 1988).

2.4. Early Detection of Recurrent Breast Cancer

CA 15-3 levels have been serially determined in patients having no evidence of disease after surgery. Stage, tumor size, or number of involved nodes before surgery showed no correlation to the postoperative episialin levels. Relapses produced significant changes in the level of circulating antigen (Colomer et al., 1989c). The same authors reported that 18 (45%) of 40 patients who suffered relapse showed elevated levels of episialin before any clinical evidence of disease. The median lead time was five months. In a large study by Omar et al. (1989), even more than 70% of the patients showed an elevated episialin level before clinical evidence of relapse. Similar results were obtained in smaller studies by other investigators (Pons-Anicet et al., 1987; Schmidt-Rhode et al., 1987; Hilkens et al., 1987; Kallioniemi et al., 1988). Pons-Anicet et al. (1987) and Colomer et al. (1989b) showed that the survival of patients in relapse with a level of episialin that had remained elevated after surgery was significantly shorter than the survival of patients with a normal episialin level after surgery. The prognostic significance of preoperative levels has not been established (Van Dalen, 1989).

In some studies the CEA level was concomitantly determined. The correlation of increased CEA levels to relapse was lower and, if the patients were positive for circulating CEA, the lead time was significantly shorter than that obtained with the CA 15-3 assay (Colomer et al., 1989a,b).

2.5. Other Clinical Applications of MAbs Against Episialin

1. Differential diagnosis: With few exceptions, MAbs against episialin are reactive only with carcinomas and therefore are useful tools for the pathologist. For instance, these MAbs can be used as single agents or in a panel with other MAbs as an aid in identification of metastases of unknown primary tumors (Hageman et al., 1987). Moreover, Zotter et al. (1987) showed that MAbs to episialin may be used to distinguish slightly dysplastic adenomas from severely dysplastic adenomas and cancer of the colon.
2. Radioimmunodetection and immunotherapy: MAbs to episialin have been used for imaging and immunotherapy of breast and other carcinomas, since they are directed to epitopes abundantly present on the cell surface (Epenetos et al. 1982a,b;

Lashford et al., 1988), although circulating antigen may affect the localization of the radiolabeled MAbs in patients. Tjandra et al. (1989) have employed MAbs directed against episialin to predict accurately lymph node involvement in approx 90% of the cases studied using immunoscintigraphy. Tumors of human xenografts in nude mice can be eradicated by treating these mice with ^{131}I-labeled antiepisialin MAbs (Ceriani and Blank, 1988; Molthoff et al., submitted). Remissions have been achieved in ovarian and lung carcinoma patients with ^{131}I-labeled MAb HMFG-2 directed against episialin (Epenetos et al., 1984; Stewart et al., 1989).

3. The Structure and Biosynthesis of Episialin

3.1. The Episialin Gene and the Deduced Structure of the Molecule

We have cloned and sequenced the episialin cDNA, and we have deduced the structure of the molecule based on the predicted amino acid sequence. The gene encodes a transmembrane molecule with a large extracellular domain, which mainly consists of repeated sequences of 20 amino acids, and a 69 amino acid cytoplasmic domain (Ligtenberg et al., 1990; Wreschner et al., 1990). The number of repeats is highly variable in the human population (Swallow et al., 1987), leading to substantial differences in the molecular weights of episialin molecules from different individuals. The repeats compose more than half of the polypeptide backbone, even in the smallest allele detected thus far. Of both the repeats and the surrounding sequences, 25% consist of serine and threonine residues, often in close proximity to proline residues. Therefore, they are potential attachment sites for O-linked glycans. The high percentage of proline residues and the extensive glycosylation give the molecule an extended and rigid structure pointing into the extracellular space.

The organization of the intron and exon sequences was determined. We have found two different splice variants leading to molecules with different signal peptides and probably to mature

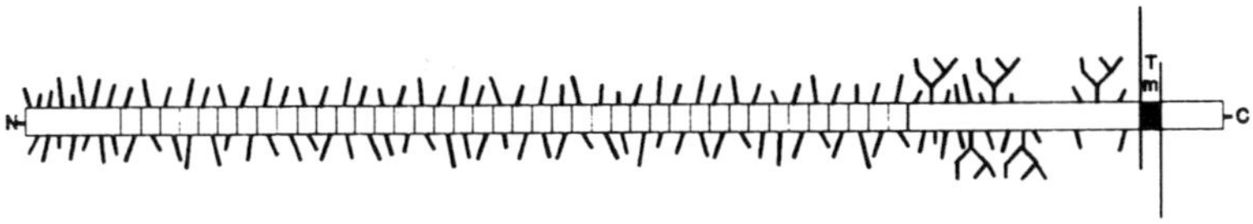

TM: Transmembrane domain

Fig. 1. A model of the episialin molecule deduced from the cDNA sequence. In this model, the protein backbone comprises 1264 amino acids and contains a tandem array of 40 repeat U (800 amino acids), which is the estimated number of repeats in the short allele of episialin in the T47D breast carcinoma cell line. The extracellular domain of the molecule is almost completely covered by O-linked glycans. Five N-linked glycans are present at the C-terminal of the repeat region. The variations in the N-terminus that result from the alternative splicing are not indicated. A typical transmembrane sequence of at least 24 amino acids is found in the C-terminal part, followed by a cytoplasmic domain of 69 amino acids.

molecules with different *N*-termini. The predicted difference between the two variants is small: 10 additional amino acids. It is not yet known if there are any differences in biological function between the splice variants. The deduced structure of episialin is shown in Fig. 1.

3.2. Biosynthesis and Carbohydrate Composition of Episialin

It has been shown by means of biosynthetic labeling followed by immunoprecipitation that episialin is synthesized as a single polypeptide chain of a relatively high molecular weight, in most cell lines approx 200 kDa or more (Hilkens and Buys, 1988; Linsley et al., 1988b). This precursor is rapidly converted to a second precursor with a molecular weight of approx 20 kDa lower, most likely by proteolysis. This processing step occurs in the endoplasmic reticulum and may be essential for further processing. The main processing of episialin occurs by the addition of numerous O-linked

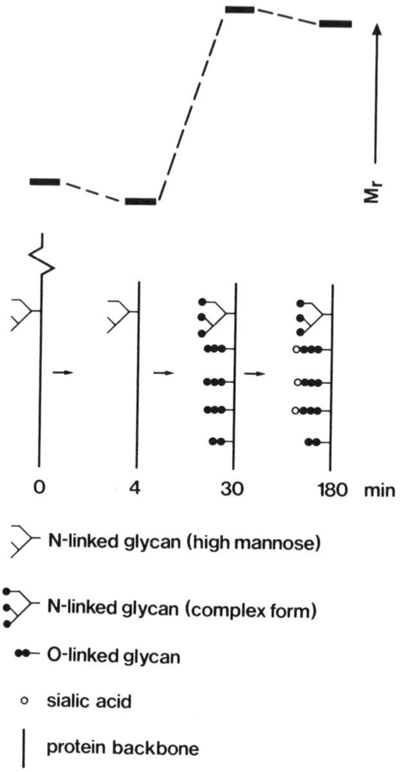

Fig. 2. Outline of the processing of episialin. The approximate time of appearance of the intermediates is indicated.

glycans, which increases the apparent molecular weight on SDS-polyacrylamide gels to more than 400 kDa. The extensive glycosylation protects the molecule against proteolytic degradation, since the precursors without O-linked sugars are degraded rapidly, whereas the mature molecule is extremely resistant to the action of proteases. The glycosylation also determines the rigid structure of the molecule, as discussed above. The last step in the processing of episialin is the addition of sialic acid to the glycans, which increases the mobility of the molecule on SDS gels. All processing steps are schematically indicated in Fig. 2.

Shimizu and Yamauchi (1982) have shown that the molecule comprises about 50% (w/w) carbohydrates, which are mainly O-linked. The structure of the most frequently present O-linked glycans on episialin purified with MAb DF3 from BT-20 breast carcinoma cells and with MAb Ca1 from HEp 2 larynx carcinoma cells were determined (Bramwell et al., 1983; Hull and Carraway, 1988). The most common glycans are relatively short (1–4 sugars) and consist of sialic acid, galactose, and galactosamine. Although the majority of the glycans on episialin are O-linked, the molecule also contains N-linked glycans, as was shown by the treatment with endoglycosidases and predicted from the cDNA sequence.

4. Glycoforms of Episialin with Different Epitope Composition

4.1. Protein and Carbohydrate Epitopes

The repetitive part of the protein backbone of episialin is very immunogenic, and most MAbs raised against episialin bind to this part of the molecule, as was shown by their reactivity with synthetic peptides (Gendler et al., 1988) and with fragments of episialin encoded by the repetitive part of the gene expressed in bacterial expression vectors. For example, MAb DF3 strongly reacts with the protein backbone. However, MAb 115D8 reacts with an epitope that involves the protein backbone, but full reactivity is dependent on the presence of carbohydrates, in particular sialic acid (Litvinov et al., submitted). Other MAbs, Ca1 (Ashall et al., 1982) and 3E1.2 (Thompson et al., 1983), seem to be directed against pure carbohydrate epitopes. However, it is difficult to prove that no amino acid residues are involved as long as the carbohydrate sequence has not been determined. The peptide sequence of the minimal epitope of some of the MAbs has been determined. Several epitopes overlap or are shifted by only one or two amino acids (Xing et al., 1989, Burchell et al., 1989). Some epitopes include a serine or threonine, which are potential glycosylation sites.

4.2. Differential Glycosylation of Episialin

Some MAbs, such as SM3 (Burchell et al., 1987), show a high preference for breast carcinomas relative to normal breast epithelium. Other MAbs, such as Om-1, show a preference for ovarian carcinomas (DeKretser et al., 1985), and MAb 202H4, recently developed in our group, reacts only with a specific subset of epithelial tissues. We have investigated the biochemical background of the preferential binding to different tissues of the various MAbs against episialin. For this purpose we used carcinoma cell lines of different tissue origin as models (Hilkens et al., 1989). The reactivity of the MAbs is complex. All MAbs against the protein backbone precipitate the precursor molecule of episialin from all cell lines expressing this epithelial sialomucin. However, some of these MAbs precipitate the mature molecule from only a restricted number of carcinoma cell lines. Even within a single cell line, some MAbs precipitate all mature molecules, others only subsets of the mature episialin molecules. The difference in reactivity of these MAbs, which are directed against the protein moiety of episialin, is caused by alterations in accessibility of the epitopes for MAbs as a result of differential glycosylation of the molecule in different cell lines. The differentially glycosylated molecules, called glycoforms, each show a restricted expression pattern resulting in positive and negative cells and cell lines. These results obtained with cell lines can be applied to explain the differential reactivity of certain MAbs with carcinomas and normal epithelial cells, and their differential reactivity with tissues of different histological origin. It is important to realize that the differential reactivity is, in most cases, not an "all-or-nothing" phenomenon, but a preferential reactivity with certain tissues or tumors. Even within one type of carcinoma, the number of epitopes accessible for a given antiepisialin MAb may vary in each individual tumor. Differential glycosylation could occur by differential initiation of the O-linked glycans or could be a result of differences in length or branching of the glycans.

5. Genetic Factors That Affect the CA 15-3 Assay Results

The apparent molecular weight of episialin from tissue specimens from each individual varies greatly (Hayes et al., 1988b; Hilkens et al., 1989). It has been shown that these differences in molecular weight are caused by genetic polymorphism (Swallow et al., 1987). Recently, it was shown that the polymorphism is the result of a variable number of tandem repeat sequences present in the gene (Ligtenberg et al., 1990; Wreschner et al., 1990). The number of tandem repeat sequences can vary from approx 40 to 90 in each allele.

MAbs 115D8 and DF3 are directed against the repetitive part of the molecule. The CA 15-3 assay uses MAb DF3 as a tracer; therefore, the result of the assay will depend mainly on the number of binding sites for MAb DF3, i.e., the number of the repeats present in the episialin molecule of each individual. This implies that the reaction level is not exactly correlated to the absolute amount of episialin molecules in the circulation.

It has been shown that, in a high percentage of breast carcinomas, one of the episialin alleles is lost (Merlo et al., 1989; Gendler et al., 1990). Therefore, the level of episialin produced by the tumor is also affected by the loss of one of the episialin alleles. Consequently, these features, together with the differences in accessibility of the epitopes recognized by the antibodies in each tumor, are among the reasons that only changes in episialin levels in patients are clinically relevant.

6. Release of Episialin from the Cell

Although episialin is released by tumor cells in vitro and in vivo, its cDNA sequence predicts that episialin has a transmembrane domain, suggesting that the molecule cannot be easily released from the membrane. There are three possible ways for the cell to release episialin: (1) release from a glycosyl phosphoinositol

(GPI) anchor, (2) removal of the transmembrane domain in the ER, and (3) proteolytic cleavage at the cell membrane. A GPI linkage is considered unlikely, based on the presence of a cytoplasmic domain, which is normally not found in this type of molecules. Furthermore, metabolic labeling studies did not support this option. The biosynthesis studies discussed in Section 3 indicate that an early proteolytic cleavage in the endoplasmic reticulum takes place. This cleavage step may remove the hydrophobic transmembrane and cytoplasmic region. As a consequence, episialin would be secreted from the cell as soon as it reaches the plasma membrane, provided that there is no association with an anchor molecule at the cell surface. There are as yet no clear indications for the presence of such a molecule. However, preliminary results in vitro suggest that most episialin is at least temporarily present in a membrane bound form, suggesting that the early proteolytic cleavage step is not directly responsible for the release of episialin from the membrane. These results suggest that episialin is most likely secreted or released from the membrane after a proteolytic cleavage step at or close to the cell surface. This is in contrast to the release of CEA into the circulation. CEA is linked to the plasma membrane by a GPI-anchor and is probably released by an extracellular phospholipase.

7. Conclusions and Future Developments

The CA 15-3 assay for the detection of episialin has been established as a reliable marker for management of breast cancer. The response to treatment of advanced cancer can be monitored in approx 70% of the patients. In the follow-up of patients with no evidence of disease, recurrent breast cancer can be detected in 45–70% of the cases with a considerable lead time before relapse is clinically detectable, but extensive prospective studies still need to be done.

Episialin is not specific for breast cancer; rather, it is also elevated in the circulation of patients with several other types of carcinomas. However, the value and frequency of elevated episialin levels is lower in these patients, as detected with the CA 15-3 assay or any other episialin detection assay developed so far. Only in patients with ovarian and a few other carcinomas does the CA 15-3 assay perform well enough to be useful.

Episialin is more frequently elevated than CEA in breast cancer. In only a few cases the CEA level is increased without an elevated CA 15-3 level. The determination of the CEA level concomitantly to the CA 15-3 assay is beneficial in only a relatively low percentage of the patients.

The CA 15-3 levels correlate strongly to those found with other episialin-detection assays, although the results deviate in some cases. With the knowledge about the different glycoforms of episialin, these differences can easily be understood. Similarly, differences in sensitivity for episialin present in sera of patients with various nonbreast carcinomas may be explained in this way. For example, the CA 15-3 assay is positive in 30–60% of sera from patients with advanced ovarian carcinomas, whereas the MAM-6 assay using 115D8 as catcher and as tracer is positive in approx 80% of the cases (Koldowsky et al., 1986; Hilkens et al., 1986). More sensitive assays for circulating episialin from other types of carcinomas could be developed by using MAbs with a high preference for episialin derived from those types of carcinomas.

Since there are MAbs avaible that preferentially react with cell-associated episialin (Litvinov et al., submitted) the problem of "spiking" could also be solved by using such MAbs in an assay system, assuming that spiking occurs as a result of entry into the circulation of cell-bound episialin from necrotic cells.

Since, in normal controls, a low, but variable in each individual, level of circulating episialin is present, early detection of breast cancer is not possible with the present assays. In order to improve the assay system, the source of these molecules has to be known. In healthy individuals, episialin is present mainly in exocrine glandular epithelial cells or in secreted material. In glandular epithelial cells, the molecule is confined to the luminal surface, and the tight junctions will prevent leakage of episialin into the circulation. Yet it is conceivable that episialin enters the circulation from slightly damaged glandular epithelium. However, it is more likely that episialin present in the serum is derived from other cell types also expressing episialin. For example, certain blast-like cells that are present in low numbers in the circulation are also episialin-positive, and could be the source of circulating antigen. If these blast-like cells are indeed the source of circulating episialin, then assays may be developed that use MAbs directed to glycoforms that are not present on these cells. Such assays may be more suitable for early detection of breast carcinomas or recurrence. Recently, we have raised such MAbs (Litvinov et al., unpublished), which will be tested for this purpose. The ratios of values from a new, more specific assay to those from the presently used CA 15-3 assay may aid in early detection of primary tumors or recurrence. For example, a high ratio of values from a tumor-preferent assay to Ca 15-3 values could be indicative of such diseases.

Acknowledgments

I thank H. Vos, M. Ligtenberg, S. Litvinov, and H. Bonfrer for fruitful discussions and critical reading of the manuscript.

References

Abe, M. and D. W. Kufe (1987), *J. Immunol.* **139,** 257–261.

Ashall, F., M. E. Bramwell, and H. Harris (1982), *Lancet* **ii,** 1–6.

Bieglmayer C., T. Szepesi, and W. Neunteufel (1988), *Cancer Lett.* **42,** 199–206.

Bieglmayer C., T. Szepesi, W. Neunteufel, and C. Nowotny (1989), *Tumor Biol.* **10,** 232–242.

Bonfrer, J. M. G. (1986), in *I Markers Tumorali in Ginecologia* (Coli, A. and G. Torre, eds.), CIC Edizioni Internazionali, Rome, pp. 271–273.

Bramwell, M. E., V. P. Bhavanandan, G. Wiseman, and H. Harris (1983), *Br. J. Cancer* **48,** 177–183, 1983.

Bray, K. R., J. E. Koda, and P. K. Gaur (1987), *Cancer Res.* **47,** 5853–5860.

Burchell, J., D. Wang, and J. Taylor-Papadimitriou (1984), *Int. J. Cancer* **34,** 763–768.

Burchell, J., S. Gendler, J. Taylor-Papadimitriou, A. Girling, A. Lewis, R. Millis, and D. Lamport (1987), *Cancer Res.* **47,** 5476–5482.

Burchell, J., J. Taylor-Papadimitriou, M. Boshell, S. Gendler, and T. Duhig (1989), *Int. J. Cancer* **44,** 691–696.

Ceriani, R. L., J. A. Peterson, J. Y. Lee, R. Moncada, and E. W. Blank (1983), *Somatic Cell Genet.* **9,** 415–427.

Ceriani, R. L. and E. W. Blank (1988), *Cancer Res.* **48,** 4664–4672.

Colomer, R., A. Ruibal, and L. Salvador (1989a), *Cancer* **64,** 1674–1681.

Colomer, R., A. Ruibal, J. Genolla, and L. Salvador (1989b), *Br. J. Cancer* **59,** 283–286.

Colomer, R., A. Ruibal, J. Genolla, D. Rubio, J. M. Del Campo, R. Bodi, and L. Salvador (1989c), *Breast Cancer Res. Treat.* **13,** 123–133.

Cordell, J., T. C. Richardson, K. A. F. Pulford, A. K. Gosh, K. C. Gatter, E. Heyderman, and D. Y. Mason (1985), *Br. J. Cancer* **52,** 347–354.

DeKretser, T. A., H. J. Thorne, D. J., Jacobs, and D. G. Jose (1985), *Eur. J. Cancer Clin. Oncol.* **21,** 1019–1035.

DeKretser, T. A., H. J. Thorne, D. Picone, and D. G. Jose (1986), *Int. J. Cancer* **37,** 705–712.

Ellis, I. O., R. A. Robins, C. W. Elston, R. W. Blamey, B. Ferry, and R. W. Baldwin (1984), *Histopathology* **8,** 501–516.

Epenetos A. A., Britton, K. E., Mather, S., Shepherd, J., Granowska, M., Taylor-Papadimitriou, J., Nimmon, C. C., Durbin, H., Hawkins, L. R., Malpas, J. S. and Bodmer, W. F. (1982a), *Lancet* **ii,** 999–1004.

Epenetos, A. A., G. Canti, J. Taylor-Papadimitriou, M. Curling, and W. F. Bodmer (1982b), *Lancet* **ii,** 1004–1006.

Epenetos, A. A, N. Courtinay Luck, K. E. Halnan, and G. Hooker (1984), *Lancet* **ii,** 1441–1443.

Gendler, S. J., J. Taylor-Papadimitriou, T. Duhig, J. Rothbard, and J. M. Burchell (1988), *J. Biol. Chem.* **263,** 12820–12823.

Gendler, S. J., E. P. Cohen, A. Craston, T. Duhig, G. Johnstone, and D. Barnes (1990), *Int. J. Cancer.* **45,** 431–435.

Hageman, Ph., J. L. Peterse, J. Hilkens, and J. Hilgers (1987), in *Application of Monoclonal Antibodies in Tumor Pathology* (Ruiter, D., S. Warnaar, and G. Fleuren, eds.), Martinus Nijhoff, Dordrecht, The Netherlands, pp. 167–190.

Hayes, D. F., V. R. Zurawski, and D. W. Kufe (1986), *J. Clin. Oncol.* **4,** 1542–1550.

Hayes, D. F., D. T. Kiang, A. H. Korzun, C. Tondini, W. C. Wood, and D. W. Kufe (1988a), *Proceedings of ASCO* **7,** 38.

Hayes, D. F., H. Sekine, D. Markus, C. A. Alper, and D. W. Kufe (1988b), *Blood* **71,** 436–440.

Hayes, D. F., H. Sekine, T. Ohno, M. Abe, K. Keefe, and D. W. Kufe (1985), *J. Clin. Invest.* **75,** 1671–1678.

Heyderman, E., I. Strudley, G. Powell, T. C. Richardson, D. L. Cordell, and D. Y. Mason (1985), *Br. J. Cancer* **52,** 355–361.

Hilkens, J. and F. Buys (1988), *J. Biol. Chem.* **263,** 4215–4222.
Hilkens, J., F. Buys, and M. Ligtenberg (1989), *Cancer Res.* **49,** 786–793.
Hilkens, J., V. Kroezen, H. Bonfrer, M. De Jong-Bakker, and P. F. Bruning (1986), *Cancer Res.* **46,** 2582–2587.
Hilkens, J., F. Buys, J. Hilgers, Ph. Hageman, J. Calafat, A. Sonnenberg, and M. Van der Valk (1984a), *Int. J. Cancer* **34,** 197–206.
Hilkens, J., V. Kroezen, H. Bonfrer, P. F. Bruning, J. Hilgers, and M. Van Eijkeren (1984b), in *Protides of the Biological Fluids,* vol. 31 (Peeterse, H., ed.), Pergamon, Oxford, pp. 651–653.
Hilkens, J., J. M. G. Bonfrer, V. Kroezen, M. Van Eijkeren, W. Nooyen, M. De Jong-Bakker, and P. F. Bruning (1987), *Int. J. Cancer* **39,** 431–435.
Hull S. R., and K. Carraway (1988), *J. Cell Biochem. [Suppl.]* **12E,** 130.
Kallioniemi, O. P., H. Oksa, R. K. Aaran, T. Hietanen, M. Lehtinen, and T. Koivula (1988), *Br. J. Cancer* **58,** 213–215.
Kerin, M. J., O. J. McAnena, V. P. O'Malley, H. Grimes, and H. F. Given (1989), *Br. J. Surg.* **76,** 838,839.
Koldowski, U., U. Wargalla, J. Hilkens, B. Feldhammer, S. Kroizin, M. Bross, and J. Hilgers (1986), *Tumor Diagnostik und Therapie* **7,** 125–128.
Kufe, D., G. Inghiriami, M. Abe, D. Hayes, H. Justi-Wheeler, and J. Schlom (1984), *Hybridoma* **3,** 223–232.
Lan, M. S., R. C. Bast, M. I. Colnaghi, R. C. Knapp, D. Colcher, J. Schlom, and R. S. Metzgar (1987), *Int. J. Cancer* **39,** 68–71.
Lashford, L. S., A. G. Davies, R. B. Richardson, S. P. Bourne, J. A. Bullimore, H. Eckert, J. T. Kemshead, and H. B. Coakham (1988), *Cancer* **61,** 857–868.
Ligtenberg, M. J. L., H. L. Vos, A. M. C. Gennissen, and J. Hilkens (1990), *J. Biol. Chem.* **265,** 5573–5578.
Linsley, P. S., J. P. Brown, J. L. Magnani, and D. Horn (1988a), *Cancer Res.* **48,** 2138–2148.
Linsley, P. S, J. C. Kallestadt, and D. Horn (1988b), *J. Biol. Chem.* **263,** 8390–8397.
Litvinor, S. L., P. Hageman, M. J. I. Ligtenberg, and J. Hilkens, submitted for publication.
Merlo, G. R., J. Siddiqui, C. S. Cropp, D. S. Liscia, R. Lidereau, R. Callahan, and D. W. Kufe (1989), *Cancer Res.* **49,** 6966–6971.
Metzgar, R. S., N. Rodriquez, O. J. Finn, M. S. Lan, V. N. Daasch, P. Fernsten, W. C. Meyers, W. F. Sindelar, R. S. Sandler, and H. F. Seigler (1984), *Proc. Natl. Acad. Sci. USA* **81,** 5242–5246.
Molthoff, C. F. M., H. M. M. Schlüper, H. M. Pinedo, and E. Boven, submitted for publication.
Omar, Y. T., A. E. Behbehani, N. Al-Naqeeb, M. M. Motawy, M. O. Foudeh, A. H. Awwad, M. Y. Nasralla, and J. J. Szymendera (1989), *Int. J. Biol. Markers* **4,** 81–86.

Papsidero, L. D. and E. A. Johnson (1986), *Int. J. Cancer* **37,** 697–701.

Papsidero, L. D., G. A. Croghan, M. J. O'Connell, L. A. Valenzuela, T. Nemoto, and T. M. Chu (1983), *Cancer Res.* **43,** 1741–1747.

Pons-Anicet, D. M. F., B. P. Krebs, R. Mira, and M. J. Namer (1987), *Br. J. Cancer* **55,** 567–569.

Pons-Anicet, D. M. F., A. Ramaldi, B. P. Krebs, and M. J. Namer (1988), *Tumor Marker Oncol.* **3,** 2.

Price, M. R., S. Edwards, R. A. Robins, J. Hilgers, J. Hilkens, and R. W. Baldwin (1986), *Eur. J. Cancer Clin. Oncol.* **22,** 115–117.

Price, M. R., G. Cocker, S. Edwards, I. S. Nagra, R. A. Robins, M. Williams, R. W. Blamey, D. M. Swallow, and R. W. Baldwin (1987), *Eur. J. Cancer Clin. Oncol.* **23,** 1169–1176.

Scambia, G., P. Benedetti, G. Panici, L. Baiocchi, S. Perrone., S. Greggi, and S. Mancuso (1988), *Gynecol. Oncol.* **30,** 265–273.

Schmidt-Rhode, P., K. D. Schulz, G. Sturm, A. Raab-Frick, and H. Prinz (1987), *Int. J. Biol. Markers.* **2,** 135–142.

Shimizu, M. and K. Yamauchi (1982), *J. Biochem.* **91,** 1741–1747.

Stacker, S. A., C. H. Thompson, C. Riglar, and I. F. C. McKenzie (1985), *J. Natl. Cancer Inst.* **75,** 801–811.

Stacker, S. A., C. H. Thompson, N. P. Sacks, J. Tjandra, M. G. Lowe, J. Bishop, and I. F. C. McKenzie (1988), *Cancer Res.* **48,** 7060–7066.

Stewart, J. S. W., V. Hird, D. Snook, M. Sullivan, G. Hooker, N. Courtenay-Luck, G. Sivolapenko, M. Griffith, M. J. Myers, H. M. Lambert, A. J. Munro, and A. A. Apenetos (1989), *Int. J. Radiat. Oncol. Biol. Phys.* **16,** 405–413.

Swallow, D. M., S. Gendler, B. Griffiths, G. Corney, J. Taylor-Papadimitriou, and M. E. Bramwell (1987), *Nature* **328,** 82–84.

Swets, J. A. (1988), *Science* **240,** 1285–1292.

Taylor-Papadimitriou, J., J. A. Peterson, J. Arklie, J. Burchell, R. L. Ceriani, and W. F. Bodmer (1981), *Int. J. Cancer* **28,** 17–21.

Thompson, C. H., S. L. Jones, R. H. Whitehead, and I. F. C. McKenzie (1983), *J. Natl. Cancer Inst.* **70,** 409–419.

Tjandra, J. J., I. S. Rusell, J. P. Collins, J. T. Andrew, M. Lichtenstein, D. Binns, and I. F. C. McKenzie (1989), *Cancer Res.* **49,** 1600–1608.

Tobias, R., C. Rothwell, J. Wagner, A. Green, and Y. S. Liu (1985), *Clin. Chem.* **31,** 986.

Tondini, C., D. F. Hayes, R. Gelman, I. C. Henderson, and D. W. Kufe (1988), *Cancer Res.* **48,** 4107–4112.

Touitou, Y., A. Darbois, A. Bogdan, A. Auzeby, and S. Keusseoglou (1989), *Br. J. Cancer* **60,** 419,420.

Van Dalen, A. (1989), *Ann. Chir. Gynaecol.* **78,** 54–64.

Van Dalen, A., J. M. G. Bonfrer, H. W. Dupree, J. Heering, D. L. van der Linde, and W. J. Nooijen (1986), in *Clinical Relevance of New Monoclonal*

Antibodies (Greten, H. and R. Klapdor, eds.), Georg Thieme, Verlag, Stuttgart, p. 185.

Wreschner, D. H., M. Hareuveni, I. Tsarfaty, N. Smorodinsky, J. Horev, J. Zaretsky, P. Kotkes, M. Weiss, R. Lathe, A. Dion, and I. Keydar (1990), *Eur. J. Biochem.* **189,** 463–473.

Xing, P. X., J. J. Tjandra, K. Reynold, P. J. McLaughlin, D. F. J. Purcell, and I. F. C. McKenzie (1989), *J. Immunol.* **142,** 3503–3509.

Zotter, S., A. Lossnitzer, Ph. Hageman, J. F. M. Delemarre, J. Hilkens, and J. Hilgers (1987), *Lab. Invest.* **57,** 193–199.

Chapter 13

Clinical Applications of CA 15-3

Daniel F. Hayes, Carlo Tondini, and Donald W. Kufe

1. Introduction

Circulating breast cancer associated tumor markers have several potential clinical uses. Although many circulating molecules have been investigated as putative breast cancer markers, only a few have been found to have sufficient sensitivity and specificity to be useful clinically. Of these, carcinoembryonic antigen (CEA) has been the most commonly used and has been considered the "gold standard."

Monoclonal antibodies have recently been developed that detect circulating breast carcinoma associated antigens. One of these, designated MAb DF3, was generated against a membrane-enriched extract of a human breast cancer metastatic to liver (Kufe et al., 1984). The antigen recognized by MAb DF3 is a high-mol-wt glycoprotein that belongs to a family of mucin-like molecules expressed on the apical surface of normal secretory glandular epithelial cells (Kufe et al., 1984; Sekine et al., 1985b; Abe and Kufe, 1987, 1989).

From: *Serological Cancer Markers* Edited by Stewart Sell ©1992 The Humana Press, Totowa, NJ

Western blot analyses of human plasma demonstrate that the DF3-reactive antigen circulates as a heterogeneous species with apparent mol wts *(M_r)* of 300–450,000 (Hayes et al., 1985; Sekine et al., 1985b). Subsequent studies have shown that this circulating antigen exhibits an electrophoretic polymorphism as a result of the expression of multiple alleles at a single genetic locus present on chromosome 1q (Swallow et al., 1987; Hayes et al., 1988b; Siddiqui et al., 1988; Merlo et al., 1989). Nucleotide sequence analysis of a partial cDNA clone that codes for the DF3 peptide core reveals a highly conserved 60-bp tandem repeat (Siddiqui et al., 1988). The polymorphism of the DF3 antigen is caused by the different numbers of these repeats in the peptide core (Merlo et al., 1989), which is a single protein of approximate M_r 160–230,000, rich in threonine, serine, proline, glycine, and alanine (Abe and Kufe, 1989).

Although the MAb DF3-reactive epitope is present within the 20 amino acid repeating segment of the peptide core (Abe and Kufe, 1989), neuraminidase treatment decreases the reactivity of the MAb with the antigen (Abe and Kufe, 1986), suggesting that recognition of the epitope is influenced by glycosylation. In this regard, the oligosaccharide pattern of DF3 antigen purified from normal human milk is substantially different from the carbohydrate composition of the antigen from cultured human breast carcinoma cells (Hull et al. 1989). The major oligosaccharides of the DF3 milk antigen are the tetrasaccharide Galβ1,4GlcNacβ1,6(Galβ1,3)GaNAC and its sialylated derivatives; those for the tumor antigen are the disaccharide Galβ1,3GalNac of the Thomsen-Friedenreich antigen. These differences could account for the specificity differences observed between assays using different MAbs that react with members of this family of antigens *(see below)*.

The physiological function of the DF3 reactive antigen is unknown. However, the widespread tissue distribution and the presence in secretory fluids of the DF3 and related glycoproteins impy an important biological role for these mucin-like molecules. In general, mucins provide lubrication and physical protection for epithelial secretory surfaces. However, recent studies have demonstrated that DF3 antigen purified from human milk or tumor suppresses human eosinophil cytoxic function by preventing adherence of eosinophils to immunoglobulin-coated targets (Hayes et al., 1990). These studies suggest that DF3 antigen serves to protect the apical portion of secretory epithelial-cell membranes from the toxic effects of activated inflammatory cells.

2. Development of the CA 15-3 Assay

Using a double-determinant radioimmunoassay (RIA) and an enzyme-linked immunoassay (EIA) with MAb DF3, we demonstrated that the DF3 antigen is elevated in approx 75% of patients with metastatic breast cancer when compared with age-matched controls and that serial DF3 antigen levels correlate to clinical course in patients with metastatic breast cancer (Hayes et al., 1985). Other investigators have developed MAbs that identify related members of the family of polymorphic, high-mol-wt, epithelial carcinoma-associated glycoproteins of which DF3 antigen is a member. One such antigen, designated MAM-6, is identified by MAb 115D8 (Hilkens et al., 1986). Studies have demonstrated that MAbs DF3 and 115D8 recognize distinct epitopes on the same antigen (Abe and Kufe, 1987). These two MAb have been used to construct a bideterminant immunoradio mimetric assay (IRMA) to identify the circulating antigen, designated CA 15-3 (Hayes et al., 1986). Several subsequent studies have demonstrated that CA 15-3 is a sensitive and relatively specific marker that has clinical utility in evaluating and monitoring patients with breast cancer.

3. Sensitivity of CA 15-3

The distribution of values of CA 15-3 in "normal" subjects and in patients with breast cancer is listed in Table 1. Although some variation exists between laboratories, the mean ± SD of CA 15-3 level in normal subjects ranges from 7 to 18 ± 3–9 U/mL and is unrelated to age or gender (Gang et al., 1985; Colomer et al., 1986; Fujino et al., 1986; Gion et al., 1986a; Hayes et al., 1986; Ogawa et al., 1986; Kikuchi et al., 1987; Ruibal et al., 1987; Sacks

Table 1
CA 15-3 Levels in Normal Subjects and in Patients with Breast Cancer

	Normal subjects			Breast cancer patients with CA 15-3 levels > cutoff, %							
				Primary stage			Metastatic[a]				
Reference	No.	CA 15-3, U/mL: M ± SD	Cutoff	I	II	III	All	ST	Bo	Li	Lu
Hayes et al., 1986	1050	13.3 ± 6.0	25	0	29	30	73	46	79	–	79
Gang et al., 1985	75	7.5 ± 3.4	15	0	41	50	75	–	–	–	–
Ogawa et al., 1986	79	9.0 ± 9.0	20	25	16	45	75	50	75	100	83
Fujino et al., 1986	228	10.3 ± 4.3	24	4	12.5	28	70	–	–	–	–
Gion et al., 1986b	81	13.8 ± 3.9	31	41	42	57	84	–	–	–	–
Colomer et al., 1986	140	14.9 ± 7.1	40	–	–	–	–	–	–	–	–
Sacks et al., 1987	30	18.0 ± 9.0	40	6	3	–	82	–	–	–	–
Maigre, 1988	–	–	25	–	1.5	–	75	–	–	–	–
Kallioniemi et al., 1988	17	–	38	7	17	64	67	–	–	–	–
Delarue et al., 1988	–	–	30	–	–	–	70	–	–	–	–
Colomer et al., 1989c	275	16.0 ± 9.0	40	–	–	–	75	–	–	–	–
Safi et al., 1989	213	–	25	5	29	32	95	22	68	71	91
Ruibal et al., 1987	–	16.5 ± 9.5	35	18	–	–	–	–	–	–	–
Pons-Anicet et al., 1987	100	–	25	9	18	27	91	–	–	–	–
Takemori et al., 1987	–	–	25	–	–	–	75	–	–	–	–
Kikuchi et al., 1987	18	8.9 ± 3.3	27	20	0	0	77	75	–	100	100
Omar et al., 1989	–	–	40	0	16	11	45	–	–	–	–
Kerin, 1989	–	–	25	5	4	10	50	–	–	–	–
Range		8.9–18.0		0–41	0–42	0–64	50–95	22–75	68–75	71–100	79–100

[a]ST, Soft tissue; Bo, Bone; Li, Liver; Lu, Lung.

et al., 1987). These data have been used to determine the appropriate "cutoff" that distinguishes normal subjects from patients with cancer. Accordingly, most authors have chosen cutoff values of 25, 30, or 40 U/mL, below which 95, 98, or 99%, respectively, of the normal population will fall.

Using these cutoffs, several investigators have reported the sensitivity of CA 15-3 levels in patients with breast cancer (Table 1). Although CA 15-3 levels are not commonly elevated in patients with stage I or II breast cancer, 30–50% of patients with stage III breast cancer (defined as locally advanced but confined to the breast) and approx 70–85% of patients with recurrent/metastatic (stage IV) breast cancer will have elevated values. CA 15-3 levels appear to be independent of histology, estrogen receptor content, or histologic grade of the primary tumors, but are related to the stage and extent of disease (Table 1) (Hayes et al., 1986; Colomer et al., 1989c; Safi et al., 1989). For example, although approx 50% of patients with local or regional recurrence have elevated CA 15-3 levels, 70–80% of patients with bone metastases and 80–90% of patients with multiple metastases, including those to liver, have levels above the chosen cutoff level (Hayes et al., 1986; Safi et al., 1989). In a recently published study, CA 15-3 levels in 80% of patients with multiple metastases were elevated compared to levels in 50% of patients with single metastases (Colomer et al., 1989c). Furthermore, when the extent of metastatic disease in each patient was estimated, CA 15-3 levels were related to more extensive disease. In patients whose disease was estimated to be of similar extent but whose major site was in different organs, or in those patients who had the same number of sites but had disease in different organs, there was no correlation to the site, even if the major site was hepatic (Colomer et al., 1989c).

4. Specificity of CA 15-3

CA 15-3 levels are commonly elevated in patients with metastatic breast cancer, but a variety of benign conditions may also result in slightly to moderately elevated levels (Table 2). Of patients with benign breast diseases, 15–20% have CA 15-3 levels

Table 2
CA 15-3 Levels in Patients with Benign Conditions

Reference	Cutoff U/mL	Patients with CA 15-3 levels above cutoff, %[a]									
		Br	Hep	GI	Res	AI	End	Hem	Ren	Gyn	Pregn/Lact
Hayes et al., 1986	25	16	50	–	–	–	–	–	–	–	0/0
Gang et al., 1985	15	18	–	–	–	–	–	–	–	–	–
Ogawa et al., 1986	20	0	0	–	0	–	0	–	0	–	–
Fujino et al., 1986	24	0	0	–	–	–	–	–	–	–	–
Gion et al., 1986a	31	22	60	–	–	–	–	–	–	–	–
Sacks et al., 1987	40	0	–	–	–	–	–	–	–	–	–
Ruibal et al., 1987	35	1.2	10	–	8.5	8.5	–	–	0	–	–
Takemori et al., 1987	25	3.7	–	–	–	–	–	–	–	–	–
Kikuchi et al., 1987	27	0	–	0	–	–	–	–	–	–	–
Maigre, 1988	25	0	71	–	–	–	–	–	–	–	–
Yedema et al., 1988	30	–	–	–	–	–	–	–	–	9	–
Kallioniemi et al., 1988	38	0	–	–	–	–	–	–	–	–	–
Safi et al., 1989	25	17	–	4–12	–	–	10	–	–	–	–
Colomer et al., 1989a	40	–	7.5	0.6	3.5	7	1	8.3	0	0.6	–
Kerin, 1989	25	5	–	–	–	–	–	–	–	–	–
Lelle et al., 1989	25	–	–	–	–	–	–	–	–	–	0/–
Touitou et al., 1989	25	–	–	–	–	–	–	–	–	0	0/–
Range		0–22	0–71	0–12	0–9	7–9	0–10	8.5	0	0–9	0

[a]Br, Breast; Hep, Hepatic, including cirrhosis amd hepatitis (acute, chronic, amd persistent); GI, Gastrointestinal, including peptic ulcer disease, gastritis, gastroenteritis, inflammatory bowel disease and colonic polyps; Res, Respiratory, including infectious and allergic pneumonitis, tuberculosis, sarcoidosis, chronic obstructive pulmonary disease, and asthma; AI, Autoimmune disease, including systemic lupus erythematosis, rheumatoid arthritis, vasculitis, and CREST syndrome; End, Endocrine, including diabetes melitus, and thyroid disease; Ren, Renal, including cystitis, nephritis, and chronic renal failure; Gyn, Gynecologic, including uterine leiomyomata, endometriotic cysts, cystadenomas (mucinous, serous), ovarian cysts, and ovarian abscesses.

≥25 U/mL. However, few if any of these conditions are associated with levels >40 U/mL. Certain studies have suggested that CA 15-3 levels are elevated only in proliferative benign breast diseases (Gion et al., 1986b; Hayes et al., 1986). In contrast, two separate investigations have suggested that the mean CA 15-3 level in patients with benign breast abnormalities is lower than that for the "normal" population (Sacks et al., 1987; Colomer et al., 1989a). However, even in these studies, elevated levels were observed in a few patients with benign breast lesions (Colomer et al., 1989a).

Several benign conditions not involving the breast have also been reported as causes of elevated CA 15-3 levels. Up to 50% of patients with acute and/or chronic inflammatory liver disease have elevated levels (Gion et al., 1986a; Hayes et al., 1986; Colomer et al., 1989a), although some authors have reported that elevated CA 15-3 levels are not associated with chronic cirrhosis (Fujino et al., 1986; Ruibal et al., 1987). Other relatively frequent but less common causes of CA 15-3 elevations include active tuberculosis, pulmonary sarcoidosis, and systemic lupus erythematosis (Colomer et al., 1989a). As with CEA, CA 15-3 levels increase slightly during later stages of pregnancy, but they rarely rise above cutoff levels (Table 2) (Hayes et al., 1986; Lelle et al., 1989; Touitou et al., 1989). In contrast, other cancer markers are frequently elevated in pregnant women. For example, tissue polypeptide antigen (TPA) may be elevated in as many as 90% of women in the third trimester, and the ovarian epithelial carcinoma marker CA 125 has been reported to be elevated in 10–40% of pregnant women (Lelle et al., 1989; Touitou et al., 1989). Although CA 15-3 levels have been reported to fluctuate by 10–15% on a daily and even hourly basis (Jager et al., 1987), levels do not appear to vary substantially with the menstrual cycle in normal women (Touitou et al., 1989). Furthermore, unlike CEA, CA 15-3 levels are not affected by smoking (Hayes, unpublished).

The etiology of elevated CA 15-3 in patients who have no history of malignancy is probably multifactoral. As noted, the antigen recognized by the CA 15-3 assay is present in most normal epithelial tissue and can be detected in normal secretions (urine, milk, and the like) and in the circulation of normal individuals (Hilkens et al., 1984; Hayes et al., 1985; Sekine et al., 1985b; Hayes et al., 1988b; Hilkens, 1988). Furthermore, the metabolism and clearance of many large circulating glycoproteins is probably through hepatic mechanisms (Thomas and Zamcheck, 1983). Since the CA 15-3 antigen is too large to be filtered through the glomerulus, the presence of this antigen in urine almost certainly represents secretion via shedding from the luminal surface of the distal collecting tubules, a location in which the antigen has been demonstrated by immunoperoxidase studies (Kufe et al., 1984; Hilkens, 1988). Hepatic clearance of the CA 15-3 antigen is further suggested by the observation of frequent and relatively high levels in patients with hepatitis and by the lack of elevated CA 15-3 levels in patients with chronic renal failure (Hayes et al., 1985,1986; Gion et al., 1986a; Ruibal et al., 1987; Colomer et al., 1989a).

5. CA 15-3 in Non-Breast Cancer Malignancies

Immunoperoxidase studies have demonstrated that MAbs DF3 and 115D8 react with a variety of normal and malignant epithelial tissues other than breast (Kufe et al., 1984; Friedman et al., 1986; Hilkens et al., 1989). Likewise, circulating CA 15-3 levels are elevated in patients with nonmammary malignancies (Table 3). Although most reports have not carefully documented the stage and extent of disease in patients with nonbreast malignancies, CA 15-3 levels appear to be most commonly elevated in gynecologic carcinomas, especially those of ovarian epithelial origin (Gang et al., 1985; Hayes et al., 1986; Ruibal et al., 1987; Yedema et al., 1988; Colomer et al., 1989b; Safi et al., 1989). Substantial and frequent (>25% of patients) elevations of CA 15-3 levels have also been reported in carcinomas of the colon, lung, stomach, pancreas, prostate, and liver (Gang et al., 1985; Hayes et al., 1986; Kikuchi et al., 1987; Takemori et al., 1987; Colomer et al., 1989b; Safi et al., 1989). As in patients with breast cancer, CA 15-3 levels are more commonly elevated in patients with more advanced disease (Hayes et al., 1986; Colomer et al., 1989b).

Table 3
CA 15-3 Levels in Patients with Nonmammary Carcinomas

Reference	Cutoff, U/mL	Patients with CA 15-3 levels above cutoff, %[a]											
		Gyn	Col	Gast	Panc	Lung	Pros	Esoph	Ren	Hem	Hep	Mel	STS
Hayes et al., 1986	25	64	53	7	80	71	100	0	75	–	28	–	–
Gang et al., 1985	15	65	–	22	63	32	33	–	–	–	–	–	–
Fujino et al., 1986	24	–	16	–	–	–	–	–	–	–	–	–	–
Gion et al., 1986a	31	–	16	–	–	21	–	–	–	–	–	–	–
Ruibal et al., 1987	35	43	20	–	–	25	–	–	–	–	–	–	–
Takemori et al., 1987	25	–	7.9	9.7	10	33	–	16.7	–	–	10	–	–
Kikuchi et al., 1987	27	–	0	50	–	0	–	–	–	–	–	–	–
Maigre, 1988	25	58	40	–	60	–	–	–	–	–	–	–	–
Yedema et al., 1988	40	50	–	–	–	–	–	–	–	–	–	–	–
Colomer et al., 1989b	25	46.6	15.5	11.5	27	26.6	11	–	–	3.8	30	0	16.6
Safi et al., 1989	25	46	15	6	26	–	–	–	–	15	–	–	33
Range		43–65	0–53	6–50	10–80	0–70	11–100	0–17	75	4–15	10–30	0	17–33

[a]Gyn, Gynecologic, including ovarian epithelial malignancies, uterine carcinoma, and cervical carcinoma; Col, Colonic carcinoma; Gast, Gastric carcinoma; Panc, Pancreatic carcinoma; Lung, Lung carcinoma, including adeno, squamous cell, and small-cell carcinoma; Pros, Prostate carcinoma; Esoph, Esophageal carcinoma; Ren, Renal carcinoma; Hem, Hematologic malignancies, including acute and chronic leukemias (myelogenous and lymphatic), and Hodgkin's and non-Hodgkin's Lymphoma; Mel, Melanoma; STS, Soft-tissue sarcoma.

Surprisingly, infrequent but substantial increases have also been reported in certain patients with nonepithelial malignancies. For example, in one study, 4% of patients with hematologic malignancies had CA 15-3 values above 40 U/mL, ranging as high as 200 U/mL (Colomer et al., 1989b). Moreover, in a small sample, 15% of patients with Hodgkin's disease and 33% of patients with soft-tissue sarcoma were found to have CA 15-3 levels >25 U/mL and two of 18 patients with soft-tissue sarcoma had CA 15-3 levels >50 U/mL (Safi et al., 1989). Elevated CA 15-3 levels have not been observed in patients with melanomas or neurologic tumors (Colomer, 1989b; Hayes, unpublished). Although this family of mucin-like antigens has been traditionally associated with epithelial tissue, these data are consistent with observations that both MAbs 115D8 and DF3 may react with hematologic and mesenchymal tissues (Hilkens, unpublished; Hayes, unpublished).

6. Comparison with Other Markers

In order to determine the clinical utility of a new circulating tumor marker, the sensitivity and specificity data must be considered in the context of previously existing markers. Several circulating substances have been proposed as potential markers for breast cancer, including

1. Tumor-associated antigens, such as CEA, TPA, gross cystic-disease fluid protein (GCDP), and other mucin-like glycoproteins (DF3 antigen, MAM-6 antigen, Mammary Serum Antigen [MSA], CA 549, Breast Cancer Mucin [BCM], and Mucinous Carcinoma Associated [MCA] antigen);
2. Certain hormones, such as calcitonin and β-HCG; and
3. Enzymes and products of certain metabolic pathways, such as β2-microglobulin, ferritin, alkaline phoshatase, hydroxyproline, and osteocalcin.

In general, only the tumor-associated antigens have had sufficient sensitivity and specificity to be of general utility in monitoring patients with breast cancer, and, of these, CEA has been the most widely accepted (Tondini et al., 1989).

Several studies have demonstrated that the CA 15-3 assay is more sensitive than that for CEA in most stages of breast cancer, and may be more specific in relationship to benign nonmammary conditions (Fujino et al., 1986; Hayes et al., 1986; Jager et al., 1987; Pons-Anicet et al., 1987; Delarue et al., 1988; Tondini et al., 1988; Colomer et al., 1989c; Omar et al., 1989; Safi et al., 1989). Although neither assay is very sensitive in patients with stage I or II breast cancer, and both antigens are very commonly elevated in patients with far-advanced metastatic breast cancer, CA 15-3 is significantly more sensitive than CEA in locally advanced primary disease and in patients with local recurrence or bone metastases (Table 4). Certain authors have also reported that CA 15-3 is more commonly elevated even in patients with liver metastases (Safi et al., 1989). Moreover, the two markers do not appear to be complementary. CA 15-3 levels are commonly elevated in patients in whom CEA levels are not, but the reverse is unusual, and the addition of CEA rarely adds additional clinical utility (Hayes et al., 1986; Pons-Anicet et al., 1987; Tondini et al., 1988; Colomer et al., 1989a; Colomer et al., 1989c; Omar et al., 1989; Safi et al., 1989). Likewise, although recent reports have suggested that the ovarian cancer marker, CA 125, is elevated in 20–40% of patients with metastatic breast cancer, elevation of CA 125 levels in the absence of elevated CA 15-3 levels is unusual (Omar et al., 1989; Perey et al., 1990).

Few data have been published regarding comparison of assays that detect different members of the sialomucin family. Early studies suggested that although antibodies against this family clearly recognize similar antigens, construction of the assays with antibodies that recognize distinct epitopes could result in different sensitivities and specificities. For example, the sensitivity of the DF3–DF3 EIA in patients with metastatic breast cancer is similar, but not identical to the CA 15-3 assay (Hayes et al., 1985,1986). However, although these assays also have similar sensitivities in patients with ovarian carcinoma, CA 15-3 levels are much more commonly elevated in patients with colorectal and lung carcinoma than are DF3–DF3 EIA levels (Hayes et al., 1986). Likewise, in a limited

Table 4
Comparision of CA 15-3 and CEA Levels in Patients with Breast Cancer[a]

Stage	No. of patients	No. of patients (%) with CA 15-3 levels >30 U/mL	No. of patients (%) with CEA levels >5.0 ng/mL	p Value[b]
Normal controls	–	(1.3)	(1.3)	–
Primary breast cancer	31	6 (19)	0	$0.005 < p < 0.01$
Metastatic breast cancer	158	99 (63)	64 (41)	<0.001
Local only	26	10 (38)	3 (12)	$0.02 < p < 0.05$
Bone only	34	24 (71)	15 (44)	0.02
Liver	24	19 (79)	18 (75)	NS

[a]Modified from Hayes et al., 1986, with permission.
[b]CA 15-3 vs CEA.

preliminary study, the sensitivity of MCA was roughly the same as that of CA 15-3 in patients with metastatic breast cancer (46 vs 51%). Furthermore, the two assays were strongly correlated in the same group of patients ($r = 0.78$) (Browning et al., 1988). The sensitivity of MSA, another assay that detects a member of the sialomucin family, is similar to that of CA 15-3 in patients with metastatic breast cancer, although in one study the combination of the two assays increased sensitivity in such patients from approx 80% to almost 100% (Sacks et al., 1987). However, the sensitivity of MSA in patients with stage I and II disease has been reported to be significantly higher than that reported for any other breast cancer marker, including CA 15-3 (68 vs 3%), whereas the specificity in patients with benign breast diseases was very similar for both assays (Sacks et al., 1987). Although the differences in performance characteristics between MSA and CA 15-3 may be a consequence of the recognition of distinct epitopic sites present on the family of breast-associated sialomucins, these data require confirmation.

7. Clinical Utility of CA 15-3

7.1. Monitoring Patients with Metastatic Disease

Potential clinical utilities for breast cancer associated tumor markers include screening the general population for the detection of new primary breast cancers, determining the differential diagnosis of suspicious breast abnormalities, determining the differential diagnosis of proven adenocarcinomas of uncertain etiology, predicting the prognosis of patients with newly diagnosed primary breast cancers or metastatic breast cancer, monitoring patients following primary and adjuvant therapy for detection of recurrences, and/or monitoring patients with known recurrent disease to determine their clinical course. Of these, the last is the most widely accepted indication (Tondini et al., 1988). For example, an early study demonstrated that serial CA 15-3 levels increased by at least 25% from baseline values in 19 of 21 patients (91%) with progressive disease and decreased by at least 50% in seven of nine patients

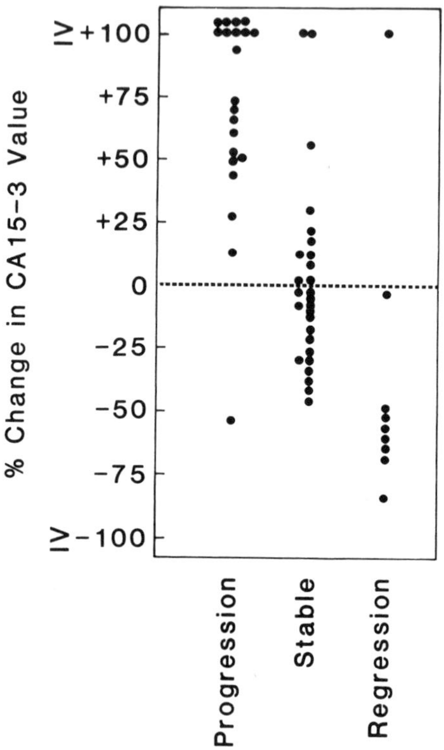

Fig. 1. Changes in CA 15-3 levels with clinical course. Serial changes in CA 15-3 levels were determined during 57 clinical courses of patients with progressive, stable, or regressive breast cancer. From Hayes et al., 1986, with permission.

(89%) with responding disease. In 16 of 27 (59%) patients with stable disease, CA 15-3 values did not differ by ±25% (Fig. 1) (Hayes et al., 1986). In a subsequent study, serial plasma sampes were collected from 53 patients with measurable metastatic disease who had a minimum of three samples drawn during a period that encompassed at least one evaluable clinical course (Tondini et al., 1988). The difference in antigen levels corresponding to a given event were determined as a percentage of change between initial levels and the level at the time of first documented clinical change, and only changes in antigen levels above the designated cutoff levels were considered to be correlative. Overall, CA 15-3 levels correlated to clinical course in 32 of 53 patients (60.3%), whereas CEA correlated in only 21 of 53 (39.6%) (Table 5). The correlation of serial CA 15-3 levels to clinical course was significantly superior to that for CEA (McNamara test $p = 0.02$). The correlation for patients with progressive disease for CA 15-3 was 75%; that for patients with responding disease was only 38%. Logistic regression models suggested that the simultaneous use of both markers failed to significantly enhance sensitivity and specificity obtained with CA 15-3 alone.

The results of this study were further analyzed to determine a "correlative value" for changes in CA 15-3 levels during clinical course. For example, for patients in whom the clinical probability of progression is low, an increase of $\geq$25% for CA 15-3 (positive correlative value) would increase the suspicion of progression to approx 75% (Table 6). Likewise, in a patient with a low probability of progression, the lack of an increase in CA 15-3 (negative correlative value) confirms the clinician's suspicion that that patient is not progressing (Table 6). In a similar manner, positive and negative correlative values for decreases in antigen levels were also determined and found to be quite useful for CA 15-3 values. In almost every situation, correlative values for CA 15-3 were equal or superior to those for either CEA alone or the combination of the two markers.

The correlation of CA 15-3 levels to clinical course has been confirmed by others (Gang et al., 1985; Fujino et al., 1986; Ogawa et al., 1986; Pons-Anicet et al., 1987; Delarue et al., 1988; Kallioniemi et al., 1988). In one study, serial CA 15-3 levels corresponded in 63 of 71 (82%) patients with metastatic disease. Furthermore, serial CA 15-3 levels were elevated and correlated to clinical course in 60% of those patients with a normal CEA (Pons-Anicet et al., 1987). Likewise, another group of investigators has suggested that the sensitivity of CA 15-3 is far superior to that of CEA, whereas the specificities are almost identical (Delarue et al.,

Table 5
Sensitivity of Changes in CA 15-3 and CEA Levels
to Monitor Clinical Course in Patients with Metastatic Breast Cancer[a]

		Number of patients (%) with changes in marker that correlated to clinical course[b]			
Disease course	No. of patients	CA 15-3	CEA	CA 15-3 and CEA	CA 15-3 or CEA
Progression	24	18 (75)	14 (58)	12 (50)	20 (83)
Regression	21	8 (38)	5 (23)	3 (16)	10 (47)
Stable disease	8	6 (75)	2 (25)	2 (25)	6 (75)
Overall	53	32 (60)	21 (39)	17 (32)	36 (67)

[a]Modified from Tondini et al., 1988, with permission.

[b]For sensitivity, the correlation of changes in antigen levels to clinical course is defined as an increase ≥25% in patients with progressive disease, as a decrease ≥25% in patients with responsive disease, and as variation of ±25% in patients with stable disease.

Table 6
Correlative Values of Increases in CA 15-3 and CEA Levels in Patients with Metastatic Breast Cancer[a]

Predictive value	Hypothetical probability of progression	Probability of progression if marker increases ≥25%	
		CA 15-3, %	CEA, %
Positive	0.3	75	51
	0.5	88	71
	0.7	94	83
Negative	0.3	89	81
	0.5	78	64
	0.7	60	44

[a]Modified from Tondini et al., 1988 with permission.

1988). They concluded that the addition of CEA was of no benefit in following patients with metastatic disease.

One important factor that must be recognized in monitoring patients with serial CA 15-3 levels is the appearance of a "spike" phenomenon, defined as a transient increase in levels following initiation of effective therapy for metastatic disease (Hayes et al., 1988a). The spike phenomenon has been described after either chemotherapy or hormone therapy, and may last as long as 20–90 d (Fig. 2). Occurrence of a "spike" in CA 15-3 levels may actually be a favorable predictor of response to therapy, but early increases in levels cannot be distinguished from progression. As in all situations, clinical judgment must be used to avoid misinterpreting increased levels of CA 15-3 as progressive disease, when in fact the patient may actually be responding to therapy.

In summary, serial CA 15-3 levels offer a reasonably sensitive and specific method of monitoring the clinical course of patients with metastatic disease. If CA 15-3 levels are elevated, serial changes correlate reliably to clinical course. Although the marker is of no value in the few patients in whom elevations are not present, CA 15-3 should be considered the current "marker of choice" for

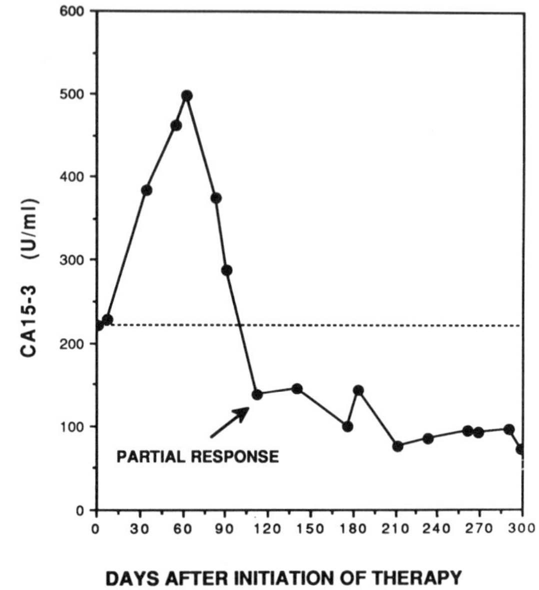

Fig. 2. CA 15-3 spike. Serial CA 15-3 levels were monitored in a patient with metastatic breast cancer treated with combination chemotherapy initiated on day 0. On day 120, clinical and radiographic evaluation determined that the patient had experienced a partial response to chemotherapy. CA 15-3 levels increased by >100% during the first 60 d of therapy and then declined to a level <50% of baseline value.

patients with metastatic disease, because of its increased sensitivity compared to CEA.

7.2. Monitoring Patients for Early Relapse After Primary Therapy

Another use of circulating breast cancer associated antigens would be to monitor patients following primary therapy in order to detect impending relapses earlier than is possible with either clinical or radiographic techniques. In this regard, the value of early diagnosis of relapse is currently controversial (Hayes and Kaplan, 1991). Early treatment of micrometastatic disease in the adjuvant setting clearly prolongs survival in certain groups of patients, but the treatment of patients with documented metastatic disease is palliative and provides little if any survival benefit. Nonetheless, few studies have addressed whether treatment early in the course of documented metastatic patients might substantially prolong their survival compared to treatment at a later, more advanced stage. A sensitive and specific tumor marker could increase the time between a reliable indication of tumor recurrence and its detection with clinical or radiographic evaluation. Approximately 75% of patients with metastatic disease will go to their physicians with symptoms referable to the specific site of relapse (Hayes and Kaplan, 1991); the remaining 25% have asymptomatic recurrences detected either by physician evaluation or by laboratory and/or radiographic testing. Earlier detection of metastases prior to the onset of symptoms may depend on the frequency of routine follow-up. Furthermore, determination of whether a marker provides a lead time prior to the detection of disease with other clinical parameters requires strict criteria for routine collection of blood samples and clinical data.

Several preliminary studies have suggested that CA 15-3 levels may rise prior to clinical detection of metastases (Table 7) (Ruibal et al., 1987; Yoshimoto et al., 1987; Kallioniemi et al., 1988; Thirion et al., 1988; Colomer et al., 1989a; Omar et al., 1989). In these studies, the incidence of elevated CA 15-3 levels prior to documentation of metastases is 25–75%. In patients in whom rising CA 15-3 levels preceeded clinical evidence of recurrence, the lead time has been reported to be from 1 to 13 mo (Kallioniemi et al., 1988; Thirion et al., 1988; Colomer et al., 1989a; Omar et al., 1989). As in patients with known metastases, CA 15-3 levels are more sensitive than CEA levels for detecting early relapses in these studies (Pons-Anicet et al., 1987; Ruibal et al., 1987; Kallioniemi et al., 1988; Thirion et al., 1988; Colomer et al., 1989a; Omar et al., 1989).

Importantly, the specificity of CA 15-3 levels in breast cancer patients after primary and adjuvant therapy appears to be satisfactory (Table 7). Specificity can be improved further if serial levels are considered elevated only if observed to rise over two consecutive months. Unfortunately, such a requirement will decrease the lead time. For example, in one study, three patients who had levels

Table 7
Prediction of Relapse by Increasing CA 15-3 Levels After Primary Therapy in Patients with Breast Cancer

Reference	Follow-up	Number of patients	Number relapsed	Cutoff, U/mL	Sens[a]	Spec[b]	True Pos[c]	False Pos[d]	Lead Time (median)[e]
Ruibal et al., 1987	14 mo	201	17	40	77	95	41	58	2–11 (7)
Thirion et al., 1988	24 mo	302	66	30	65	98	91.5	8.5	1–13 (4)
Maigre, 1988	9–18 mo	302	66	25	77	NA[f]	NA	NA	NA
Kallioniemi et al., 1988	1–3 yr	NA	NA	38	NA	NA	NA	NA	1–13 (NA)
Colomer et al., 1989a	12.9 mo	337	40	40	45	96	45	40	1–12 (5)
Safi et al., 1989	51 mo	671	205	25	73	94	NA	NA	1–18 (6)
Range					45–77	94–98	41–92	9–58	1–18 (4–7)

[a]Sensitivity, % of patients with clinically or radiographically documented metastases with elevated CA 15-3.

[b]Specificity, % of patients without clinically or radiographically documented metastases with nonelevated CA 15-3.

[c]Pos, Positive; % of patients with elevated CA 15-3 after primary therapy who subsequently developed clinically or radiographically documented metastases during follow-up.

[d]Percentage of patients with elevated CA 15-3 after primary therapy who did not subsequently develop clinically or radiographically documented metastases during follow-up.

[e]Time (months) from first elevation of CA 15-3 until clinically or radiographically documented metastases were identified.

[f]NA, not available.

over 40 U/mL during routine follow-up, but whose levels returned to normal, did not subsequently relapse. In contrast, all other patients, whose values rose and remained elevated, did relapse within the succeeding 7 mo (Omar et al., 1989). In a larger study, 12 of 350 patients (4%) who were free of disease after primary therapy had elevated CA 15-3 levels, between 40 and 60 U/mL. In eight of these, a subsequent sample drawn within a month after the initially elevated level demonstrated a return to normal, and none of these patients relapsed. In three others, the elevated level could be explained by the presence of a benign condition known to cause low levels of elevations. Therefore, in only one patient (0.3%) was a persistently elevated CA 15-3 level not associated with a benign condition or a subsequent relapse (Colomer et al., 1989a).

These preliminary results are encouraging, but none of these studies has been performed in a prospective manner with rigid criteria for routine follow-up. Although a large multicenter trial is currently ongoing in the United States, data will not be available for several years. In the meantime, serial tumor markers should be used to monitor patients after primary therapy with the understanding that the clinical utility of such early detection has not been established. Furthermore, the performance characteristics of CA 15-3 specifically in this setting have not been determined.

7.3. Determining Prognosis

Tumor-marker levels at the time of diagnosis might be prognostic of the ultimate clinical outcome. For example, results of a few studies suggest that elevated CEA levels are associated with a worse prognosis (Krebs et al., 1976; Bezwoda et al., 1981; De Jong-Bakker et al., 1981). However, several other studies have failed to show a correlation between perioperative CEA levels and clinical outcome (Koch et al., 1980; Doyle et al., 1981; Mughal et al., 1983; Loprinzi et al., 1986; Theriault et al., 1989). Immunoperoxidase and immunoblot studies have suggested that high expression of the sialo-mucin antigen family in primary breast tissues may be associated with improved prognosis (Wilkinson et al., 1984; Ellis et al., 1985, 1987; Angus et al., 1986; Helle, 1986; Rasmussen et al., 1986).

A large study from the Cancer and Leukemia Group B (CALGB) has demonstrated that patients whose tumors exhibit high immunoperoxidase-staining scores with MAb DF3, presumably associated with superior differentiation, have a significantly better disease-free and overall survival when compared to those whose staining scores are low (Hayes, et al., 1991b). However, elevated circulating CA 15-3 levels at the time of diagnosis appear to predict a worse prognosis (Ruibal et al., 1987; Kallioniemi et al., 1988; Colomer et al., 1989a,c). For example, Colomer et al. (1989a) have reported that patients with postoperative CA 15-3 levels >40 U/mL have a disease-free survival almost half that of those with normal levels, and significantly shorter overall survival (18.3 vs 25 mo, $p < 0.0001$). Similarly, high postoperative CEA levels were also associated with shorter disease-free and overall survival differences, although the differences were not as significant as those seen with CA 15-3 (Colomer et al., 1989a). The contradiction between evaluation of antigen expression in primary tumors and detection of high levels of antigen in plasma may be attributable to the lack of staging data in the studies that determine prognosis with circulating CA 15-3 levels. None of these studies has determined whether elevated CA 15-3 levels are independent of stage as prognostic factors. Since CA 15-3 levels are associated with more advanced stages of both primary and metastatic disease, elevated CA 15-3 levels may simply reflect the presence of micrometastatic disease and may not be a predictor of biological behavior. A large, multiinstitutional prospec-tive trial assessing this question is currently underway.

7.4. Other Uses in Breast Cancer

CA 15-3 is either less well-studied or less useful for other utilities. For example, the low sensitivity and relatively poor specificity of detection of early primary breast cancers in the normal population precludes use of this assay for screening or in the evaluation of suspicious breast masses or mammographic results (*see* Tables 1 and 2). Likewise, since CA 15-3 is elevated in several different types of adenocarcinomas, and may even be elevated in nonepithelial malignancies, circulating CA 15-3 levels are of little value in the differential diagnosis of carcinomas of unknown origin.

8. Use of CA 15-3 in Monitoring Patients with Nonbreast Malignancies

Since CA 15-3 is commonly elevated in nonbreast malignancies, this assay could potentially be useful to monitor such patients (*see* Table 3). One early study has suggested that the DF3–DF3 EIA is elevated in 25–60% of patients with all histological types of ovarian cancer (Sekine et al., 1985a). Furthermore, although not as sensitive, DF3–DF3 EIA is complementary to CA 125. Of 45 patients with ovarian epithelial malignancies, 36 (80%) had elevated CA 125 levels, 21 (47%) had elevated DF3 levels, and 41 (91%) had elevations of one or the other. Moreover, several patients with nonmalignant gynecological disorders who had elevated CA 125 levels had normal DF3 levels (Sekine et al., 1985a). In a similar fashion, Yedema et al. have published that CA 15-3 and CA 125 are complementary in evaluating patients with benign and malignant ovarian tumors. They have reported that the predictive value for malignancy if both markers are elevated may approach 100% (Yedema et al., 1988). The utility of CA 15-3 in other malignancies is essentially unknown. However, recently MAb have been produced against a lung cancer associated sialomucin (Maimonis et al., 1990). These MAbs have been used to construct a double-determinant assay that detects a circulating lung cancer associated sialomucin. The sensitivity of this assay in patients with all histological types of lung cancer is 50–70% (Hayes et al., 1991a).

9. Miscellaneous Uses

Evaluation of CA 15-3 levels in effusions has been proposed as one means of determining their etiology. For example, one recent study reported that CA 15-3 levels were above 16 U/mL in 38% of malignant effusions, and were less than that cutoff in all of

40 tuberculous effusions (Shimokata et al., 1988). Although the negative predictive value of a CA 15-3 effusion level <16 U/mL was low, they suggested that the positive predictive value of an elevation >16 U/mL approached 100%. This study did not include effusions attributable to breast cancer (Shimokata et al., 1988). Recently, amniotic fluid and umbilical-cord blood were evaluated for the presence of several tumor markers. CEA and CA 125 levels were frequently elevated in such patients, but CA 15-3 levels could not be detected in either (Lelle et al., 1989). The clinical significance of these findings is not clear.

10. Summary

In summary, the CA 15-3 assay detects a high-mol-wt circulating glycoprotein that is produced by normal epithelial tissues and that can be detected in the plasma from normal subjects. This antigen is frequently elevated in plasmas from patients with epithelial malignancies, and the sensitivity of the CA 15-3 assay in patients with metastatic breast cancer is between 75 and 90%. Although the assay is not useful in distinguishing benign from malignant conditions, especially when levels are only moderately elevated, and also cannot be used to distinguish different types of epithelial malignancies, it is a sensitive and reliable marker for monitoring clinical course in patients with metastatic breast cancer. Furthermore, preliminary data suggests that it may also play a role in detecting early recurrences in patients following primary and adjuvant therapy for breast cancer. Large ongoing multicenter prospective trials should further define the clinical utility of the CA 15-3 assay.

References

Abe, M. and D. W. Kufe (1986), *J. Cell. Physiol.* **126,** 126–132.
Abe, M. and D. W. Kufe (1987), *J. Immunol.* **139,** 257–261.
Abe, M., and D. W. Kufe (1989), *Cancer Res.* **49,** 2834–2839.
Angus, B., J. Napier, J. Purvis, I. Ellis, R. Hawkins, F. Carpenter, and C. Horne (1986), *J. Pathol.* **149,** 301–306.

Bezwoda, W., D. Derman, and T. Bothwell (1981), *Cancer* **48,** 1623–1628.
Browning, M., N. McFarlane, J. Horobin, P. Preece, and R. Wood (1988), *Ann. Clin. Biochem.* **25,** 54–56.
Colomer, R., A. Ruibal, and L. Salvador (1989c), *Cancer* **64,** 1674–1681.
Colomer, R., A. Ruibal, J. Genolla, and L. Salvador (1989b), *Br. J. Cancer* **59,** 283–286.
Colomer, R., A. Ruibal, J. Genolla, D. Rubio, C. J. M. Del, R. Bodi, and L. Salvador (1989a), *Breast Cancer Res. Treat.* **13,** 123–133.
Colomer, R., A. Ruibal, M. Navarro, G. Encabo, L. A. Sole, and L. Salvador (1986), *Int. J. Biol. Markers* **1,** 89–92.
De Jong-Bakker, M., A. Hart, and J. Persijn (1981), *Eur. J. Cancer Clin. Oncol.* **17,** 1307–1313.
Delarue, J. C., H. Mouriesse, F. Dubois, S. Friedman, and L. F. May (1988), *Breast Cancer Res. Treat.* **11,** 273–276.
Doyle, P., R. Nicholson, and G. Groome (1981), *Clin. Oncol.* **7,** 53–58.
Ellis, I., J. Bell, J. Todd, M. Williams, C. Dowle, A. Robins, C. Elston, R. Blamey, and R. Baldwin (1987), *Br. J. Cancer* **56,** 295–299.
Ellis I., C. Hinton, J. MacNay, C. Elston, A. Robins, A. Owalnati, R. Blamey, R. Baldwin, and B. Ferry (1985), *Br. Med. J.* **290,** 881–883.
Friedman, E. L., D. F. Hayes, and D. W. Kufe (1986), *Cancer Res.* **46,** 5189–5194.
Fujino, N., Y. Haga, K. Sakamoto, H. Egami, M. Kimura, R Nishimura and M. Akagi (1986), *Jpn. J. Clin. Oncol.* **16,** 335–346.
Gang, Y., I. Adachi, H. Ohkura, H. Yamamoto, Y. Mizuguchi, and K. Abe (1985), *Gan To Kagaku Ryoho* **12,** 2379–2386.
Gion, M., R. Mione, R. Dittadi, S. Fasan, A. Pallini, and G. Bruscagnin (1986a), *J. Nucl. Med. Allied Sci.* **3,** 29–36.
Gion, M., R. Mione, R. Dittadi, L. Griggio, G. Munegato, M. Valsecchi, M. O. Del, and G. Bruscagnin (1986b), *Int. J. Biol. Markers* **1,** 33–38.
Hayes, D. F., V. R. J. Zurawski, and D. W. Kufe (1986), *J. Clin. Oncol.* **4,** 1542–1550.
Hayes, D. F. and W. Kaplan (1991), in *Breast Diseases* (Harris, J., S. Hellman, I. Henderson, and D. Kinne, eds.), Lippincott, Philadelphia, PA, pp. 505–525.
Hayes, D. F., D. S. Silberstein, S. Rodrique, and D. W. Kufe (1990), *J. Immunol.* **145,** 962–970.
Hayes, D. F., D. T. Kiang, A. Korzun, C. Tondini, W. Wood, and et al. (1988a), *Proc. Am. Soc. Clin. Oncol.* **7,** 38a.
Hayes, D. F., H. Sekine, D. Marcus, C. A. Alper, and D. W. Kufe (1988b), *Blood* **71,** 436–440.
Hayes, D. F., H. Sekine, T. Ohno, M. Abe, K. Keefe, and D. W. Kufe (1985), *J. Clin. Invest.* **75,** 1671–1678.

Hayes, D. F., P. Maimonis, V. Wood, M. Bornstein, S. Schaffel, A. Skarin, and D. W. Kufe (1991a), *Proceedings of the American Society of Clinical Oncology* **10,** 36a.

Hayes, D. F., R. Mesa-Tejada, L. Papsidero, G. Croghan, A. Korzun, L. Norton, W. Wood, J. Strauchen, M. Grimes, R. Weiss, H. Ree, A. Thor, F. Koerner, M. Rice, M. Barcos, and D. W. Kufe (1991b), *J. Clin. Oncol.* **9,** 1–10.

Helle, M. (1986), *Acta Pathol. Microbiol. Immunol. Scand.* **94,** 375–380.

Hilkens, J. (1988), *Cancer Rev.* **11–12,** 25–54.

Hilkens, J., F. Buijs, and M. Ligtenberg (1989), *Cancer Res.* **49,** 786–793.

Hilkens, J., F. Buijs, J. Hilgers, P. Hageman, J. Calafat, A. Sonnenberg and M. van der Valk (1984), *Int. J. Cancer* **34,** 197–206.

Hilkens J., V. Kroezen, J. M. Bonfrer, J. B. M. De and P. F. Bruning (1986), *Cancer Res.* **46,** 2582–2587.

Hull, S., A. Bright, K. Carraway, M. Abe, D. Hayes, and D. W Kufe (1989), *Cancer Commun.* **1,** 261–267.

Jager, W., W. Sauerbrei, M. Diedrich, B. Krempel, and L. Wildt (1987), *Onkologie* **10,** 290–293.

Kallioniemi, O., H. Oksa, R. Aaran, T. Hietanen, M. Lehtinen, and T. Koivula (1988), *Br. J. Cancer* **58,** 213–215.

Kerin, M. J., O. J. McAnena, V. P. OMalley, H. Grimes, and H. F. Given (1989), *Br. J. Surg.* **76,** 838–839.

Kikuchi, K., Y. Uematsu, Y. Takada, E. Kurihara, T. Suito, M. Fujisaki, R. Takahashi, and T. Tamura (1987), *Gan To Kagaku Ryoho* **14,** 3095–3100.

Koch, M., A. Paterson, and T. McPherson (1980), *Clin. Oncol.* **6,** 323–327.

Krebs, B., R. Lupo, and M. Namer (1976), *Bull. Cancer* **63,** 485–488.

Kufe, D., G. Inghirami, M. Abe, D. Hayes, W. H. Justi, and J. Schlom (1984), *Hybridoma* **3,** 223–232.

Lelle, R. J., E. Henkel, D. Leinemann, and K. Goeschen (1989), *Gynecol. Obstet. Invest.* **27,** 137–142.

Loprinzi, C. L., D. C. Tormey, P. Rasmussen, G. Falkson, T. E. Davis, H. C. Falkson, and A. Y. Chang (1986), *J. Clin. Oncol.* **4,** 46–56.

Maigre, M., P. Fumoleau, G. Ricolleau, Y. Guillard, A. Cussac, J. Vignoud, and V. Ahkong (1988), *Sem Hop Paris.* **64,** 9–13.

Maimonis, P., D. F. Hayes, C. O'Hara, and D. Kufe (1990), *Cancer Res.* **50,** 6738–6743.

Merlo, G., J. Siddiqui, C. Cropp, D. Liscia, R. Lidereau, R. Callahan, and D. Kufe (1989), *Cancer Res.* **49,** 6966–6971.

Mughal, A. W., G. N. Hortobagyi, H. A. Fritsche, A. U. Buzdar, H. Y. Yap, and G. R. Blumenschein (1983), *JAMA* **249,** 1881–1886.

Ogawa, T., M. Izumio, H. Morita, T. Ishida, Y. Iino, K. Hoshino, T. Yokoe, H. Suzuki, S. Murata, S. Matsuzaki, and M. Suzuku (1986), *Gan No Rinsho* **32,** 27–32.

Omar, Y., A. Behbehani, N. Al-Naqeeb, M. Motawy, M. Foudeh, A. Awwad, M. Nasralla, and J. Szymendera (1989), *Int. J. Biol. Markers* **4,** 81–86.

Perey, L., D. Hayes, C. Tondini, G. van Melle, J. Bauer, T. Lemarchand, M. Reymond, J. Mach, and S. Leyvraz (1990), *Br. J. Cancer* **62,** 668–670.

Pons-Anicet, D. M., B. P. Krebs, R. Mira, and M. Namer (1987), *Br. J. Cancer* **55,** 567–569.

Rasmussen, B., C. Rose, J. Hilkens, and J. Hilgers (1986), *Virchows Arch. (Pathol. Anat.)*, **409,** 497–505.

Ruibal, A., R. Colomer, and J. Genolla (1987), *Horm. Metab.* **1,** 11–15.

Sacks, N. P., S. A. Stacker, C. H. Thompson, J. P. Collins, I. S. Russell, J. A. Sullivan, and I. F. McKenzie (1987), *Br. J. Cancer* **56,** 820–824.

Safi F., I. Kohler, E. Rottinger, P. Suhr, and H. G. Beger (1989), *Int. J. Biol. Markers* **4,** 207–214.

Sekine, H., D. F. Hayes, T. Ohno, K. A. Keefe, E. Schaetzl, R. C. Bast, R. Knapp, and D. W. Kufe (1985a), *J. Clin. Oncol.* **3,** 1355–1363.

Sekine, H., T. Ohno, and D. W. Kufe (1985b), *J. Immunol.* **135,** 3610–3615.

Shimokata, K., Y. Totani, K. Nakanishi, M. Yamamoto, Y. Hasegawa, H. Kawatsu, H. Sasou, T. Murate, S. Ichiyama, T- Kurasawa (1988), *Eur. Respir. J.* **1,** 341–344.

Siddiqui J., M. Abe, D. Hayes, E. Shani, E. Yunis, and D. Kufe (1988), *Proc. Natl. Acad. Sci. USA* **85,** 2320–2323.

Swallow, D., S. Gendler, B. Griffiths, G. Corney, J. Taylor-Papadimitriou, and M. Bramwell (1987), *Nature* **328,** 82–84.

Takemori, Y., H. Odani, H. Watanabe, H. Ohta, Y. Satomura, T. Okai, N. Sawabu, M. Mai, N. Hatori, and T. Hashimoto (1987), *Jpn. J. Cancer Chemother.* **14,** 114–118.

Theriault, R. L., G. N. Hortobagyi, H. A. Fritsche, D. Frye, R. Martinez, and A. U. Buzdar (1989), *Cancer* **63,** 828–835.

Thirion, B., G. Ricolleay, and P. Fumoleau (1988), *Third International Workshop on Monoclonal Antibodies and Breast Cancer,* abstract.

Thomas, P. and N. Zamcheck (1983), *Dig. Dis. Sci.* **28,** 215–224.

Tondini, C., D. F. Hayes, R. Gelman, I. C. Henderson, and D. W. Kufe (1988), *Cancer Res.* **48,** 4107–4112.

Tondini, C., D. F. Hayes, and D. Kufe (1989), in *Diagnosis and Therapy of Breast Cancer* (Henderson, I. C., ed.), Saunders, Philadelphia, PA, pp. 653–674.

Touitou, Y., Y. Darbois, A. Bogdan, A. Auzeby, and S. Keusseoglou (1989), *Br. J. Cancer* **60,** 419, 420.

Wilkinson, M., A. Howell, M. Harris, J. Taylor-Papadimitriou, R. Swindell, and R. Sellwood (1984), *Int. J. Cancer* **33,** 299–304.

Yedema, C., L. Massuger, J. Hilgers, J. Servaas, L. Poels, and et al. (1988), *Int. J. Cancer Suppl.* **3,** 6–67.

Yoshimoto, M., F. Akiyama, S. Watanabe, F. Kasumi, A. Fukami, T. Nakajima, M. Nishi, T. Kajitani, and S. Takahashi (1987), *Gan To Kagaku Ryoho* **14,** 2310–2315.

Chapter 14

CA 19-9, GICA (Gastrointestinal Cancer Antigen)

Rolf Lamerz

1. Introduction

Following the detection and clinical exploitation of alpha-fetoprotein (AFP), calcinoembryonic antigen (CEA), and human chorionic genadotropin (HCG) as first and basic tumor markers, the discovery of blood group-related carbohydrate structures on glycoproteins and glycolipids as indicators of malignancy has opened a wide array of scientific and clinical work (Lloyd, 1987). This has only become fully assessable by the introduction of hybridoma technique and the development of murine monoclonal antibodies (Köhler and Milstein, 1975), which made possible the differentiation of even narrow-related substances of protein/carbohydrate/lipid nature. Blood group antigens can also be defined as markers of normal differentiation whose control of malignant transformation becomes disarranged leading to an altered expression (overproduction, synthesis of precursor structures, fetal or inappropriate tissue expression, dis/activation of secretory genes, and so on). In this respect, the detection of circulating sialyl-Le^{a}/CA 19-9 presents a

From: *Serological Cancer Markers* Edited by Stewart Sell ©1992 The Humana Press, Totowa, NJ

landmark in recent clinical tumor immunology. In the following, a review is given on the immunohistochemical and clinical significance of the antigen.

2. Definition and Characterization of CA 19-9

In 1979, first experiences were reported about a murine monoclonal antibody (MAb) called 1116NS 19-9 (MAb 19-9, IgG_1 immunoglobulin), which had been generated against a human colorectal carcinoma cell line (SW1116) (Koprowski et al., 1979). The corresponding antigen detected by the MAb was determined by isolation studies as a molecule of 36 kDa and termed CA 19-9 or GICA (gastrointestinal cancer antigen). Biochemically, CA 19-9 corresponds to a monosialoganglioside (glycoplipid) that could be identified as sialolylated lacto-*N*-fucopentaose II, a hapten of human Lewis^a blood group determinant (Magnani et al., 1982; Falk et al., 1983; Hansson and Zopf, 1985). Its immunochemical demonstration is abolished by neuraminidase treatment (Magnani et al., 1982) consistent with a conformational analysis by which neuraminic acid seems to be incorporated in the epitope-creating unit responsible for the antibody binding site (Bechtel et al., 1990).

CA 19-9 (sialyl-Le^a) is derived like Le^x, sialyl-Le^x and Le^y from Lewis blood group system (Le$^{a/b}$); it may occur as monosialoganglioside/glycolipid in tissue (Magnani et al., 1982) or as circulating mucin in serum (Magnani et al., 1983) and contains neuraminic acid and fucose. Biosynthetically, it develops via a precursor carbohydrate chain (type I) by means of an α-3-sialyltransferase that binds *N*-acetyl neuraminic acid to a terminal galactose residue in α-2-3-position as a precursor antigen (CA 50), and by fucosylation in α-1-4-position at *N*-acetylglucosamine (Hansson and Zopf, 1985). The reaction is encoded by the Lewis^a gene (Lloyd, 1987). The purification of a human gastrointestinal tumor-associated antigen expressing CA 19-9 from the colorectal carcinoma cell line SW1116 revealed a glycoprotein of apparent mol mass 210 kDa, which aggregated without detergents to a mass of 600–2000 kDa (main amino acids serine, threonine, proline; mucin-like structure with 85% of carbohydrates) (Klug et al., 1988).

3. Tissue Expression of CA 19-9

3.1. General Appearance

By means of immunofluorescence and immunoperoxidase techniques using MAb 19-9, antigen CA 19-9 could be detected in colonic (59%), gastric (89%), and pancreatic adenocarcinoma (77–88%); in carcinomas of the liver, papilla of Vater (Kimura and Ohtsubo, 1988), gallbladder, lung, kidney, breast, and ovary (mucinous type); and in benign and malignant tumors of the parotid (Atkinson et al., 1982; Charpin et al., 1982; Dietel et al., 1986; Haglund et al., 1986a; Ouyang et al., 1987; Pour et al., 1988; Prantl, 1987). Furthermore, it was found in fetal epithelia of the stomach (41%), colon (69%), small bowel (89%), liver, and pancreas (Raux et al., 1983), as well as in traces in normal adult organs like pancreas (up to 32%), stomach, liver, colon, gallbladder, ductus choledochus, ducts of esophagus glands, in epithelia of the larynx, trachea, bronchus, lung (epithelial cells, near to the cell membrane and luminal site), conjunctiva, tear and saliva glands, ovary (15%), in ovarian nontumorous mucus epithelium, fallopian tube, in the goblet cells, and in mucus-producing columnar cells of the endocervix (Atkinson et al., 1982; Bra et al., 1986; Dietel et al., 1986; Olding et al., 1984). Therefore, CA 19-9 is regarded as a normal constituent of gastrointestinal and cervical mucosa.

The immunohistologic distribution of CA 19-9 in tissues is consistent with the quantitative determination of higher CA 19-9 concentrations in cancer than in normal or inflamed tissues like pancreatic cancer (340–79,755 U/mg protein), chronic pancreatitis (11–921 U/mg protein), normal adult pancreas (3–409 U/mg protein), fetal pancreas (1–434 U/mg protein); metastatic liver cancer, cholangiocarcinoma (104–1643 U/mg protein), benign liver disease (4–1416 U/mg protein), fetal liver, gallbladder (cancer about 10,000

U/mg protein; benign biliary disease: 5–8272 U/mg protein), stomach (benign: 9–84 U/mg protein; cancer: 7–987 U/mg protein), and colon cancer (124 U/mg protein) (Nishida et al., 1988a).

3.2. Pancreas

CA 19-9 (and Le^a as well as disialosyl-Le^a and CA 50; Itzkowitz et al., 1988; Schwenk et al., 1989) was present only in the ducts (apical surface and on supranuclear cytoplasm) of fetal (including acinar cells), normal (72%), or inflamed (96%) pancreas (focally and weakly), in acute (92%) or chronic pancreatitis without stromal type staining (Haglund et al., 1986a; Itzkowitz et al., 1988; Schwenk et al., 1989; Shimizu et al., 1990); in hyperplastic epithelium, the antigen was not only localized at the basolateral plasma membrance, but also in cytoplasm (Ichihara et al., 1988). In pancreatic ductular adenocarcinoma, CA 19-9 was detected in 77–85% of tumor cells with a clear correlation to the degree of differentiation with more stained cells in well-differentiated areas than in poorly differentiated or anaplastic lesions (Haglund et al., 1986a; Pour et al., 1988; Schwenk et al., 1989) in addition to some pancreatic acinar cells or ductal cells; in cancerous glands, it was distributed over the entire surface and cytoplasm loosing polar distribution pattern of the antigen and at the surrounding stroma adjacent to the cancer cells (Ichihara et al., 1988). No correlation (Nishida et al., 1988a), or a weak (Haglund et al., 1986a) or a strong correlation (Takasaki et al., 1988), was found between tissue expression of CA 19-9 and its serum concentration.

Concerning $Lewis^{a/b}$ phenotype and CA 19-9 expression, negative findings were reported for all cases of $Le^{a-/b-}$ in contrast to predominantly positive findings in $Le^{a+/b-}$ and $Le^{a-/b+}$ phenotype cases (Pour et al., 1988; Schwenk et al., 1989).

3.3. Stomach and Colon–Rectum

In addition, CA 19-9 could be found in gastric cancer (58–62% positive; Hirohashi et al., 1984), in normal stomach surface epithelium (foveolary type), or in mediastinal metaplasia (goblet cell type), and in rising distribution with increasing atrophy and metaplasia (43%), as in benign ulcer disease (48%) (Lindgren and Sipponen, 1985; Sipponen and Lindgren, 1986).

Concerning colonic tissue (Gong et al., 1985), CA 19-9 was not expressed in normal colonic mucosa in contrast to a positive expression of Le^a and disialosyl-Le^a (Itzkowitz et al., 1988), only weakly expressed in the vicinity of carcinoma, and expressed in 80.6% of cases with adenomas showing a correlation with the extent of atypical cells/grade of dysplasia and without relation to histologic type (Enblad et al., 1988); in rectal adenomas, CA 19-9 appeared only in few foci of upper crypts adjacent to carcinoma and only rarely in normal mucosa in contrast to CA 50 frequently expressed in normal epithelium (Enblad et al., 1988). Furthermore, a focal expression of CA 19-9 was detected in regenerating dysplastic and cancerous mucosa of ulcerative colitis, leaving negative normal hyperplastic epithelia or inflammatory regions without dysplasia (Olding et al., 1985; Allen et al., 1987).

In focal carcinoma within an adenoma, CA 19-9 was strongly expressed as well as diffusely in 50% of cases, and in 71–82.2% of cases in progressive carcinoma of homogenous or heterogenous type (Gong et al., 1985; Afdhal et al., 1987; Lorenz et al., 1987), in 11% as strong and in 53% as focal staining (Arends et al., 1983); only as apical in 50% and as combined apical and cytoplasmic staining in 20% (Lorenz et al., 1987), and more frequently in Duke's stage C/D and in poorly differentiated carcinomas (Afdhal et al., 1987). There was no correlation between CA 19-9 expression in tumor and bowel region, staging, grading (Arends et al., 1983; Lorenz et al., 1987), ploidy (Arends et al., 1983), or clinical course between CA 19-9 positive/negative cases (Arends et al., 1984), but a good correlation between the intensity of CA 19-9 staining or percentage of stained cells and serum CA 19-9 level (Lorenz et al., 1987), for adenomas to tumor size, strong dysplasia, and the villous type (Afdhal et al., 1987).

Increasing tissue concentrations of CA 19-9 were observed from normal colonic mucosa (37–5800 U/g wet wt) through adenoma to carcinoma (120–72,660 U/g wet wt), whereas in adenomas, different histologies and dysplasias showed no differences in contrast to a clear correlation between CA 19-9 tissue concentration and size of adenoma (Fischbach and Mössner, 1988) and in adenocarcinoma with increasing tumor stage (Quentmeier et al., 1987; Fischbach and Mössner, 1988).

3.4. Breast and Gynecologic Organs

CA 19-9 expression in human breast tissues showed variable activity in ductal and acinar epithelium of normal and hyperplastic tissues and an overall incidence of 62% in breast carcinoma with only a small number of cell positivity in half of cases, and a significant relationship between CA 19-9 and poor differentiation, and not with local lymph node status (Walker and Day, 1986).

In ovarian tumors, CA 19-9 was mainly detected in serous tumors together with CA 125, and predominantly in mucinous tumors (Macdonald et al., 1988; Neunteufel and Breitenecker, 1989b) with poor correlation between tissue expression and circulating CA 19-9 levels in contrast to a good correlation for CA 125 (Breitenecker et al., 1989). In borderline ovarian tumors, CA 19-9 was detected more often in mucinous (89% vs 44% for CEA and none for CA 125) than in serous borderline ones (52% vs 62% for CA 125 and 19% for CEA) (Neunteufel et al., 1989c). A complementary staining pattern of CA 19-9 and CA 125 was found in ovarian tumors for different areas of the same primary and between primary tumors and their metastases with a strong staining of CA 19-9 in gastric, pancreatic, and lung primaries and negative staining in CA 125 positive ovarian secondaries (Macdonald et al., 1988).

In the decidua and fetal membrane, CA 19-9 and CA 125 were present in the cytoplasm of decidual cells and amnion epithelial cells (cytosolic fractions) (Kobayashi et al., 1989). In contrast to CA 125 levels decreasing with gestational week in the amniotic fluid, CA 19-9 levels increased and correlated with amnion tissue levels.

In the uterine cervix, CA 125 was detected in glandular cells of normal cervix and microglandular hyperplasia in contrast to no reactivity for CEA or CA 19-9 (Nanbu et al., 1988). In neoplastic glandular cells (adenocarcinoma), CA 125 was negative or not at the luminal surface in contrast to a positive reaction for CEA and CA 19-9 in 78/0% of adenocarcinoma *in situ*, 80/40% of less invasive and 84/56% of frankly invasive adenocarcinoma. In the normal endometrial mucosa, CA 19-9 (mid phase of secretion) and CA 125 (mid and late phases) were detected as secretion products of the normal endometrium (Neunteufel and Breitenecker, 1989a). Higher positivity rates were found in atypical hyperplasia (CA 19-9: 57%; CA 125: 48%; CEA: 5%). In endometrial carcinoma (n = 40), the percentage of CA 19-9 positive cases was highest (93%) with staining of >50% of tumor cells and increased with increasing differentiation (CA 125: 65%, CEA: 58%). There was no significant correlation between tumor markers and estrogen or progesteron receptor content, but for CA 19-9 a correlation with histological grading.

4. Measurement of Circulating CA 19-9

CA 19-9 is determined by means of radio- or enzyme immunoassays using MAb 1116NS 19-9 (IgG_1 murine immunoglobulin) as capture and tracer antibody. Meanwhile, CA 19-9 kits are commercially available from different companies (Stieber et al., 1985).

4.1. CA 19-9 in Serum

4.1.1. Healthy Subjects

As serum reference range, values between 0 and 35–40 U/mL are reported (1 U = 0.8 ng). Following extensive investigations, CA 19-9 serum levels ≤37 U/mL were found in healthy subjects (n = 2700) (Del Villano et al., 1983a). There was no correlation with age or smoking but there was with sex, women having slightly higher levels than men (Green et al., 1986). In this respect, it is important that in healthy as well as in ill subjects belonging to the rare blood group constellation of negative Lewis$^{a/b}$ (about 3–7% of the population), CA 19-9 is not expressed because of lack of an essential sialyl-transferase and a fucosylated precursor (Brockhaus et al., 1985; Tempero et al., 1987). During menses and pregnancy, slight elevations of CA 19-9 have been encountered in about 14% of nonpregnant (43–65 U/mL) and 10% of pregnant women from different gestational weeks (38–117 U/mL) without apparent relation to the stage of pregnancy (Touitou et al., 1989). Others (Lellé et al., 1989) found only slight elevations of serum CA 19-9 during gestation (2.8%), some higher values during delivery (19%), and very high levels in amniotic fluid during the second trimester (16–18th gestational week: 80%, maximal 1533 U/mL), as confirmed by others (Kobayashi et al., 1989), and to a similar degree in umbilical cord blood.

4.1.2. Benign Diseases (Fig. 1)

Elevated serum levels of CA 19-9 (>37 U/mL) were reported in benign nongastrointestinal diseases in about 1% of cases as well as in benign gastrointestinal diseases in 3–4% of cases (Del Villano et al., 1983a; Kuusela et al., 1984), but later more extensive studies gave a higher incidence generally in benign disease (9.8–13%), in patients with chocolate (91 U/mL) or dermoid cysts (340/794 U/mL) (Nagata et al., 1989), in cholecystitis and obstructive jaundice (20%; Benamouzig et al., 1989; Barone et al., 1988), cholelithiasis (16–44%; Touitou and Bogdan, 1988), choledocholithiasis (Klapdor, 1986), cholecystolithiasis (33%; Harmenberg et al., 1988), sclerotic cholangitis (14%; Harmenberg et al., 1988), acute cholangitis (Albert et al., 1988), hepatitis (2.6–23.0%; Touitou and Bogdan, 1988), toxic hepatitis (14%), chronic active hepatitis (33%), liver cirrhosis (16.7–19.4%), primary biliary cirrhosis (16%), massive liver cell necrosis (up to 60%) (Del Villano and Zurawski, 1983b; Ruibal et al., 1983; Heptner et al., 1985; Olsson et al., 1985; Satake et al., 1985b; Andriulli et al., 1986; Encabo and Ruibal, 1986; Kew et al., 1987; Harmenberg et al., 1988; Paganuzzi et al., 1988; Touitou and Bogdan, 1988; Benamouzig et al., 1989; Safi et al., 1989), benign lung disease (chronic obstructive, acute pneumonia, allergy: 13.3% >25 U/mL; Marechal et al., 1988); furthermore, in cystic fibrosis with a sensitivity of 67% ($n = 57$) and a specificity of 92% (Duffy et al., 1985; Buamah et al., 1986; Roberts et al., 1986;

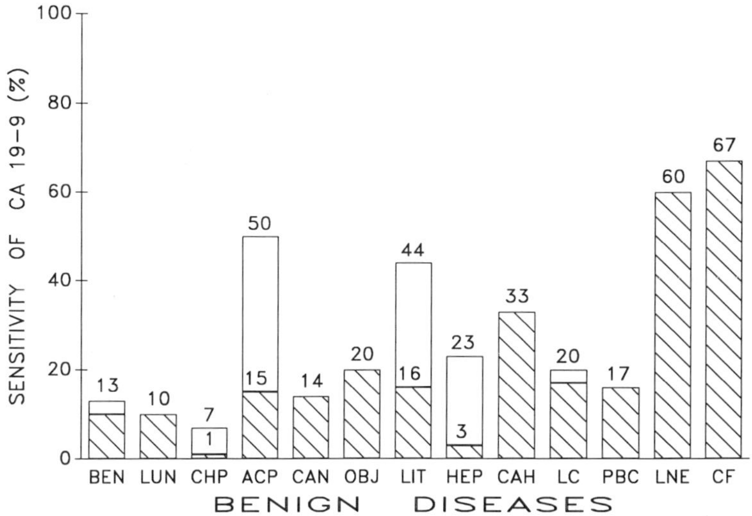

Fig. 1. Diagnostic sensitivity (false positives, reduction in specificity) of serum CA 19-9 in patients with benign diseases (summary statistics from the literature as lower and upper range value or mean). BEN = general benign diseases; LUN = benign lung diseases; CHP/ACP = chronic/acute pancreatitis; CAN = cholangitis; OBJ = obstructive jaundice; LIT = cholelithiasis; HEP = hepatitis; CAH = chronic active hepatitis; LC = liver cirrhosis; PBC = primary biliary cirrhosis; LNE = liver cell necrosis; CF = cystic fibrosis.

Uhlenbruck et al., 1988). In addition, increased levels were observed in 0–27% of cases with chronic active pancreatitis, whereas higher incidence rates of 15–50% were reported for acute pancreatitis or an acute exacerbation of chronic pancreatitis disclosing values mostly below 100 to maximal 500 U/mL (Farini et al., 1985; Heptner et al., 1985; Klapdor et al., 1985b; Satake et al., 1985a,b; Andriulli et al., 1986; Pasquali et al., 1987; Safi et al., 1987). Especially high serum CA 19-9 concentrations were observed in benign biliary tract disease complicated by acute cholangitis (190–32,000 U/mL) that was best differentiated at a higher cutoff of 75 U/mL vs malignant groups despite similar cholestasis and high CA 19-9

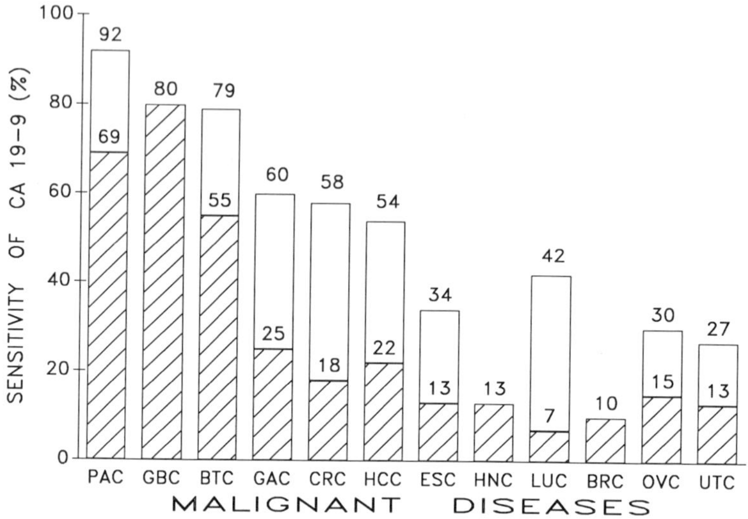

Fig. 2. Diagnostic sensitivity (right positives) of serum CA 19-9 in patients with malignant diseases (summary statistics from the literature as lower and upper range value or mean). PAC = excretory ductular pancreatic carcinoma; GBC = gallbladder cancer; BTC = biliary tract cancer; GAC = gastric cancer; CRC = colorectal cancer; HCC = hepatocellular cancer; ESC = esophagal cancer; HNC = head-and-neck cancer; LUC = lung cancer; BRC = breast cancer; OVC = epithelial ovarian cancer; UTC = uterine (endometrial/cervical) cancer.

levels in gallbladder or common duct bile ($7.3 \times 10^4 - 2.3 \times 10^9$ U/mL) (Albert et al., 1988). The levels returned to normal after treatment of cholangitis.

4.1.3. Malignant Diseases (Fig. 2)

4.1.3.1. Pancreatic Cancer. Highest incidence rates of elevated CA 19-9 levels were reported for excretory ductular pancreatic cancer (incidence rate 8/100,000 inhabitants/yr) with a sensitivity of 67.6–92% and maximal values up to >100,000 U/mL (Malesci et al., 1981; Herlyn et al., 1982; Del Villano et al., 1983a; Klapdor et al., 1984a,b; Ritts et al., 1984; Savarino et al., 1984; Farini et al., 1985; Gupta et al., 1985; Heptner et al., 1985; Satake et al., 1985a,b; Staab et al., 1985; Tatsuta et al., 1985; Yoshikawa et al., 1985; Andriulli et al., 1986; Del Favero et al., 1986a,b; Haglund et al., 1986b; Safi et al., 1986a, 1987, 1989; Sakahara et al., 1986; Venot et al., 1986; Wang et al., 1986; Buamah et al., 1987; Pasquali et al., 1987; Basso et al., 1988; Benini et al., 1988; Charneau et al., 1988; Glenn et al., 1988; Harmenberg et al., 1988; Hayakawa et al., 1988; Paganuzzi et al., 1988; Röthlin et al., 1988; Takasaki et al., 1988), a specificity of 64.6–92.4% (Wang et al., 1986; Pasquali et al., 1987; Safi et al., 1987; Basso et al., 1988; Benini et al., 1988; Charneau et al., 1988; Paganuzzi et al., 1988; Röthlin et al., 1988) and an accuracy of 61% (Basso et al., 1988). These sensitivity rates were about twice that of CEA (70% vs 43%: Ritts et al., 1984; 89% vs 37%: Staab, 1986) and superior to CEA (Staab et al., 1985; Safi et al., 1986a; Fabris et al., 1988) and tissue polypeptide antigen (TPA) (Basso et al., 1988; Fabris et al., 1988) in receiver operating characteristic (ROC) analysis. For pancreatic cancer, the height and frequency of pathologic CA 19-9 levels correlated with tumor location (head, 59–80%, corpus/tail, 57–85%; Hayakawa et al., 1988; Tatsuta et al., 1985), tumor extent (Röthlin et al., 1988; e.g., <2 cm diameter: 30%: Manabe et al., 1988; <3/3–6 cm/>6 cm diameter: 57/80/100%: Tatsuta et al., 1985; <3/3–5 cm/>5 cm diameter: 13/90/92%, Sakahara et al., 1986), resectability (56–77%; Hayakawa et al., 1988), metastasis (Röthlin et al., 1988), cholestasis (Röthlin et al., 1988), with stromal staining of cancer tissues (Röthlin et al., 1988), but not with histologic differentiation (Klapdor and Greten, 1984a), except two communications about false negative findings in patients with poorly differentiated pancreatic carcinoma (Malesci et al., 1987) and higher positivity rates in moderately differentiated cancer (Röthlin et al., 1988).

The significance of serum CA 19-9 was documented at a higher cutoff (70 U/mL) also for the diagnosis of pancreatic cancer (s = 70%, sp = 87%, pos./neg. pred. value = 59/92%), in addition to conventional physical methods without difference in sensitivity between patients with local/regional or metastatic disease (50 vs 71%; $n = 6/14$; Pleskow et al., 1989). Nevertheless, the marker analysis does not seem to replace physical methods and fine needle biopsy for proof of diagnosis (Dunn and McKinstry, 1989). A further study (Richter et al., 1989) corroborated the clinical utility of CA 19-9 (c.o. 70 U/mL) for diagnosis of pancreatic cancer in symptomatic patients presenting with pain and/or weight loss by starting with CA 19-9-RIA or abdominal ultrasonography. Equivalent positive and negative predictive values were observed at a prevalence range for pancreatic cancer of 0.02–0.15, and led to the recommendation of the CA 19-9 RIA as a useful and cost-effective initial test for suspected pancreatic cancer. Other authors (Wang et al., 1986) favored the combination of ultrasonography and CA 19-9 serum determination for noninvasive diagnosis of advanced pancreatic cancer (diagnostic $s = 95.8\%$, sp = 84.5%, accuracy = 86.4%).

Finally, the prognostic value of the preoperative CA 19-9 level for resectable pancreatic adenocarcinoma was demonstrated by observing more frequent pathologic levels ≤1000 U/mL (53%, n = 20/38) than >1000 U/mL (1/9 = 11%) and during follow-up, a longer disease-free interval and survival than in nonresectable cases (Glenn et al., 1988). Furthermore, follow-up cases with normalization of CA 19-9 disclosed a longer survival (7/8 >18 mo) than patients with nonnormalizing values (6/6 <12 mo).

4.1.3.2. Hepatobiliary Cancer. For primary liver cancer (hepatocellular and cholangiocellular), a sensitivity between 22 and 51% (Malesci et al., 1981; Klapdor et al., 1985a; Stieber et al., 1985; Andriulli et al., 1986; Kew et al., 1987; Leandro et al., 1989) was reported, with a higher sensitivity for AFP (s = 84%, sp = 83%) compared to CA 19-9 (s = 44%, sp = 76%), which was not of complementary usefulness (Leandro et al., 1989). In addition, elevated CA 19-9 serum levels were found in gallbladder (>80%; Satake et al., 1985b; Harmenberg et al., 1988; Nishino et al., 1988; Strom et al., 1989), bile duct (100%; Satake et al., 1985b; Harmenberg et al., 1988), and biliary tract cancer (55–79%; Malesci et al., 1981; Klapdor et al., 1985a; Stieber et al., 1985; Andriulli et al., 1986; Paganuzzi et al., 1988). For discrimination between benign and malignant disease with obstructive jaundice, a sensitivity for CA 19-9 of 82.8–90% (c.o. 37 U/mL) and a poor specificity of only about 45% were observed (Barone et al., 1988; Benamouzig et al., 1989); a better discrimination was obtained by a higher cut-off at 200 U/mL (*s* = 65%, sp = 91%), because CA 19-9 levels were more increased in patients with malignant than benign biliary obstruction. In comparison with individuals showing a normal gall-bladder function, patients with invasive adenocarcinoma disclosed similar bile CA 19-9 concentrations (normal median 165.5 U/mL vs carcinoma with 277.2 U/mL) but significant differences in serum CA 19-9 levels (6.6 U/mL in benign disease vs 59.1 U/mL in cancer) (Strom et al., 1989).

4.1.3.3. Stomach Cancer. In gastric cancer, elevated levels of CA 19-9 were found in 25–60% of cases (Malesci et al., 1981; Staab et al., 1984; Gupta et al., 1985; Satake et al., 1985b; Stieber et al., 1985; Yoshikawa et al., 1985; Andriulli et al., 1986) with a clear dependence on tumor stage (I–IV: 31%, 43%, 67%, 72%; Safi et al., 1985). In this disease, a complementary sensitivity with CEA was observed leading to doubling of rates with combined use of both markers (CA 19–9/CEA: 25/21%, together: 38%; Staab et al., 1984,1985, 1986).

4.1.3.4. Colorectal Cancer. In colorectal cancer, the total positivity rate varied from 18 to 58% (Herlyn et al., 1982; Del Villano et al., 1983a; Heptner et al., 1984; Kuusela et al., 1984; Ritts et al., 1984; Staab et al., 1984, 1985, 1986; Klapdor et al., 1985a; Olsson et al., 1985; Satake et al., 1985b; Schröck et al., 1985; Stieber et al., 1985; Andriulli et al., 1986; Novis et al., 1986; Polterauer et al., 1986), and showed a correlation to tumor stage (Duke's A–D: 7%, 17%, 47%, 75%). In comparison with CEA (total sensitivity 38%; Duke's D 65%; Ritts et al., 1984), CA 19-9 was less sensitive (18 vs 29%: Ritts et al., 1984; 31 vs 58%: Roberts, 1988; recurrence 50 vs 88%: Novis et al., 1986) in contrast to a higher specificity of up to 99% (100 vs 79%; Roberts et al., 1988). These findings were also confirmed by other investigators (Duke's C/D: CA 19-9 *s* = 45% vs CEA *s* = 88%; Duke's D with liver metastasis: 48 vs 94%: Safi et al., 1988; 59 vs 88%: Lorenz et al., 1989) (Jalanko et al., 1984; Kuusela et al., 1984; Staab et al., 1984) with one exception of equal low sensitivity and high specificity (*s* = 23%, sp = 95%; Goldberg et al., 1989). For this reason CA 19-9 should only be used as second marker following the first marker CEA or in CEA-negative cases of colorectal carcinoma (Kuusela et al., 1984; Staab et al., 1984, 1985, 1986; Szymendera et al., 1985; Polterauer et al., 1986; Roberts, 1988). Like for CEA, gastrointestinal tumors with liver metastasis seem to express higher CA 19-9 levels (Lorenz et al., 1989; Novis et al., 1986).

In addition, no differences of elevated CA 19-9 levels (>37 U/mL) were observed in colorectal cancer patients between draining or peripheral blood (29.5 vs 29.5%), in contrast to significantly higher CEA levels (>5 ng/mL) in the draining blood (60.2 vs 28.9%). This was consistent with a more diffuse immunohistochemical staining for CEA and a more sporadic distribution of CA 19-9, as well as a predominant draining of CEA by the hematogenous portal system and of CA 19-9 by the thoracic duct lymphatic system (Tabuchi et al., 1988).

4.1.3.5. Lung Cancer. Obviously lower sensitivity rates of less diagnostic utility have been reported for CA 19-9 in bronchial carcinoma (7–42%: Del Villano et al., 1983a; Ritts et al., 1984; Bisset et al., 1985; Glaubitt and Cordoni-Voutsus, 1985; Molina et al., 1985; Vindimian et al., 1987). The simultaneous determination of CA 19-9 (c.o. 37 U/mL) and CA 125 (c.o. 35 U/mL) disclosed normal levels in healthy subjects and patients with NED (n = 15) in contrast to 25% in MO patients (n = 87) and 40.3% in metastatic lung cancer (MT, n = 72) for CA 19-9 in comparison with 18.7 and 22.9% for CA 125 (Molina et al., 1989). Of large cell undifferentiated cases, 50% were positive for CA 19-9 (other types 30%) compared with 60% (15.4%) for CA 125.

4.1.3.6. Breast and Gynecologic Cancer. In breast cancer, sensitivities of about only 10% were reported (Del Villano et al., 1983a; Pfeiffer et al., 1984; Ritts et al., 1984). In ovarian cancer, elevated CA 19-9 levels were mainly reported for epithelial ovarian carcinoma (15–37.5%) with higher values for the mucinous type (nonmucinous 25–28.9% vs mucinous with 68.2–87.5%: Fioretti et al., 1988; Neghishi et al., 1987) (Bast et al., 1984; Canney et al., 1985; Schröck et al., 1985; Hoffmann et al., 1986; Fioretti et al., 1988; Göcze et al., 1988; Koelbl et al., 1989), in contrast to no elevations in malignant nonepithelial or benign ovarian tumors (Göcze et al., 1988).

For uterine carcinoma, a sensitivity of 13–27% (Schröck et al., 1985; Göcze et al., 1988) was reported for endometrial adenocarcinoma and of 7.3–13% for squamous carcinoma of the cervix, in contrast to CA 125 (31.9%) and CA 15-3 (23.1%) with more frequently elevated levels of CA 19-9 (c.o. 37 U/mL) only in advanced stages ($n = 91$; stage III: 16.7%/$n = 12$; stage IV: 33.3%/$n = 3$) (Benedetti-Panici et al., 1989; Göcze et al., 1988).

4.1.3.7. Other Malignant Diseases. For head-and-neck neoplasms ($n = 125$) elevated concentrations of CA 19-9 (>37 U/mL) were found in patients with squamous cell carcinomas (13%) and malignant (22%) but not benign salivary gland tumors (Gustafsson et al., 1988); furthermore, in squamous cell carcinoma of the esophagus ($s = 13$–34%) (Munck-Wikland et al., 1988; McKnight et al., 1989), and finally in a case of endocrine pancreatic cancer (glucagonoma) metastatic to the liver (Archambeaud-Mouveroux et al., 1986).

4.1.4. Follow-up in Malignant Disease

During follow-up, benign diseases may show a transitory elevation of CA 19-9 or constantly low pathologic levels mostly below 100–200 U/mL. In contrast, malignant diseases before treatment may develop constantly or exponentially rising levels up to more than 10,000 U/mL. In pancreatic, hepatobiliary, gastric, and colonic carcinoma, there is generally a good correlation between CA 19-9 and clinical course of disease following surgical, radio- or cytostatic therapy (Sears et al., 1982; Polterauer et al., 1986; Harmenberg et al., 1988; Roberts, 1988; Safi et al., 1989), during which the level changes may anticipate the clinical outcome by a lead time of up to seven months in about half of the cases (Glenn et al., 1988; Röthlin et al., 1988). A normalization of CA 19-9 levels was reported within 2–4 wk following complete tumor removal (stage I), only a transitory fall of the CA 19-9 level without normalization on palliative treatment, and a new increase with the development of local recurrence or metastases on progression (Klapdor et al., 1985a; Safi et al., 1985). In patients operated radically for pancreatic carcinoma (pancreaticoduodenectomy), the postoperative normalization of CA 19-9 was classified as a prognostically favorable index (survival >7 mo) and its new increase as an early indicator of liver involvement rather than abdominal sonography (lead time ≥2 mo) (Beretta et al., 1987). CA 19-9 level changes with clinical follow-up were also useful for the after-care of gastric (*s* = 38–70%, sp = 89–91%) and colorectal cancer (*s* = 53–73%, sp = 91–94%; Safi et al., 1985,1988; Schmid et al., 1985) and showed an increase in sensitivity, specificity, and accuracy in combination with CEA (Safi et al., 1986b). In pancreatic and hepatobiliary cancer, the CA 19-9 level changes during follow-up appear in up to 90% of cases and seem also to happen more quickly and reliably than by morphological imaging techniques (Klapdor et al., 1985a). In addition, CA 19-9 seems to be a good parameter for monitoring intraarterial chemotherapy of liver metastases (Lorenz et al., 1985,1989; Sears et al., 1985; Safi et al., 1988).

4.2. CA 19-9 in Effusions

An investigation on tumor-associated antigens in serous effusions (Mezger et al., 1988) showed that CA 19-9 (cutoff 30 U/mL) discriminated well between benign and malignant serous effusions. In pleural effusions, CA 19-9 showed only a global sensitivity of 24% (sp/pos. pred. value = 100%, neg. pred. value = 31%, prevalence = 78%), but better values in ascitic effusions (*s* = 52%, sp/pos. pred. value = 100%, neg. pred. value = 50%, prevalence = 68%). The sensitivity was varying for CA 19-9 between 17 and 100% (median 49%), with low sensitivity in lymphoma/leukemia and sarcoma and higher rates in gastrointestinal and nonsmall cell lung cancer. For immunocytology, anti-CA 19-9 antibodies did not stain mesothelial cells, granulocytes, lymphocytes, and macrophages, but only tumor cells in effusions from patients with breast, gastrointestinal, ovarian, and nonsmall cell lung cancer in 20–56% of cases despite a large heterogeneity of expression in different tumor cells. Furthermore, by the combination of circulating and cell-bound tumor marker determinations with conventional cytology, the detection rate was increased from 31% through 36% (+immunocytology) to 44% (+circulating marker).

4.3. CA 19-9 in Secretions

For clinical purposes, the determination of CA 19-9 is mainly useful in serum and serum-dependent body fluids like ascitic and pleural effusions in contrast to its use in all kinds of secretions, because even in healthy individuals belonging to the positive blood group Lewis$^{a/b}$, very high levels of CA 19-9 are encountered in sputum and saliva (Pak et al., 1984; Brockhaus et al., 1985; Ura et al., 1985), milk (Hanisch et al., 1985b), seminal plasma (Uhlenbruck et al., 1984,1985; Hanisch et al., 1985a; Panidis et al., 1988), gastric secretions (Farinati et al., 1988), amniotic fluid, urine (Tizzani et al., 1987), ovarian secretion, feces (Ura et al., 1985), bronchial secretions (Vindimian et al., 1984), and others. In some respect, this holds true also for CA 19-9 determinations in biliary/duodenal/pancreatic secretions (Heptner et al., 1985; Schmiegel et al., 1985b).

Mostly elevated CA 19-9 levels have been reported even under normal conditions for pancreatic juice with levels between 250–400,000 U/mL in pancreatic cancer (n = 68) and between 17–150,000 U/mL in chronic pancreatitis (n = 71), in which it was not possible to discriminate between benign and malignant pancreatic disease in contrast to the respective serum samples (s = 80%, sp = 91.5%) (Heptner et al., 1985; Schmiegel et al., 1985a,b). CA 19-9 secreted in pancreatic fluids of benign or malignant provenance was identified as the same mucin form (mol wt 2×10^6) (Kalthoff et al., 1986). Following other authors (Malesci et al., 1988; Nishida et al., 1988b), CA 19-9 measurement in pure pancreatic juices (as U/μg protein or U/mL) discriminated patients with early and resectable pancreatic cancer better (Malesci et al., 1987,1988) than or equal (Nishida et al., 1988b) to serum CA 19-9, whereas others (Tappero and Piantino, 1987) did not disclose a better differential diagnosis by duodenal juice CA 19-9 (U/μg protein) between pancreatic cancer and chronic calcifying pancreatitis.

In pancreatic cyst fluids, other authors (Nishida et al., 1989) were able to differentiate pancreatic cystadenocarcinoma from cystadenoma by means of CA 19-9 determination with very high levels in the cancer cysts (100,000/320,000 U/mL) and serum (83/6200 U/mL), in contrast to normal marker levels in serum and cyst fluid of cystadenoma. This is consistent with findings of abnormally high CA 19-9 concentrations >10,000 U/mL in pancreatic cyst fluids of malignant origin in combination with CEA elevations of about 1000 ng/mL (Tatsuta et al., 1986).

The immunohistochemical and quantitative investigation of CA 19-9, CA 125, and CEA in normal bronchial mucus yielded a positive expression in epithelial cells lining the central airways (trachea, bronchi, bronchioli) and respiratory glands for all three markers (Matsuoka et al., 1990). Most bronchial mucus contained remarkably high levels of all markers ranging from 210 to 95,000 U/mL (294–197,917 U/mg protein; CA 19-9),190–41,000 U/mL (CA 125), and 6–940 ng/mL (CEA), in contrast to normal concentrations in serum.

Similar findings were obtained in bronchogenic cysts (benign tumors of ventral foregut origin), in which a strong expression of CA 19-9 and CEA was found in pulmonary sequestration, mediastinal bronchogenic cysts, and mediastinal mature teratomas with high levels of CA 19-9 (>200,000–6,200,000 U/mL) and CEA (388–4850 ng/mL) in the cyst fluid that returned to normal range after operation (Uyama et al., 1989). This is in agreement with a reported case of highly elevated serum CA 19-9 and a cystic mass with purulent hemorrhagic material in the lung without evidence of malignancy (cyst fluid CA 19-9: 1,162,100 U/mL) (Okubo et al., 1989).

Concerning cervical mucus, extremely high levels of CA 125 (luteal phase: mean 53,000 U/mL; follicular phase: 126,100 U/mL) were found together with relatively low levels of CEA (luteal 2100, follicular 3600 ng/mL) and CA 19-9 (luteal 3100, follicular 3400 U/mL) in cervical mucus of healthy women, in contrast to relatively low CA 125 (mean 63,100 U/mL) levels and extremely high levels of CEA (165,400 ng/mL) or CA 19-9 (116,400 U/mL) in mucus of patients with cervical adenocarcinoma (Fujii et al., 1988).

The ratio (CEA + CA 19-9)/CA 125 was <0.5 in patients without gynecologic disorders or with leiomyoma and ≥0.5 in patients with cervical adenocarcinoma and seemed clinically useful.

CA 19-9 determination in gastric juice of patients with gastric cancer ($n = 23$), chronic atrophic gastritis ($n = 57$), and healthy controls ($n = 55$; upper reference cutoff: 450 U/mL) showed significantly increased levels in chronic atrophic gastritis (495.9 ± 364.9 U/mL), but still higher values in gastric cancer ($s = 65\%$, sp = 71%), recommending the test for identifying patients at risk for gastric cancer (Farinati et al., 1988).

Finally, CA 19-9 qualified as a useful urinary marker for bladder cancer ($s = 71.6\%$, sp = 91.6%, pos. pred. value = 90.5%, accuray = 81%) (Tizzani et al., 1987).

5. Use of Anti-CA 19-9 Antibodies in Immunoscintigraphy

The monoclonal antibody 19-9 has also been used for immunoscintigraphy. In the first study (Chatal et al., 1982) for the detection of gastrointestinal carcinoma, a sensitivity of 77% was obtained by an immunococktail of CEA and CA 19-9 antibodies. Since this pilot study, the commercially available kit (IMACIS 1) has also been used by other groups (Baum et al., 1988). For lowering the nonspecific binding of complement, these antibodies (CA 19-9, IgG_1, affinity 3×10^7; CEA IgG_1, affinity 1.1×10^9; labeled with ^{131}I) were used as $F(ab')_2$ fragments (mol wt 100,000). In a retrospective study ($n = 32$) the sensitivity/specificity/ pos./neg. pred. value ratings were 77/88/82/81% and even increased in a prospective study ($n = 60$) to 87/92/86/92% for tumor detection in the pelvis, liver, peritoneal/abdominal, lung, bone, and other regions (Baum et al., 1988). These findings are in contrast to other results (Hölting et al., 1989) using the same immunococktail, in which 42 patients with recurrent colorectal cancer were investigated and yielded an overall sensitivity by immunoscintigraphy of only 23% (pos./neg. pred. value 33/37%) in contrast to higher values by conventional methods ($s = 77\%$, pos./neg. pred. val. = 94/79%). Concerning isolated pancreatic cancer immunoscintigraphy using CEA/CA 19-9 immunococktail, successful imaging has been reported by Montz et al. (1985) in 13/21 (62%) cases. Nevertheless the detection rate for pancreatic cancer is still low (about 70%) and the size of tumors detected (mostly >2 cm in diameter) not yet satisfactory (Baum, 1989).

6. Comparison of CA 19-9 with Other Carbohydrate Markers

The main tumor markers related to CA 19-9 are CA 50 (*see* Chapter 17), DU-PAN-2 (*see* Chapter 16), and CA 125 (*see* Chapter 19).

Quite recently, a new carbohydrate marker called CA-195 has been detected and commercialized as immunoradiometric sandwich assay using the murine monoclonal antibody CC3C195 as capture and tracer antibody. This antibody not only reacts with sialylated Le^a antigen equivalent to CA 19-9, but also at lower affinity with nonsialylated Le^a antigen itself (Bray and Gaur, 1988). In comparison with CA 19-9 (c.o. 37 U/mL), CA-195 (c.o. 10 U/mL) showed similar low positivity rates for normal subjects (5.8%), a lower one in benign diseases (15.4 vs 23.2%), and a higher sensitivity for colorectal (47.0 vs 35.6%, $n = 149$) and upper gastrointestinal malignant disease (pancreas, stomach, esophagus, gallbladder, liver, and so on: 53.0 vs 45.4%, $n = 119$) (Bhargava et al., 1989). This also held true for active colorectal (82 vs 63%, $n = 79$), and upper gastrointestinal disease (71.6 vs 61.4%, $n = 88$). There was a significant correlation between CA 19-9 and CA 195 ($r = 0.67$), but no significant complementarity by the use of both tests.

On the other hand, a comparative study on carbohydrate markers CA 19-9, CA 195, and CA 50 yielded marked differences in sensitivity for different malignant disease groups after correction of cutoff values by ROC analysis for a similar specificity vs benign diseases (Lamerz et al., 1990). At specificity rates between 89 and 97%, CA 19-9 as well as CA-195 showed only marginal sensitivity ($s = 23/22\%$) at high cutoffs (80–100 U/mL) for hepatocellular cancer ($n = 74$), and for pancreatic cancer ($n = 36$), only minor differences ($s = 61/56\%$/CA 50: 58%) between all three markers at different cutoffs. In stomach cancer CA 19-9 disclosed highest sensitivity ($s = 71\%$, cutoff 15 U/mL) followed by CA 50/CA 195 ($s = 60/54\%$, cutoff 25/15 U/mL), and for colorectal cancer ($n = 32$) CA 19-9 showed a similar sensitivity of 72% (cutoff 15 U/mL) vs CA 50/CA 195 ($s = 63/56\%$, cutoff = 25/15 U/mL).

Finally, as further anti-CA 19-9 related monoclonal antibodies shall be mentioned, the monoclonal antibody AR-3, which detects a human carcinoma-associated CAR-3-epitope on a high molecular weight mucin (mol wt > 400,000) strictly related to Le^a and Le^b antigens (Prat et al., 1989), another monoclonal antibody (121 SLE, IgM) being associated with the same molecular sialylated Le^a structure but recognizing an epitope different from MAb 19-9 (Herrero-Zabaleta et al., 1987), and furthermore, two monoclonal antibodies against mucin-like glycoproteins called YPAN (Yvan et al., 1985) and SPAN-1 (Chung et al., 1987) that share biological properties with CA 19-9 but seem to appear also in $Le^{a-/b-}$ individuals (Ho et al., 1988).

7. Final Comment

CA 19-9 represents the most important and basic carbohydrate tumor marker whose discovery initialized the era of monoclonal antibody technique for tumor marker research. As Lewis blood group related substance (sialyl-Lewis^a), it is regarded as a normal constituent of gastrointestinal and cervical tissue that may occur in normal secretions but usually only in marginal concentration <37–40 U/mL in normal blood, where it appears in high concentrations on tissue damage mostly of malignant origin. Besides a limited usefulness in immunohistochemistry and a developing significance in immunoimaging, its main indication is the determination in serum and strictly serum-dependent body fluids mainly for monitoring therapy of malignant gastrointestinal diseases and detection of recurrence because of its lead time effect in half of cases. CA 19-9 is actually qualified as first choice marker in pancreatic and hepatobiliary cancer, as useful additional marker with CEA in gastric cancer because of additive and complementary sensitivity, and as second choice marker after CEA for colorectal cancer, whereas in hepatocellular and nongastrointestinal cancer, it is of limited or lacking usefulness. For pancreatic cancer, its additional application for diagnosis and prognosis seems promising. Finally, its determination in serum is negative in Lewis$^{a-/b-}$ phenotypic individuals, doubtful in those with Lewis$^{a-/b+}$ or Lewis$^{a+/b-}$ phenotype, and critical in secretions.

References

Afdhal, N. H., A. Long, I. Tobbia, A. Cullen, and D. P. O'Donoghue (1987), *Gut* **28,** 594.

Albert, M. B., W. M. Steinberg, and J. P. Henry (1988), *Dig. Dis. Sci.* **33,** 1223–1225.

Allen, D. C., H. Foster, J. C. Orchin, and J. D. Biggart (1987), *J. Clin. Pathol.* **40,** 157–162.

Andriulli, A., T. Gindro, P. Piantino, R. Farini, G. Cavallini, L. Piazzi, R. Naccarato, G. Dobrilla, G. Verme, and L. A. Scuro (1986), *Digestion* **33,** 26–33.

Archambeaud-Mouveroux, F., F. Cardinaud, J. Venot, Ph. Benard, and J. M. Bonnet Blanc (1986), *N. Engl. J. Med.* **315,** 1555.

Arends, J. W., T. Wiggers, B. Schutte, C. T. Thijs, C. Verstijnen, J. Hilgers, G.-H. Blijham, and F. T. Bosman (1983), *Int. J. Cancer* **32,** 289–293.

Arends, J. W., T. Wiggers, C. Verstijnen, J. Hilgers, and F. T. Bosman (1984), *Int. J. Cancer* **34,** 193–196.

Atkinson, B. F., C. S. Ernst, M. Herlyn, Z. Steplewski, H. F. Sears, and H. Koprowski (1982), *Cancer Res.* **42,** 4280–4283.

Barone, D., M. Onetto, M. Conio, M. Paganuzzi, S. Saccomanno, H. Aste, and V. Pugliese (1988), *Int. J. Biol. Markers* **3,** 95–100.

Basso, D., C. Fabris, G. Del Favero, A. Panucci, M. Plebani, C. Angonese, G. Leandro, G. Dodi, A. Burlina, and R. Naccarato (1988), *Oncology* **45,** 24–29.

Bast, R. C., T. L. Klug, E. Schaetzl, P. Lavin, J. M. Niloff, T. J. Greber, V. R. Zurawski, and R. C. Knapp (1984), *Am. J. Obstet. Gynecol.* **149,** 553–559.

Baum, R. P., M. Lorenz, C. Hottenrott, M. Albrecht, R. Senekowitsch, J. Happ, A. Hertel, J. Spitz, and G. Hör (1988), *Int. J. Biol. Markers* **3,** 177–184.

Baum, R. P. (1989), *Hepatogastroenterology* **36,** 459–461.

Bechtel, B., A. J. Wand, K. Wroblewski, H. Koprowski, and J. Thurin (1990), *J. Biol. Chem.* **265,** 2028–2037.

Benamouzig, R., C. Buffet, C. Fourre, O. Ink, F. Moati, and J. P. Etienne (1989), *Dig. Dis. Sci.* **34,** 1640–1642.

Benedetti-Panici, P., G. Scambia, G. Baiocchi, C. Sonsini, S. Greggi, F. Battaglia, and S. Mancuso (1989), *Tumor Biol.* **10,** 109–116.

Benini, L., G. Cavallini, D. Zordam, P. Rizotti, L. Brigo, G. Brocco, L. Perobelli, M. Zanchetta, P. Pederzoli, and L. A. Scuro (1988), *Pancreas* **3,** 61–66.

Beretta, E., A. Malesci, A. Zerbi, A. Mariani, M. Carlucci, C. Bonato, A. M. Ferrari, and V. Di Carlo (1987), *Cancer* **60,** 2428–2431.

Bhargava, A. K., N. J. Petrelli, A. Karna, P. L. Parshall, J. E. Fitzpatrick, H. O. Douglass, L. Herrera, K. Bray, and P. Gaur (1989), *J. Clin. Lab. Anal.* **3,** 370–377.

Bisset, J. P., J. P. Kleisbauer, F. Roux, and M. J. Treffot (1985), *Pathol. Biol.* **33,** 672–676.

Bra, J., E. H. Zavaleta, R. Mollicone, M. Nap, and P. Burtin (1986), *Am. J. Clin. Pathol.* **85,** 152–159.

Bray, K. R., and P. K. Gaur (1988), *J. Clin. Lab. Anal.* **2,** 187–193.

Breitenecker, G., W. Neunteufel, C. Bieglmayer, H. Kölbl, and K. Schieder (1989), *Int. J. Gynecol. Pathol.* **8,** 97–102.

Brockhaus, M., M. Wysocka, J. L. Magnani, Z. Steplewski, H. Koprowski, and V. Ginsburg (1985), *Vox Sang.* **48,** 34–38.

Buamah, P. K., C. Cornell, A. J. Cassels-Smith, and A. McGill (1986), *Clin. Chem.* **32,** 913.

Buamah P., C. Cornell, C. W. Venables, and A. W. Skillen (1987), *Eur. J. Cancer Clin. Oncol.* **23,** 87–91.

Canney, P. A., P. M. Wilkinson, R. D. James, and M. Moore (1985), *Br. J. Cancer* **52,** 131–133.

Charneau, J., O. Douay, A. Daver, and J. Boyer (1988), *Gastroentérol. Clin. Biol.* **12,** 548–552.

Charpin, C., A. K. Bhan, V. R. Zurawski, and R. E. Scully (1982), *Int. J. Gynecol. Pathol.* **1,** 231–245.

Chatal, J. F., J. C. Saccavini, P. Fumoleau, A. Baudy, J. Y. Douillard, J. Aubry, and B. Le Mevel (1982), *J. Nucl. Med.* **23,** 8.

Chung, Y. S., J. J. L. Ho, Y. S. Kim, H. Tanaka, B. Nakata, A. Hiura, H. Motoyoshi, K. Satake, and K. Umeyama (1987), *Cancer* **60,** 1636–1643.

Del Favero, G., C. Fabris, A. Panucci, D. Basso, M. Plebani, U Baccaglini, G. Leandro, A. Burlina, and R. Naccarato (1986a), *Bull. Cancer (Paris)* **73,** 251–255.

Del Favero, G., C. Fabris, M. Plebani, A. Panucci, A. Piccoli, L. Perobelli, S. Pedrazzoli, U. Baccalini, A. Burlina, and R. Naccarato (1986b), *Cancer* **57,** 1576–1579.

Del Villano, B. C., S. Brennan, P. Brock, C. Bucher, V. Liu, M. McClure, B. Rake, S. Space, B. Westrick, H. Shoemaker, and V. R. Zurawski (1983a), *Clin. Chem.* **29,** 549–552.

Del Villano, B. C. and V. R. Zurawski (1983b), in *Laboratory Research Methods in Biological Medicine, vo. 8: Immunodiagnostics* (Aliosi, R. M., ed.), Liss, New York, pp. 269–282.

Dietel, M., H. Arps, R. Klapdor, S. Müller-Hagen, M. Sieck, and L. Hoffmann (1986), *J. Cancer Res. Clin. Oncol.* **111,** 257–265.

Duffy, M. J., F. O'Sullivan, T. J. McDonnell, and M. X. Fitzgerald (1985), *Clin. Chem.* **31,** 1245, 1246.

Dunn, P. M. and M. McKinstry (1989), *Ann. Intern. Med.* **111,** 343.

Enblad, P., C. Busch, U. Carlsson, G. Ekelund, B. Glimelius, C. Lindström, J. Ponten, and L. Pahlman (1988), *Am. J. Clin. Pathol.* **90,** 121–130.

Encabo, G. and A. Ruibal (1986), *Bull. Cancer (Paris)* **73,** 256–259.

Fabris, C., G. Del Favero, D. Basso, A. Piccoli, T. Meggiato, C. Angonese, M. Plebani, G. Leandro, A. Burlina, and R. Naccarato (1988), *Am. J. Gastroenterol.* **83,** 549–553.

Falk, K. E., K. A. Karlsson, G. Larson, J. Thurin, M. Blaszczyk, Z. Steplewski, and H. Koprowski (1983), *Biochem. Biophys. Res. Commun.* **110,** 383–391.

Farinati, F., D. Nitti, F. Cardin, F. Di Mario, F. Costa, C. Rossi, A. Marchett, M. Lise, and R. Naccarato (1988), *Eur. J. Cancer Clin. Oncol.* **14,** 923–927.

Farini, R., C. Fabris, P. Bonvicini, A. Piccoli, G. Del Favero, R. Venturini, A. Panucci, and R. Naccarato (1985), *Eur. J. Cancer Clin. Oncol.* **21,** 429–432.

Fioretti, P., A. Gadducci, M. Ferdeghini, T. Bartolini, V. Fontana, and V. Facchini (1988), *Eur. J. Gynaecol. Oncol.* **9,** 291–294.

Fischbach, W. and J. Mössner (1988), *Res. Exp. Med.* **188,** 101–114.

Fujii, S., I. Konishi, Y. Nanbu, H. Nonogaki, F. Kobayashi, N. Sagawa, T. Mori, and K. Endo (1988), *Cancer* **62,** 541–547.

Glaubitt, D. and M. Cordoni-Voutsus (1985), in *Neue tumorassoziierte Antigene* (Greten, H. and R. Klapdor, eds.), Thieme-Verlag Stuttgart, NY, pp. 254–260.

Glenn, J., W. M. Steinberg, S. H. Kurtzman, S. M. Steinberg, and W. F. Sindelar (1988), *J. Clin. Oncol.* **6,** 462–468.

Göcze, P. M., D. G. Szabo, G. N. Than, I. F. Csaba, and K. F. Krommer (1988), *Gynecol. Obstet. Invest.* **25,** 268–272.

Goldberg, E. M., L. M. Simunovic, S. L. Drake, W. F. Mueller, and H. L. Verrill (1989), *Hybridoma* **8,** 569–575.

Gong, E., S. Hirohashi, Y. Shimosato, M. Watanabe, Y. Ino, S. Toshima, and S. Kodaira (1985), *J. Natl. Cancer Inst.* **75,** 447–454.

Green, P. J., S. K. Ballas, P. Westkaemper, H. G. Schwartz, T. L. Klug, and V. R. Zurawski (1986), *J. Natl. Cancer Inst.* **77,** 337–341.

Gupta, M. K., R. Arciaga, L. Bocci, R. Tubbs, R. Bukowski, and S. D. Deodhar (1985), *Cancer* **56,** 277–283.

Gustafsson, H., L. Franzen, K. Grankvist, M. Anniko, and R. Henriksson (1988), *J. Cancer Res. Clin. Oncol.* **114,** 394–398.

Haglund, C., J. Lindgren, P. J. Roberts, and S. Nordling (1986a), *Br. J. Cancer* **53,** 189–195.

Haglund, C., P. J. Roberts, P. Kuusela, T. M. Scheinin, O. Mäkelä, and H. Jalanko (1986b), *Br. J. Cancer* **53,** 197–202.

Hanisch, F. G., H. Egge, J. Peter-Karalinic, G. Uhlenbruck, C. Dienst, and R. Fangmann (1985a), *Eur. J. Biochem.* **152,** 343–351.

Hanisch, F. G., G. Uhlenbruck, C. Dienst, M. Stottrop, and E. Hippauf (1985b), *Eur. J. Biochem.* **149,** 323–330.

Hansson, G. C., and D. Zopf (1985), *J. Biol. Chem.* **260,** 9388–9392.

Harmenberg, U., B. Wahren, and K. L. Wiechel (1988), *Cancer Res.* **48,** 1985–1988.

Hayakawa, T., T. Kondo, T. Shibata, H. Hamano, M. Kitagawa, Y. Sakai, and H. Ono (1988), *Cancer* **61,** 1827–1831.

Heptner, G., S. Domschke, F. Krapf, M. U. Schneider, H. Iro, and W. Domschke (1984), *Dtsch. Med. Wochenschr.* **109,** 1309–1312.

Heptner, G., S. Domschke, M. U. Schneider, and W. Domschke (1985), *Dtsch. Med. Wochenschr.* **110,** 624–628.

Herlyn, M., H. F. Sears, Z. Steplewski, and H. Koprowski (1982), *J. Clin. Immunol.* **2,** 135–140.

Herrero-Zabaleta, M. E., R. Gautier, P. Burtin, N. Daher, and J. Bara (1987), *Bull. Cancer* **74,** 387–396.

Hirohashi, S., Y. Shimosato, Y. Ino, Y. Tome, M. Watanabe, T. Hirota, and M. Itabashi (1984), *Gann* **75,** 540–547.

Ho, J. J. L., Y. Chung, Y. Fujimkoto, N. Bi, W. Ryan, S. Yuan, J. C. Byrd, and Y. S. Kim (1988), *Cancer Res.* **48,** 3924–3928.

Hoffmann, L., S. Müller-Hagen, R. Klapdor, M. Dietel, H. Arps, and E. Schäfer (1986), *J. Cancer Res. Clin. Oncol.* (Suppl.)**111,** 134.

Hölting, T., P. Schlag, M. Steinbächer, U. Kretzschmar, P. Georgi, and Ch. Herfarth (1989), *Cancer* **64,** 830–833.

Ichihara, T., H. Nagura, A. Nakao, J. Sakamoto, T. Watanabe, and H. Takagi (1988), *Cancer* **61,** 324–333.

Itzkowitz, S. H., M. Yuan, Y. Fukushi, H. Lee, Z. Shi, V. R. Zurawski, and S. Hakomori (1988), *Cancer Res.* **48,** 3834–3842.

Jalanko, H., P. Kuusela, P. Roberts, P. Sipponnen, C. A. Haglund, and O. Mäkkelä (1984), *J. Clin. Pathol.* **37,** 218–222.

Kalthoff, H., Ch. Kreiker, W. H. Schmiegel, H. Greten, and H. G. Thiele (1986), *Cancer Res.* **46,** 3605–3607.

Kew, M. C., E. L. Berger, and H. Koprowski (1987), *Br. J. Cancer* **56,** 86–88.

Kimura, W. and K. Ohtsubo (1988), *Cancer* **61,** 1394–1402.

Klapdor, R. and H. Greten (1984a), *Dtsch. Med. Wochenschr.* **109,** 1935–1939.

Klapdor, R., U. Klapdor, M. Bahlo, and H. Greten (1984b), *Tumor Diagn Ther.* **5,** 161–165.

Klapdor, R., U. Klapdor, M. Bahlo, B. Schmieding, B. Kremer, M. Dallek, L. Hoffmann, H. V. Ackeren, H. W. Schreiber, and H. Greten (1985a), in *Neue tumorassoziierte Antigene* (Greten, H. and R. Klapdor, eds.), Thieme-Verlag, Stuttgart, NY, pp. 58–67.

Klapdor, U., R. Klapdor, G. Helferich, D. Striefler, M. Bahlo, H. G. Bützow, N. Soehendra, and H. Greten (1985b), in *Neue tumorassoziierte Antigene* (Greten, H. and R. Klapdor, eds.), Thieme-Verlag, Stuttgart, NY, pp. 86–94.

Klapdor, R. (1986), *Dtsch. Med. Wochenschr.* **111,** 1039.

Klug, T. L., N. C. LeDonne, T. F. Greber, and V. R. Zurawski (1988), *Cancer Res.* **48,** 1505–1511.

Kobayashi, F., N. Sagawa, Y. Nanbu, K. Nakamura, M. Nonogaki, Ch. Ban, S. Fujii, and T. Mori (1989), *Am. J. Obstet. Gynecol.* **160,** 1232–1238.

Köhler, G. and C. Milstein (1975), *Nature* **256,** 495, 496.

Koelbel, H., K. Schieder, W. Neunteufel, and Ch. Bieglmayer (1989), *Neoplasma* **36,** 473–478.

Koprowski, H., Z. Steplewski, K. Mitchell, M. Herlyn, D. Herlyn, and P. Fuhrer (1979), *Somatic Cell Genet.* **5,** 957–972.

Kuusela, P., H. Jalanko, P. Roberts, P. Sipponen, J. P. Mecklin, R. Pitkänen, and O. Mäkelä (1984), *Br. J. Cancer* **49,** 135–139.

Lamerz, R., S. Hueck, P. Stieber, E. Segura, and A. Fateh-Moghadam (1990), in *Recent Results in Tumor Diagnosis and Therapy* (Klapdor R., ed.), Zuckschwerdt-Verlag München, San Francisco, pp. 69–74.

Leandro, G., S. Zizzari, C. Fabris, D. Basso, S. Elba, G. Del Favero, T. Meggiato, C. Angonese, F. Di Mario, O. G. Manghisi, and R. Naccarato (1989), *Oncology* **46,** 381–385.

Lellé, R. J., E. Henkel, D. Leinemann, and K. Goeschen (1989), *Gynecol. Obstet. Invest.* **27,** 137–142.

Lindgren, J. and P. Sipponen (1985), *Tumour Biol.* **6,** 389.

Lloyd, K. O. (1987), *Am. J. Clin. Pathol.* **87,** 129–139.

Lorenz, M., C. Hottenrott, J. Happ, M. Reimann-Kirkowa, F. D. Maul, A. Enke, and G. Hör (1985), in *Neue tumorassoziierte Antigene* (Greten, H. and R. Klapdor, eds.), Thieme-Verlag, Stuttgart, NY, pp. 112–128.

Lorenz, M., G. Herrmann, R. P. Baum, M. Schulz, G. Hör, C. Hottenrott, and A. Encke (1987), *Nuc Compact* **18,** 102–108.

Lorenz, M., R. P. Baum, G. Oremek, R. Inglis, M. Reimann-Kirkowa, G. Hör, U. Seiffert, and C. Hottenrott (1989), *Int. J. Biol. Markers* **4,** 18–26.

Macdonald, F., R. Bird, H. Stokes, B. Russell, and J. Crocker (1988), *J. Clin. Pathol.* **41,** 260–264.

Magnani, J. L., B. Nilsson, M. Brockhaus, D. Zopf, Z. Steplewski, H. Koprowski, and V. Ginsburg (1982), *J. Biol. Chem.* **257,** 14365–14369.

Magnani, J. L., Z. Steplewski, H. Koprowski, and V. Ginsburg (1983), *Cancer Res.* **43,** 5489–5492.

Malesci, A., M. A. Tommasini, P. Bocchia, A. Zerbi, E. Beretta, M. Vecchi, and V. di Carlo (1981), *La Ricerca Clin. Lab.* **11,** 303–306.

Malesci, A., M. A. Tommasini, C. Bonato, P. Bocchia, M. Bersani, A. Zerbi, E. Beretta, and V. di Carlo (1987), *Gastroenterology* **92,** 60–67.

Malesci, A., A. Evangelista, A. Mariani, M. Bersanti, C. Bonato, M. Basilico, M. Montorsi, and E. Beretta (1988), *Int. J. Pancreatol.* **3 (Suppl. 1),** S119–S123.

Manabe, T., T. Miyashita, G. Ohshio, A. Nonaka, T. Suzuki, K. Endo, M. Takahashi, and T. Tobe (1988), *Cancer* **62,** 135–141.

Marechal, F., G. Berthot, and G. Deltour (1988), *Anticancer Res.* **8,** 677–680.

Matsuoka, Y., K. Endo, Y. Kawamura, T. Yoshida, T. Saga, Y. Watanabe, M. Koizumi, T. Nakashima, J. Konishi, N. Yamaguchi, and R. Yatani (1990), *Cancer* **65,** 506–510.

McKnight, A., A. Mannell, I. Shperling (1989), *Br. J. Cancer* **60,** 249–251.

Mezger, J., W. Permanetter, A. L. Gerbes, W. Wilmanns, and R. Lamerz (1988), *J. Clin. Pathol.* **41,** 633–643.

Molina, R., A. M. Ballesta, E. Letang, J. L. Marin, E. Casals, M. Elena, J. Sanchez-Lloret, and A. Balague (1985), *Tumour Biol.* **6,** 394.

Molina, R., P. Santabarbara, X. Filella, P. Mengual, A. M. Ballesta, and A. Balague (1989), *Int. J. Biol. Markers* **4,** 215–220.

Montz, R., R. Klapdor, B. Kremer, and B. Rothe (1985), *Nucl. Med.* **24,** 232–237.

Munck-Wikland, E., R. Kuyelenstierna, B. Wahren, J. Lindholm, and S. Haglund (1988), *Cancer* **62,** 2281–2286.

Nagata, H., K. Takahashi, Y. Yamane, K. Yoshino, T. Shibukawa, and M. Kitao (1989), *Gynecol. Obstet. Invest.* **28,** 165–168.

Nanbu, Y., S. Fujii, I. Konishi, H. Nonogaki, and T. Mori (1988), *Cancer* **62,** 2580–2588.

Neghishi, Y., T. Furukawa, T. Oka, M. Sakamoto, T. Hirata, K. Okabe, K. Matayoshi, K. Akiya, and H. Soma (1987), *Gynecol. Obstet. Invest.* **23,** 200–207.

Neunteufel, W. and G. Breitenecker (1989a), *Cancer Lett.* **48,** 77–83.

Neunteufel, W. and G. Breitenecker (1989b), *Gynecol. Oncol.* **32,** 297–302.

Neunteufel W., G. Gitsch, K. Schieder, H. Kölbl, and G. Breitenecker (1989c), *Anticancer Res.* **9,** 993–997.

Nishida, K., H. Miyagawa, T. Yoshikawa, and M. Kondo (1988a), *Oncology* **45,** 166–171.

Nishida, K., N. Tasaki, H. Miyagawa, T. Yoshikawa, and M. Kondo (1988b), *Am. J. Gastroenterol.* **83,** 126–129.

Nishida, K., K. Shiga, K. Kato, K. Kunihiro, T. Fijii, T. Tomii, H. Yamamoto, E. Yamane, B. Nishioka, T. Yoshikawa, and M. Kondo (1989), *Hepato-gastroenterology* **36,** 442–445.

Nishino, H., K. Satake, E. C. Kim, A. Hiura, O. Arai, T. Kubo, and K. Umeyama (1988), *Am. Surg.* **54,** 487–491.

Novis, B. H., E. Gluck, P. Thomas, G. D. Steele, V. R. Zurawski, R. Stewart, P. T. Lavin, and N. Zamcheck (1986), *J. Clin. Oncol.* **4,** 987–993.

Okubo, A., S. Sone, F. Ogushi, T. Ogura, T. Uyama, Y. Monden, and I. I. Kunio (1989), *Cancer* **63,** 1994–1997.

Olding, L. B., J. Thurin, C. Svalander, and H. Koprowski (1984), *Int. J. Cancer* **34,** 187–192.

Olding, L. B., C. Ahren, J. Thurin, K. A. Karlsson, C. Svalander, and H. Koprowski (1985), *Int. J. Cancer* **36,** 131–136.

Olsson, N. O., D. Crimet-Montange, and F. Martin (1985), *Gastroentérol. Clin. Biol.* **9,** 206–211.

Ouyang, Q., M. Vilien, B. R. Juhl, L. G. Larsen, and V. Binder (1987), *Acta Pathol. Microbiol. Scand. [A]* **95,** 177–183.

Paganuzzi, M., M. Onetto, P. Marroni, D. Barone, M. Conio, H. Aste, V. Pugliese (1988), *Cancer* **61,** 2100–2108.

Pak, K. Y., M. Blaszczyk, M. Herlyn, Z. Steplewski, and H. Koprowski (1984), *Hybridoma* **3,** 1–10.

Panidis, D. K., G. D. Vlassis, B. A. Papameletiou, J. M. Matalliotakis, and A. P. Palogeropoulos (1988), *Arch. Androl.* **21,** 51–58.

Pasquali, C., C. Sperti, A. A. D'Andrea, B. Bonadimani, G. Del Favero, P. Petrin, and S. Pedrazzoli (1987), *Pancreas* **2,** 34–37.

Pfeiffer, R., K. Dimitriadis, K. Balzer, U. Giesche, E. Aulbert, B. Hoffmann, and C. G. Schmidt (1984), *Tumor Diagn. Ther.* **5,** 196–200.

Pleskow, D. K., H. J. Berger, J. Gyves, E. Allen, A. McLean, and D. K. Podolsky (1989), *Ann. Intern. Med.* **110,** 704–709.

Polterauer, P., M. Havel, and M. M. Müller (1986), *Tumor Diagn. Ther.* **7,** 17–20.

Pour, P. M., M. Tempero, H. Takasaki, E. Uchida, Y. Takiyama, D. A. Burnett, and Z. Steplewski (1988), *Cancer Res.* **48,** 5422–5426.

Prantl, F. (1987), *Tumor Diagn. Ther.* **8,** 64–68.

Prat, M., E. Medico, P. Rossino, C. Garrino, and P. M. Comoglio (1989), *Cancer Res.* **49,** 1415–1421.

Quentmeier, A., P. Müller, V. Schwarz, U. Abel, and P. Schlag (1987), *Cancer* **60,** 2261–2226.

Raux, H., F. Labbe, M. C. Fondaneche, H. Koprowski, and P. Burtin (1983), *Int. J. Cancer* **32,** 315–319.

Richter, J. M., M. R. Christensen, A. K. Rustgi, and M. D. Silverstein (1989), *Arch. Intern. Med.* **149,** 2292–2297.
Ritts, R. E., B. C. Del Villano, V. L. W. Go, R. B. Herberman, T. L. Klug, and V. R. Zurawski (1984), *Int. J. Cancer* **33,** 339–345.
Roberts, D. D., D. L. Monsein, R. C. Frates, M. S. Chernick, and V. Ginsburg (1986), *Arch. Biochem. Biophys.* **245,** 292–294.
Roberts, P. J. (1988), *Scand. J. Gastroenterol.* (suppl.) **149,** 50–58.
Röthlin, M., U. Metzger, J. Joller, and F. Largiadèr (1988), *Schweiz. Med. Wochenschr.* **118,** 924–929.
Ruibal, A., G. Encabo, R. Geffaell, E. Martinez-Miralles, J. M. Fort, and J. Fernandez-Llamazares (1983), *Bull. Cancer (Paris)* **70,** 438–440.
Safi, F., R. Bittner, and H. G. Beger (1985), in *Neue tumorassoziierte Antigene* (Greten, H. and R. Klapdor, eds.), Thieme-Verlag, Stuttgart, NY, pp. 19–27.
Safi, F., H. G. Beger, R. Bittner, M. Büchler, and U. Krautzberger (1986a), *Cancer* **57,** 779–783.
Safi F., B. Rappenecker, R. Roscher, and H. G. Beger (1986b), *Med. Klin.* **81,** 12–14.
Safi F., R. Roscher, R. Bittner, B. Schenkluhn, H. P. Dopfer, and H. G. Beger (1987), *Pancreas* **2,** 398–403.
Safi F., R. Roscher, R. Bittner, and H. G. Beger (1988), *Int. J. Biol. Markers* **3,** 101–106.
Safi F., R. Roscher, and H. G. Beger (1989), *Hepatogastroenterology* **35,** 419–423.
Sakahara, H., K. Endo, K. Nakajima, T. Nakashima, M. Koizumi, H. Ohta, A. Hidaka, S. Kohno, Y. Nakano, A. Naito, T. Suzuki, and K. Torizuka (1986), *Cancer* **57,** 1324–1326.
Satake, K., G. Kananzawa, I. Kho, Y. Chung, and K. Umeyama (1985a), *Am. J. Gastroenterol.* **80,** 630–636.
Satake, K., G. Kananzawa, I. Kho, Y. S. Chung, and K. Umeyama (1985b), *J. Surg. Oncol.* **29,** 15–21.
Savarino, V., C. Mansi, V. Pugliese, G. B. Ferrara, V. Arcuri, and G. Celle (1984), *Digestion* **29,** 1–4.
Schmid, L., A. Magacz, K. Zellmann, M. Oberdorfer, and H. Langhammer (1985), in *Neue tumorassoziierte Antigene* (Greten, H. and R. Klapdor, eds.), Thieme-Verlag, Stuttgart, NY, pp. 45–49.
Schmiegel, W. H., W. Eberl, C. Kreiker, H. Kalthoff, G. H. Bützow, K. Jessen, R. Klapdor, N. Soehendra, M. Wargenau, M. Classen, H. Greten, and H. G. Thiele (1985a), *Hepatogastroenterology* **32,** 141–149.
Schmiegel, W. H., C. Kreiker, W. Eberl, R. Arndt, M. Classen, H. Greten, K. Jessen, H. Kalthoff, N. Soehendra, and H. G. Thiele (1985b), *Gut* **26,** 456–460.

Schröck, R., R. Hafter, K. Jürgensmeyer, A. Hünichen, L. Schmid, and H. Graeff (1985), in *Neue tumorassoziierte Antigene* (Greten, H. and R. Klapdor, eds.), Thieme-Verlag, Stuttgart, NY, pp. 186–196.

Schwenk, J. and J. Makovitzky (1989), *Virchows Arch. [A]* **414,** 465–476.

Sears, H. F., M. Herlyn, B. Del Villano, Z. Steplewski, and H. Korprowski (1982), *J. Clin. Immunol.* **2,** 141–149.

Sears, H. F., J. W. Shen, B. Atkinson, P. F. Engstrom, and H. Koprowski (1985), *Am. J. Clin. Oncol.* **8,** 108–117.

Shimizu, M., Y. Saitoh, H. Ohyanagi, and H. Itoh (1990), *Arch. Pathol. Lab. Med.* **114,** 195–200.

Sipponen, P. and J. Lindgren (1986), *Acta Pathol. Microbiol. Immunol. Scand. [A]* **94,** 305–311.

Staab, H. J., A. Hornung, F. A. Anderer, and G. Kieninger (1984), *Dtsch. Med. Wochenschr.* **109,** 1141–1147.

Staab, H. J., T. Brümmendorf, A. Hornung, F. A. Anderer, and G. Kieninger (1985), *Klin. Wochenschr.* **63,** 106–115.

Staab, H. J. (1986), GIT Lab. Med **9,** 553–557.

Stieber, P., R. Lamerz, and A. Fateh-Moghadam (1985), *Tumour Biol.* **6,** 388.

Strom, B. L., D. Iliopoulos, B. Atkinson, M. Herlyn, S. L. West, G. Maislin, S. Saul, M. A. Varello, H. A. Rodrigez-Martinez, J. Rios-Dalenz, and R. D. Solowy (1989), *J. Natl. Cancer Inst.* **81,** 1575–1580.

Szymendera, J. J., M. P. Nowacki, 1. Kozlowiczgudzinska, and M. Kowalska (1985), *Dis. Colon Rect.* **28,** 895–899.

Tabuchi, Y., H. Deguchi, and Y. Saitoh (1988), *Cancer* **62,** 1605–1613.

Takasaki, H., E. Uchida, M. A. Tempero, D. A. Burnett, R. S. Metzgar, and P. M. Pour (1988), *Cancer Res.* **48,** 1435–1438.

Tappero, G. and P. Piantino (1987), *Int. J. Biol. Markers* **2,** 191–196.

Tatsuta, M., H. Yamamura, H. Ishi, M. Ichii, S. Noguchi, R. Yamamoto, and S. Okuda (1985), *Cancer* **56,** 2669–2673.

Tatsuta, M., H. Ishii, M. Ichii, S. Noguchi, R. Yamamoto, H. Yamamura, and S. Okuda (1986), *Cancer* **57,** 1836–1839.

Tempero, M. A., E. Uchida, H. Takasaki, D. A. Burnett, Z. Steplewski, and P. M. Pour (1987), *Cancer Res.* **47,** 5501–5503.

Tizzani, A., G. Cassetta, A. Cicigoi, P. Piana, A. Cerchier, F. Pecchio, and P. Piantino (1987), *Int. J. Biol. Markers* **2,** 121–124.

Touitou, Y. and A. Bogdan (1988), *Eur. J. Cancer Clin. Oncol.* **24,** 1083–1091.

Touitou, Y., Y. Darbois, A. Bogdan, A. Auzéby, and S. Keusseoglou (1989), *Br. J. Cancer* **60,** 419–420.

Uhlenbruck, G., U. V. Meensel-Maene, F. G. Hanisch, and C. Dienst (1984), *Hoppe Seylers Z. Physiol. Chem.* **365,** 613–617.

Uhlenbruck, G., U. Höller, J. Heising, A. van Mill, and C. Dienst (1985), *Urol. Res.* **13,** 223–226.

Uhlenbruck, G., U. Scheuring, C. Dienst, D. Kaiser, B. Roth, and H. Skopnik (1988), *Klin. Pädiatr.* **200,** 89–95.

Ura, Y., M. Ishida, and Y. Ochi (1985), *Tumour Biol.* **6,** 392.

Uyama, T., Y. Monden, M. Sumitomo, K. Miura, and S. Kimura (1989), *J. Surg. Oncol.* **41,** 103–108.

Venot, J., D. Vincent, A. Gainant, B. Descottes, F. Cessot, and C. Beck (1986), *Gastroenterol. Clin. Biol.* **10,** 208–210.

Vindimian, M., J. J. Lafitte, D. Duriez, and P. Wattre (1984), *Presse Med.* **13,** 1787.

Vindimian, M., J. J. Lafitte, and P. Wattre (1987), *Biomed. Pharmacother.* **41,** 191–195.

Walker, R. A. and S. J. Day (1986), *Virchows Arch. [A]* **409,** 375–383.

Wang, T. H., J. T. Lin, D. S. Chem, J. C. Sheu, and J. L. Sung (1986), *Pancreas* **1,** 219–223.

Yoshikawa, T., K. Nishida, M. Tanigawa, K. Fukumoto, and M. Kondo (1985), *Digestion* **31,** 67–76.

Yvan, S., J. J. L. Ho, M. Yvan, and Y. S. Kim (1985), *Cancer Res.* **45,** 6179–6187.

Chapter 15

Mucin-Like Cancer-Associated Antigen (MCA) as Available Circulating Tumor Marker for Breast Cancer

Emilio Bombardieri
and Massimo Gion

1. Introduction

Laboratory tests have demonstrated, during the past years, the existence of several breast cancer associated antigens. Recently, the development and the application of monoclonal antibody (MAb) techniques have facilitated the identification of various breast cancer associated antigens (Kufe et al., 1984; Hilkens et al., 1985; Iacobelli et al., 1985; White et al., 1985; Bray et al., 1987; Cohen et al., 1987). The different epitopes are usually carried by mucinous substances, which belong to a polymorphic family of glycoproteins produced by the glandular mucinous epitelia (Smets and Van Beek, 1984; Feizi, 1985; Hakomori, 1989).

From: *Serological Cancer Markers* Edited by Stewart Sell ©1992 The Humana Press, Totowa, NJ

The main characteristic of these high-mol-wt molecules is that, during neoplastic transformation, they are released in detectable amounts into the bloodstream and thus become suitable for cancer detection and monitoring. Another important aspect of their biology is their highly heterogeneous distribution in different tissues and tumor types. This leads to the general observation that the available tumor-associated epitopes are not tumor-specific (they are present also in normal tissues). Moreover, their specificity is not restricted to one particular histotype. Nevertheless, some of the epitopes, especially those recognized by MAbs generated against breast cancer tissue and breast carcinoma cell lines, are present in the breast tissues and may be detectable in the sera of cancer patients as a signal of breast cancer (Bombardieri et al., 1990).

MCA (mucin-like carcinoma-associated antigen) is a new member of the family of circulating tumor markers of breast cancer. The antibody that identifies MCA, MAb b-12, was obtained against a mixture of different human breast carcinoma cell lines (ZR-75-1, MCF-7, MDA-MB-231). The MCA molecule is a mucin-like glycoprotein with a mol wt of 350 kDa and has been studied in the ZR-75 breast cancer cell line (Stahli et al., 1985, 1988). Treatment of MCA with *O*-glycanase and periodate seemed to demonstrate that the MCA b-12 epitope is presumably of peptide nature (Stahli et al., 1988). MCA reactivity was also observed in human milk; the antigen obtained from milk gave a band with an apparent molecular size of 450 kDa. MAb b-12 proved to be suitable for immunobiological assays and was therefore used to carry out immunohistochemical studies and to develop an enzyme immunoassay (EIA) method (Stahli et al., 1985; 1988; Zenklusen et al., 1988; Bombardieri et al., 1989).

2. MCA Tissue Presence and Distribution

By means of a two-site solid-phase EIA in which MAb b-12 was used both as a catcher antibody (coated to polystyrene beads) and as a tracer antibody (conjugated to horseradish peroxidase), high levels of MCA were demonstrated in the cytosol of many breast

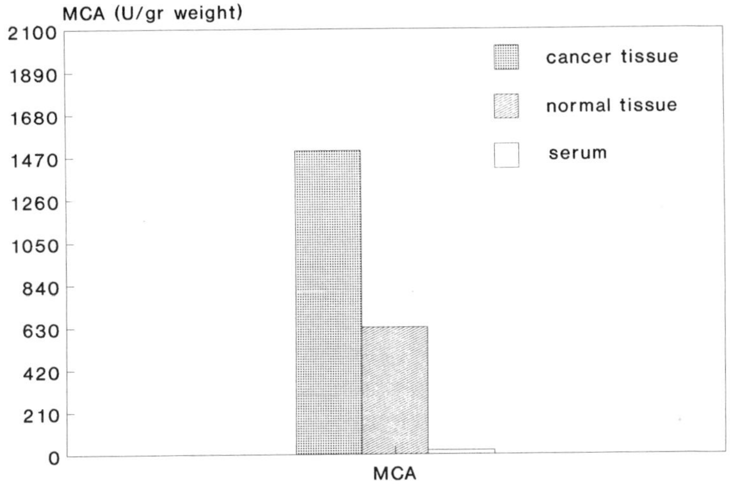

Fig. 1. MCA concentrations expressed in U/g tissue weight in breast cancer (dotted histogram), in normal breast (hatched histogram), and in serum (white histogram). The difference between breast cancer and normal tissue is based only on the quantity of the antigen.

cancer cell lines (range 30–126 U/mg cytosol proteins) (Bombardieri et al., 1989). In 21 of 24 patients (84%), the MCA cytosol concentrations were significantly higher in breast cancer cells than in normal tissue. The mean MCA concentration in the cytosol of breast cancer cells was higher than the mean MCA concentration in the cytosol of the corresponding normal tissues. This observation explains the fact that MCA is detectable also in normal breast tissues, although the antigen is, of course, more clearly expressed in breast cancer tissues (Fig. 1). We also found MCA in metastases, since these do not lose their capability to produce the antigen.

Zenklusen et al. (1988) demonstrated the immunoreactivity of MAb b-12 on 122 breast carcinoma samples. They found that all breast cancers were stained by MAb b-12, and noted 36.9% of high reactivity, 31.1% of intermediate reactivity, and 32.0% of low reactivity. These authors demonstrated the presence of MCA also in other nonbreast cancer tissues, though with minor frequency and with minor staining intensity. The same phenomenon was observed in some normal mucinous epithelia, but in these cases the positive staining, when present, was limited to a line surrounding the apical cell surface around the glandular lumina and to the mucinous secretions inside the lumina (Zenklusen et al., 1988).

Martinazzi and coworkers (1990) obtained similar results in 108 cases of breast cancer. A positivity rate of 100% was obtained in all the histotypes they evaluated; the various histotypes differed only in their staining patterns. However, there is a lot of controversy over the evaluation criteria of staining positivity. The immunoreactivity for MCA was described also in a series of cancers in sites other than the breast. The highest positivity rate was observed in lung cancer. In a previous study, we could not demonstrate any correlation between MCA and cytosol levels of estrogen receptors, progesterone receptors, and other tumor markers (CEA, ferritin, and TPA) (Bombardieri et al., 1989). These findings were confirmed in this new immunohistochemical study, except for the proliferative index (as shown by the immunoreactivity with the Ki67 antibody). No statistical correlation was found between MAb b-12 staining and the antibody's reactivity with estrogen receptors, progesterone receptors, epidermal growth factor receptor, and p53 proteins. By contrast, there was a statistically significant correlation between proliferative fraction (Ki67) and MCA presence ($p = 0.001$) (Martinazzi et al., 1990).

3. MCA Serum Levels in Cancer Patients

The mean MCA serum concentration in the control group of healthy subjects in our first study was 6.2 U/mL, with a standard deviation of 3 U/mL. The 95th centile value was chosen as positive/negative cutoff (Bombardieri et al., 1989). Table 1 shows the positivity rate in the series of patients that we observed. Other authors using the same positive/negative cutoff obtained more favorable results (Molina et al., 1990). Molina et al. examined 247 patients with cancer; among the breast cancer patients they found 19.8% serum positivity in patients with locoregional disease and

Table 1
MCA Serum Levels (U/mL) in Breast Cancer Patients[a]

Group	Number of cases	Mean	Range	Positivity rate, % (> 11.0 U/mL)
Stage 1	10	7.7	3.4–12.8	20.0
Stage 2	55	8.6	2.4–32.9	21.8
Stage 3	14	10.7	2.4–27.6	35.7
Tl	19	8.2	3.4–14.3	21.0
T2	44	8.7	2.4–32.9	22.7
T3	11	11.2	2.4–27.6	45.4
T4	5	8.5	5.1–11.8	1/5
No	35	8.2	2.6–14.3	20.0
N1	38	9.3	2.4–32.9	28.9
N2	6	12.2	5.1–27.6	2/6
0 Ln[b]	82	7.9	1.8–20.1	15.8
1–3 Ln	33	8.8	1.5–27.6	27.3
4–10 Ln	24	11.0	2.4–27.8	50.6
>10 Ln	6	15.1	5.0–32.9	3/6
Overall	147	9.0	1.5–32.9	26.5

[a]From Bombardieri et al., 1989, partially modified.
[b]Ln = number of lymph nodes involved.

77.7% in cases with distant metastases (Table 2). In patients without distant metastases, MCA was able to discriminate between T1–T2 and T3–T4 (tumor size), but not between N^+/N^-. Conversely, CEA was able to discriminate between N^+/N^-. The frequency of serum positivity in patients with different sites of metastasis was highest for the liver (100%), followed by bone (82%) and lung (80%), and lowest for the kidney (50%). Other cancers showed high MCA levels. We wish to point out that, in particular, advanced colorectal cancer (20%), advanced lung cancer (40%), and ovarian cancer (44.4%) caused a relevant frequency of positivity (Koelbl et al., 1989; Scheithauer and Mairinger, 1989; Molina et al., 1990).

Table 2
MCA Serum Levels (U/mL) in Patients with Breast Diseases[a]

Group	Number of cases	Mean	Range	Positivity rate, % (> 11.0 U/mL)
Benign	42	6.4	1.5–15	9.5
Cancer locoregional	96	7.5	1–37	19.8
Metastatic	85	27.7	1–120	77.7

[a]From Molina et al., 1990, modified.

Table 3
MCA Serum Levels (U/mL) in Patients with Benign Diseases[a]

Group	Number of cases	Mean	Range	Positivity rate, % (> 11.0 U/mL)
Liver cirrhosis	20	9.6	2.0–21.0	40.0
Renal failure	12	7.4	1.0–14.0	16.0
Autoimmune	10	5.3	1.6–8.9	–
Gastrointestinal	13	4.5	1.1–13.0	7.0
Lung	20	7.2	3.0–17.5	20.0
Breast	42	6.4	1.0–15.0	9.5

[a]From Molina et al., 1990, modified.

4. MCA Serum Levels in Benign Disease

Many benign diseases, such as liver cirrhosis, renal failure, autoimmune disease, chronic lung diseases, and the like, can induce MCA serum-level elevation (Molina et al., 1990; Soriano et al., 1990). Table 3 list the results obtained by Molina's group. Certain physiological conditions affect the MCA serum levels, for instance, pregnancy, especially during the third trimester. Our data confirm those reported by Bieglmayer et al. (1989), who found high MCA concentrations in the sera of pregnant women as well as in the amniotic fluid. After parturition, the serum concentrations demonstrated a final increase: A complete normalization can be observed one or two months after parturition. These changes in the course of a pregnancy can be explained by the fact that MCA is normally present in milk, and during the transformation and differentiation of the mammary gland induced by pregnancy, the antigen is overexpressed and its presence is detectable at high levels, just as during neoplastic progression.

5. MCA Test in Association with Other Tumor Markers

Regarding the simultaneous determination of MCA in association with other breast cancer tumor markers, many papers compare the sensitivity of the different breast cancer mucin determinations (Martinazzi et al., 1990; Molina et al., 1990; Soriano et al., 1990; Koelbl et al., 1989). In the study by Molina et al., the sensitivity of CA 15-3 seemed slightly lower than that described for MCA. Nevertheless, it is well known that the results depend on the criteria of evaluation. Molina et al. adopted a positive/negative cutoff of 11 U/mL for MCA and 40 U/mL for CA 15-3. Rasoul-Rockenschaub et al. (1989) adopted different thresholds: 14.4 for MCA and 20.4 for CA 15-3. In this case the overall sensitivity of the tests indicates a superiority of the CA 15-3 test in comparison to MCA. The true positive results and the false negative results during follow-up in the Rasoul-Rockenschaub study were superior to those described for MCA. This study showed the diagnostic sensitivity of MCA and CA 15-3 determination in comparison to that of the CEA test, which was considered as the reference tumor marker. Table 4 displays the different sensitivities of the single tumor-marker determination compared to the multimarker determination. Generally the use of the association of different tumor-marker tests leads to an increase in diagnostic sensitivity with a loss of specificity. In addition, the cost/benefit balance is to be taken into consideration, because a diagnostic gain does not always imply acceptable costs.

Table 4
MCA and CA 15.3 Diagnostic Sensitivity in Comparison to CEA in Breast Cancer and Metastatic Lesions[a]

Skeletal lesions	
CEA	57.7%
MCA	60.0%
CA 15-3	66.66%
CEA + MCA	77.77%
CEA + CA 15-3	75.75%
CEA + MCA + CA 15-3	81.81%
Visceral lesions	
CEA	19.44%
MCA	58.43%
CA 15-3	66.66%
CEA + MCA	61.11%
CEA + CA 15-3	69.44%
CEA + MCA + CA 15-3	72.22%
Diffuse metastatic breast cancer	
CEA	66.66%
MCA	90.47%
CA 15-3	95.23%
CEA + MCA	95.23%
CEA + CA 15-3	100.0%
CEA + MCA + CA 15-3	100.0%

[a]From Rasoul-Rockenschaub et al., 1989, modified.

6. Follow-Up and Monitoring Studies

During follow-up after radical surgery, MCA levels decrease to between 15 and 10 U/mL in about 2 wk (Fig. 2). Complete normalization takes approx 3 mo.

Bieglmayer, Cooper, Steger, and other authors published good papers about serial determination of MCA after or during breast cancer treatments (Bieglmayer et al., 1988; Eskelinen et al., 1988; Cooper et al., 1989; Steger et al., 1989; Novakovic et al., 1989). In

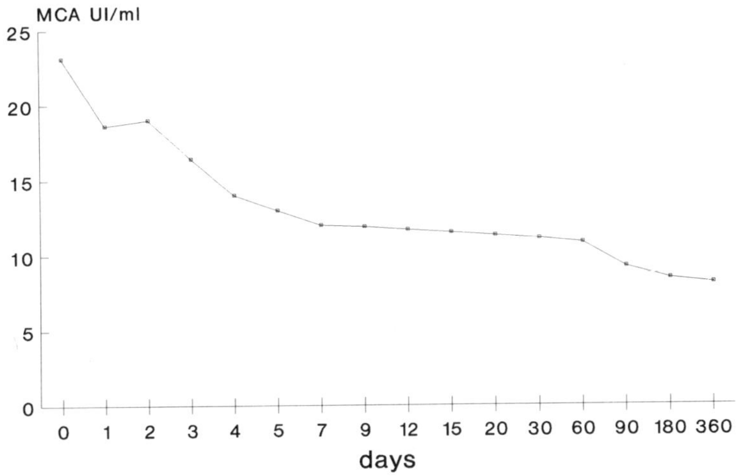

Fig. 2. Curve representing serum MCA disappearance in a breast cancer patient (stage pT3 N1 NO) after radical resection. Within 2 wk levels between 10 and 15 U/mL are reached and within 2 mo the levels are below the cutoff (personal data).

many cases, MCA demonstrated its clinical utility as a laboratory test available to indicate disease relapse or response to treatment. Also, CEA and other tumor markers proved to be valid for this clinical application. The performance of each tumor marker in terms of diagnostic sensitivity was quite different in the various series of patients studied.

The study by Cooper et al. (1989) has particular relevance because the authors established different upper limits of normality in premenopausal women (16.4 U/mL) and in postmenopausal women (19.6 U/mL). The levels at presentation in stages I, II, and III were not significantly different from the postmenopausal controls. Longitudinal studies over 5–9 yr in 20 patients with stage I and II disease who had remained tumor-free showed a narrow MCA range for each individual patient. Rising MCA levels occurred in 12/14 of patients who developed metastases 2–8 yr after surgery, but local recurrence was not associated with a rise in MCA. MCA levels fell during clinical response to therapy in patients with metastatic cancer.

Bieglmayer et al. (1989) reported that in several patients at risk a clinical diagnosis of metastases was preceded by elevated MCA levels for several months.

7. Relationship Between MCA and CA 15-3

In our study, we found a highly significant correlation between MCA and CA 15-3 cytosol concentrations ($p = 0.004$) (Bombardieri et al., 1989). Other authors reported a statistically significant correlation between MCA and CA 15-3 serum levels (Koelbl, 1989). We also noted a certain correlation between serum levels of MCA and CA 15-3 in the same series of samples (Fig. 3). This is probably because all three epitopes identified by b-12, DF3, and 115.D8 coexist on the mucinous molecule that carries the antigenic reactivity. Nevertheless, the antibodies may have different spectra of reactivity because of a diversity in affinity and in the number of repetitive binding sites.

The problem of the crossreactivity of two tumor markers has not yet been solved. It is important to realize that the information from these two mucins has different meanings and that their determinations can be associated and considered as complementary to each other. From the clinical point of view, we and other authors have described cases negative for MCA and positive for CA 15-3 and vice versa, and this observation is a valid support for all those who suggest adopting a simultaneous test for different tumor markers to improve their clinical efficacy.

8. Prognostic Applications

The last point is the prognostic application of MCA determination. Prior studies confirmed the relationship among CEA, CA 15-3, and other prognostic factors in breast cancer, such as tumor size and nodal involvement. An immunohistochemical evaluation

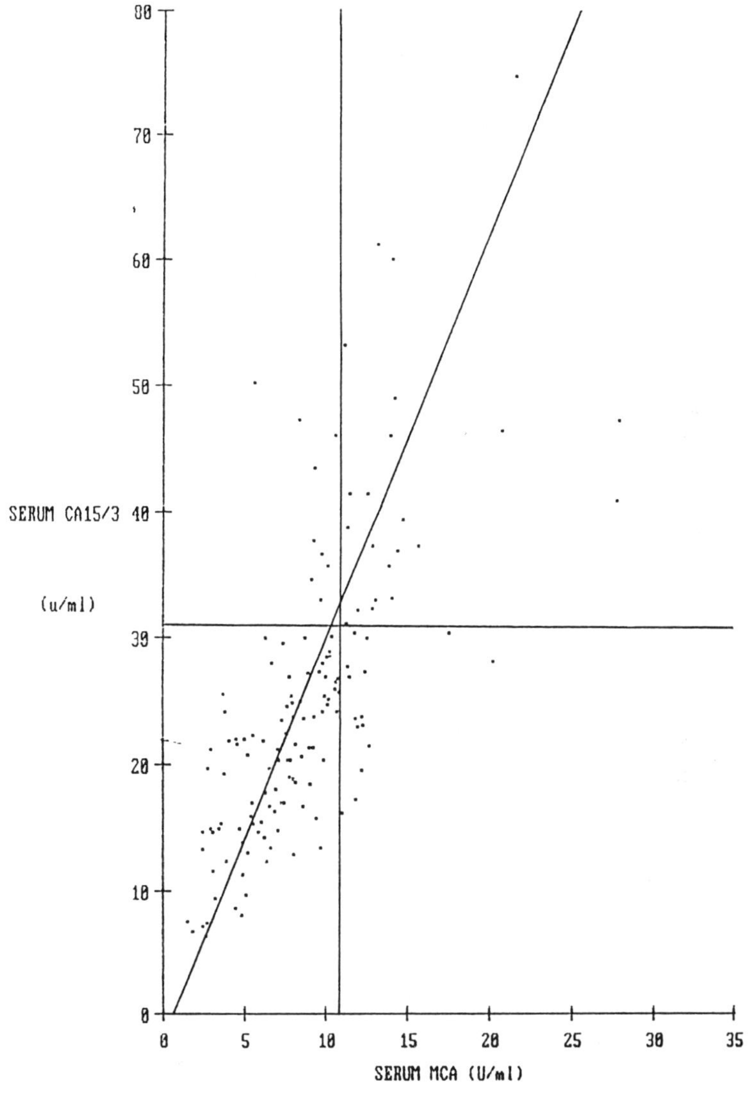

Fig. 3. Correlation between MCA and CA 15-3 in serum of 145 patients with primary breast cancer (linear regression analysis: $n = 145$; $y = 0.33x - 3.3$; $r = 0.66$; $p < 0.00001$). Vertical line: MCA negative/positive cutoff; horizontal line: CA 15-3 negative/positive cutoff; upper left area: MCA negative, CA 15-3 positive; upper right area: MCA positive, CA 15-3 positive; lower right area: MCA positive, CA 15-3 negative.

showed a strong relationship between MCA staining and proliferative activity of the cancer tissue. A recent paper compares the prognostic value of CEA, MCA, and CA 15-3 in discriminating a group of high-risk patients (Molina et al., 1990). In patients with breast cancer without metastases, Molina et al. found a relation between positivity of MCA and prognostic factors (tumor size, nodal involvement). The disease-free interval in patients with locoregional breast cancer was shorter in cases with abnormal presurgical MCA levels ($p = 0.002$) (Molina et al., 1990).

9. Conclusions

Among all the different possibilities of studying breast cancer in the laboratory, the measurement of circulating tumor-marker levels is still a field of investigation and effort.

Tumors often produce substances that are secreted into the bloodstream and can be tested as a dynamic signal of (a) the presence of a tumor; (b) the stage; (c) the changes in number of tumor cells.

This is the correct definition of *circulating tumor markers,* which are, today, the object of interest of many physicians, because it is easy to draw blood from a patient by intravenous injection in order to obtain information on a tumor.

MCA is a breast cancer associated mucin that is often detectable in the blood of breast cancer patients. It therefore seems to have good characteristics to be proposed as a reliable laboratory test for studying breast cancer:

1. It has a good correlation to the stage of the disease and lymph-node invasion.
2. Its changes in serum levels indicate the development of the disease or the efficacy of therapy.
3. Serum levels can be a biological parameter for prognostic evaluation.

Acknowledgment

The authors are grateful to Elisabetta Baldini and Marije de Jager for editorial and secretarial assistance.

References

Bieglmayer, C., T. Szepesi, and W. Neunteufel (1988), *Cancer Lett.* **42,** 199–206.

Bieglmayer, C., T. Szepesi, W. Neunteufel, and C. Nowotny (1989), *Tumor Biol.* **10,** 232–242.

Bombardieri, E., E. Seregni, and P. Veronesi (1990), *Minerva Biotec.* **2,** 8–17.

Bombardieri, E., M., Gion, R. Mione, R. Dittadi, M. Bruscagnin, and G. Buraggi (1989), *Cancer* **3,** 490–495.

Bray, K. R., J. E. Koda, and P. K. Gaur (1987), *Cancer Res.* **47,** 5853–5860.

Cohen, C., F. E. Sharkey, G. Shulman, E. O. Uthman, and L. R. Budgeon (1987), *Cancer* **60,** 1294–1305.

Cooper, E. H., M. A. Forbes, A. K. Hancock, J. J. Price, and D. Parker (1989), *Br. J. Cancer* **59,** 797–800.

Eskelinen, M., S. Tikanoa, and Y. Collan (1988), *Anticancer Res.* **8,** 665–668.

Feizi, T. (1985), *Cancer Surveys* **4,** 245–269.

Hakomori, S. I. (1989), *Adv. Cancer Res.* **52,** 257–319.

Hilkens, J., V. Kroezen, J. M. G. Bonfrer, P. F. Bruning, J. Hilgers, and A. van Eijkeren (1985), *Protides of the Biological Fluids,* XXXI (Peeters, H., ed.), Pergamon, Oxford, pp. 651–653.

Iacobelli, S., V. Natoli, G. Scambia, G. Santeusanio, R. Negrini, and C. Natoli (1985), *Cancer Res.* **45,** 4434–4438.

Koelbl, H., K. Schieder, W. Neunteufel, and Ch. Bieglmayer (1989), *Neoplasma* **36,** 4.

Kufe, D., G. Inghirami, M. Abe, D. Hayes, G. Justi-Wheeler, H. and J. Schlom (1984), *Hybridoma* **3,** 223–232.

Martinazzi, M., F. Crivelli, C. Grassi, and C. Zampatti (1990), *Int. J. Biol. Markers* **5,** 138–144.

Molina, R., X. Filella, P. Mengual, M. Prats, G. Zanon, M. Daniels and A. M. Ballesta (1990), *Int. J. Biol. Markers* **5,** n. 1, 14–21.

Novakovic, S., G. Krosl and S. Plesnicar (1989), *Tumor Diagn. Ther.* **10,** 136–141.

Rasoul-Rockenschaub, S., C. C. Zielinski, E. Kubista, V. Vavra, E. Pospischil, A. Staffen, K. Czerwenka, P. Aginger, and J. Spona (1989), *Eur. J. Cancer Clin. Oncol.* **25,** 7, 1067–1072.

Scheithauer, W. and D. Mairinger (1989), *J. Cancer Res. Clin. Oncol.* **115,** 474, 475.

Smets, L. A. and W. P. Van Beek (1984), *Biochim. Biophys. Acta* **738,** 237–249.

Soriano, A., M. T. Allende, F. Vizoso, J. Fdez Garcia, J. Vivanco, and A. Ruibal (1990), *Int. J. Biol. Markers* **5,** n. 1, pp. 46,47.

Stahli, C., B. Takacs, V. Miggiano, T. Staehelin, and H. Carman (1985), *Experientia* **41,** 1377–1381.

Stahli, C., M. Caravatti, M. Aeschbacher, C. Kocyba, B. Takacs, and H. Carmann (1988), *Cancer Res.* **48,** 6799–6802.

Steger, G. G., R. Mader, K. Derfler, K. Moser, and C. Dittrich (1989), *Klin. Wochenschr.* **67,** 813–817.

White, C. A., R. Dulbecco, R. Allen, M. Bowman, and B. Armstrong (1985), *Cancer Res.* **45,** 1337–1343.

Zenklusen, H. R., C. Stahli, F. Gudat, J.V. Overbeck, J. Rolink, and Ph.U. Hietz (1988), *Virchows Arch.* [A] **413,** 3–10.

Chapter 16

DU-PAN-2, A Clinically Useful Mucin Marker of Differentiation of Pancreatic and Other Ductal Cells and Their Tumors

Richard S. Metzgar, Norio Sawabu, and Michael A. Hollingsworth

1. The Diagnostic and Therapeutic Challenge of Pancreatic Cancer

There are a number of distinguishing and unique clinical and biological aspects of exocrine pancreatic cancer that make diagnosis difficult. The disease is rarely diagnosed at an early stage. This is the major factor in the poor prognosis of this malignancy. Symptoms, when they occur, are vague and include anorexia, weight loss, abdominal pain, vomiting, nausea, and jaundice. Patients with tumors of the head of the pancreas often have symptoms related to tumor invasion and compression of the common bile duct. Tumor

From: *Serological Cancer Markers* Edited by Stewart Sell ©1992 The Humana Press, Totowa, NJ

involvement in the head of the pancreas is found in 80–90% of patients with exocrine pancreatic tumors. The remaining 10–20% of patients have tumors in the tail of the pancreas and are not likely to have early jaundice because of slight involvement of the biliary duct system.

Routine clinical laboratory testes usually do not distinguish benign from malignant pancreatic disease. Therefore, a variety of both invasive and noninvasive techniques have been applied to facilitate this diagnosis. These methods include computed tomography, ultrasound, angiography, percutaneous needle biopsy and endoscopy. However, even when a definitive diagnosis of pancreatic adenocarcinoma is reached using these methods, the tumor has generally reached a stage at which surgical resection has little effect on the patient's survival. The tumor is also not very responsive to chemotherapy, and radiation is used predominantly as a palliative treatment.

Exocrine pancreatic tumors are predominantly (>80%) of the ductal-cell type and are usually classified ultrastructurally as well-differentiated or moderately well-differentiated. A few are classified as poorly differentiated or undifferentiated. Because the long-term survival rate in this disease is low (approx 5% of patients survive 5 yr with surgical resection), there has been little correlation of disease stage and differentiation grade to survival. A distinguishing histological feature of pancreatic tumors is their marked ability to induce formation of stromal elements in their local environment. This could be a result of the tumor's secretion of growth factors that stimulate fibroblast and connective-tissue growth.

Cellular, molecular, and genetic research on pancreatic tumors has been difficult and relatively slow for several reasons. The tumor exists in an organ that has as one of its major functions the secretion of enzymes that degrade proteins, lipids, carbohydrates, and nucleic acids. The rapid degradation of RNA by *in situ* pancreatic ribonucleases has made molecular genetic studies extremely difficult. In addition to problems with autolytic enzymatic digestion, the predominance of stromal elements in many tumors makes it difficult to obtain adequate quantities of pure populations of tumor cells for reaearch studies. Research on pancreatic tumors is also hampered by the lack of availability of normal pancreatic ductal cells. Although short-term cultures of enriched duct populations have been prepared from animals, including primates, little work has been done on human pancreatic-duct-cell cultures. The most productive research studies have used tissue-culture cell lines derived from pancreatic tumors.

2. Mucins as Tumor Markers of Pancreatic Adenocarcinomas

Pancreatic adenocarcinomas of ductal-cell origin are often characterized by their secretion and release of mucins and other membranous material into tumor ducts. The mucin molecules often enter blood, lymph, and pancreatic secretions, and have been excellent candidates for tumor markers that can be quantified in various body fluids. Retrospective analysis of numerous murine monoclonal antibodies reactive with pancreatic tumors has shown them to be reactive with epitopes on mucin molecules. Some of these antibodies are described in this volume. Since many terminal sugars on mucin oligosaccharide side chains are blood group antigens, some antibodies were reactive with ABO or various forms of the Lewis blood group antigens and will be discussed in Dr. Hakamori's chapter in this volume on carbohydrate epitopes of tumors. As will be discussed later in this review, antibodies to breast-tumor mucins, which are less glycosylated than pancreatic-tumor mucins, often react with peptide epitopes on deglycosylated tumor apomucin. Other monoclonal antibodies, such as DU-PAN-2, detect epitopes that were less well-defined and may be reactive with conformational epitopes that consist of both peptide and carbohydrate determinants. Since mucin molecules demonstrate heterogeneity in their oligosaccharide structure, not all the mucin determinants defined by monoclonal antibodies are present on every mucin molecule. For example, a DU-PAN-2 antibody affinity column (Lan et al., 1987b) was used to demonstrate that some, but not all, molecules expressing the DU-PAN-2 epitope coexpressed the CA 19-9 epitope. Moreover, since the CA 19-9 epitope is a sialylated Lewis A antigen, it was not detected in Lewis A negative donors whose tumors were able to express the DU-PAN-2 epitope (Tempero et al., 1989). We are only now beginning to appreciate the heterogeneity of different mucin molecules and the specificity of their expression in the individual secretory epithelial cells of different organs and tissues. The functional role of mucins is usually lubrication and protection of secretory epithelial cells from the harsh environment of the cavities that they line and form. Thus, it is tempting to speculate that mucin expression on tumor cells may influence the recognition of tumor antigens by the afferent or efferent arm of the immune system. Most studies on the immune response to pancreatic-tumor mucins have been concerned with epitopes recognized by B cells that may have involved T-cell help in generating a humoral response. However, in recent collaborative and independent studies with Dr. Olivera Finn and her colleagues at Duke University, we have obtained evidence that cytotoxic T cells from patients with pancreatic cancer can recognize mucin-peptide epitopes (Barnd et al., 1989; Wahab and Metzgar, 1991). The clinical and biological significance of this finding will be discussed in section 8 of this chapter, which is concerned with future perspectives. However, the data suggest that mucin-peptide epitopes may be recognized by human T cells and that this recognition may be related to the unique amino acid sequence repetition that seems to be characteristic of mucin genes.

3. Molecular and Genetic Characterizations of Pancreatic Mucin

The properties of molecules bearing the DU PAN-2 epitope have been well defined (Lan et al., 1985,1987a,1990a). In summary, the molecule shows all the hallmarks of a mucin. Analysis of amino acid composition showed that the sum of serine, threonine, proline, alanine, and glycine composed >50% of the amino acid residues. Saccharide units were *O*-glycosidically linked to the peptide via GalNAc and contained fucose, galactose, GlcNAc, GalNAc, and sialic acid. The total carbohydrate content by weight was about

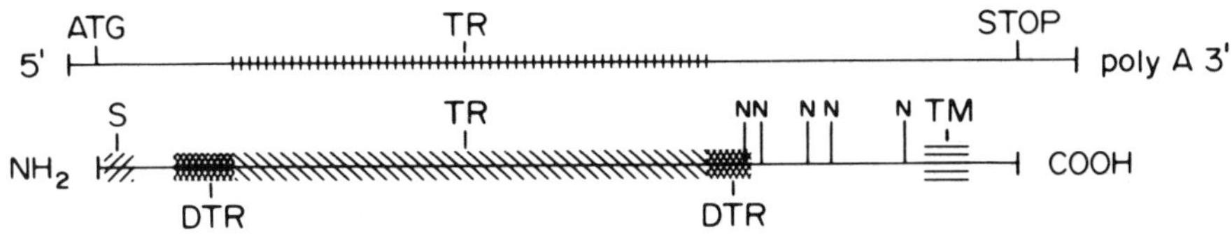

Fig. 1. Molecular structure of a human pancreatic-tumor-mucin gene. A diagram of the cDNA nucleotide sequence is shown at the top. ATG, start codon; TR, tandem repeat; STOP, termination codon. A diagram based on the translated protein sequence is shown at the bottom. S, putative signal peptide; DTR, degenerate tandem repeat; N, putative *N*-glycosylation site; TM, putative transmembrane region.

80%. The total mol wt of the molecule was $>1 \times 10^6$, with some species upward of 5×10^6 dalton, as determined by analytical equilibrium sedimentation. Characterization of the DU-PAN-2 epitope was difficult, since most efforts to fractionate the molecule resulted in loss of the ability of the mucin subunits to bind antibody. However, recent studies by Dr. John Magnani of Biocarb, Inc. (Gaithersburg, MD) using synthetic oligosaccharide-protein conjugates, have shown that the epitope recognized by the DU-PAN-2 antibody was only present on the oligosaccharide LsTa: Neu Ac α 2–3 Gal β 1–3 Glc NAc β 1–3 Gal β 1–4 Glc (Bodmer et al., 1991). This finding confirms a previous report by Khorrami et al. (1989) who reported a similar oligosaccharide structure on purified pancreatic tumor mucin expressing the DU-PAN-2 epitope.

We have recently cloned and sequenced the cDNA for the core protein of the human pancreatic mucin that expressed the DU-PAN-2 epitope (Lan et al., 1990b; Hollingsworth et al., 1990). This was accomplished by screening a λgt11 cDNA library from the HPAF pancreatic-tumor cell line with rabbit and chimpanzee antisera against purified deglycosylated pancreatic-tumor mucin. A schematic diagram of the cDNA sequence and the translated protein sequence is shown in Fig. 1. The cDNA sequence revealed an mRNA with a 72-bp 5' untranslated region and a 307-bp 3' untranslated region, which contained a polyadenylation signal 22 bp to the 5' side of the poly A tail. The total length of the cDNA was just over 4.3 kbp. Over 2500 bp of this sequence consisted of 42 tandemly repeated 60 nt sequence units identical to those previously reported for a human breast mucin cDNA (Gendler et al., 1988; Siddiqui et al., 1988). The predicted amino acid sequence from the mucin cDNA revealed a protein of 126 kDa containing 1295 amino acid residues with 42 tandem repeats. The deduced amino acid composition of the protein was consistent with that expected for mucin, with serine, threonine, proline, alanine, and glycine together constituting over 60% of the residues. Approximately 30% of the predicted protein sequence was outside the tandem repeat.

There were 126 amino acids on the amino-terminal side of the tandem repeats and 329 amino acids on the carboxy-terminal side. Immediately adjoining the tandem repeat sequences on both the amino-terminal and carboxy-terminal sides were sequences with substantial homology to the tandem repeat, which became progressively degenerate from that sequence as one moved away from the tandem repeat in either direction. Although there were similarities, the degeneracy did not follow an identical pattern on both sides of the tandem repeat.

The derived amino acid sequence could represent a membrane-bound molecule, since there was a putative 13 amino acid signal sequence near the amino-terminal end and a 31 amino acid hydrophobic region 69 amino acids from the carboxy terminus. There was an alternative splice site in the mRNA just inside the signal sequence that resulted in the production of proteins with alternative amino termini (Ligtenberg et al., 1990). One laboratory has reported the isolation of a cDNA for a putative secreted form of this mucin from a breast tumor cell line (Williams et al, 1990), which contained an insertion 3' of the tandem repeat that introduced a stop codon into the sequence prior to the putative transmembrane region. However, our laboratory, as well as others working on identical breast-tumor mucins, have not yet detected a cDNA sequence representing a secreted form of mucin. Therefore, the mechanism of secretion or release of the molecule from the cell has not been definitively established.

Two other features of the protein sequence were worth noting. One, there were five potential *N*-linked glycosylation sites between the tandem repeat and the carboxy terminus, one of which occurred near the end of a degenerate repeat sequence. This confirmed previous reports of *N*-linked glycosylation in mucin (Hilkens and Buijs, 1988; Gum et al., 1989; Abe and Kufe, 1989). Two, a very high percentage of the residues outside the tandem repeat were serine and threonine (27%), demonstrating that many potential *O*-linked glycosylation sites exist outside the tandem repeat portion of the molecule.

Previous work in our laboratory demonstrated immunological crossreactivity between lysates of pancreatic and breast tumor cell lines, deglycosylated purified pancreatic mucin, and peptides based on the cloned breast mucin tandem repeat sequence (Lan et al., 1990a). More recent work (Lan et al., 1990b; Gendler et al., 1990; Ligtenberg et al., 1990) has demonstrated >99% homology between this pancreatic mucin cDNA sequence and human breast mucin cDNA sequence. However, these mucins showed no significant homology to a partial cDNA sequence for human intestinal mucin (Gum et al., 1989). The identity between the breast and pancreatic tumor mucin cDNA sequences was somewhat surprising, given the previously described biochemical properties of these molecules. The purified glycosylated breast form of this mucin has consistently been shown to have an M_r in the range of 250–450 kDa, whereas the pancreatic mucin showed a larger M_r of >1000 kDa. The breast mucin was typically 50% carbohydrate by weight (Shimizu and Yamauchi, 1982), whereas the pancreatic mucin was 80% carbohydrate by weight (Lan et al., 1987a). Monoclonal antibodies that recognized peptides corresponding to the breast mucin tandem repeat also reacted with native breast mucin, but did not react with native pancreatic mucin until it was deglycosylated (Lan et al., 1990a). The data indicated that the core peptide for this mucin molecule has been glycosylated in distinct ways by tumors and normal tissues of breast and pancreas. Other unpublished data from our laboratory showed that the mRNA for this mucin was also expressed in epithelial cells found in normal and malignant tracheobronchial tissues. However, pancreatic mucin mRNA was not detected in some poorly differentiated pancreatic tumor cell lines (Lan et al., 1990a). Thus, it appeared that mucin molecules could be expressed in a differentiation-related manner in pancreatic tumors.

One other structural feature of the mucin gene is worth noting. It has been reported that there is a considerable amount of allelic variation in the length of the tandem repeat portion of the mucin gene, to such an extent that this gene may be considered a variable-number-of-tandem-repeat (VNTR) locus (Gendler et al., 1988). This is unusual, since most VNTR loci in humans are not expressed as proteins. A recent study found 30 distinct mucin alleles in 69 individuals (Gendler et al., 1990). VNTR loci are useful genetic markers for chromosome linkage mapping and genetic fingerprinting (Nakamura et al., 1987). In addition, the breast/pancreatic mucin gene has been localized to chromosome 1q21 (Swallow et al., 1987), a region that has been found to be affected by loss of heterozygosity, trisomy, translocation, and other alterations in tumor cells. Thus, further characterization of this mucin gene may improve its diagnostic utility and extend its usefulness beyond applications to cancer.

4. Tissue Distribution and Cellular Localization of the DU-PAN-2 Pancreatic Tumor Mucin

Retrospective analysis of the tissue- and tumor-distribution studies of the DU-PAN-2 antigen that were completed prior to the recent molecular and genetic studies (Borowitz et al., 1984) suggested that the original findings were commensurate with those expected for an epitope of a pancreatic ductal-cell mucin. There was strong expression of the DU-PAN-2 antigen in a significant percentage of glandular epithelia along the pancreatic, biliary, breast, and bronchial duct systems. A lower level of expression of the antigen was noted in a few cells in salivary glands, stomach, colon, and intestine. There was a commensurate quantitative difference in the expression of the DU-PAN-2 epitope on tumors derived from the secretory epithelial cells of these tissues.

Table 1
Detection by Immunohistochemical Analysis of DU-PAN-2 Antigen in Various Cancers of the Digestive Tract

		Intensity of positive reactions[b]				
Tumor	Negative[a]	+	++	+++	Total tested	Incidence (%)
Pancreas	3	4	8	14	29	26/29 (90)
Biliary tract	2	0	2	7	11	9/11 (81)
Papilloma	2	0	0	3	5	3/5 (60)
Gallbladder	1	1	1	1	4	3/4 (75)
Liver (hepatocellular)	3	2	1	2	8	5/8 (63)
Stomach	25	16	7	2	50	25/50 (50)
Colon	14	0	6	6	26	12/26 (46)

[a]Negative = no antigen-positive cells.
[b]+ = approx 10–30% antigen-positive cells; ++ = approx 30–60% antigen-positive cells; +++ = >60% antigen-positive cells.

Preliminary data obtained by Borowitz et al. (1984) demonstrated that DU-PAN-2 antigen was detected in 100% of pancreatic cancers (16/16) and biliary cancer (5/5); among other cancers, the antigen was present in 86% of stomach cancers (18/21), 38% of colon cancers (5/13), 60% of ovarian cancers (9/15), 36% of lung cancers (4/11), and 21% of breast cancers (3/14). The antigen was absent in renal cancers (0/6). A more recent immunohistochemical study, in Japan, of the distribution of DU-PAN-2 antigen in tumors of the gastrointestinal tract reported similar findings, except for a decreased incidence in gastric cancer and reactivity with hepatocellular carcinomas (Satomura et al., 1986, and Table 1).

A comparison of the cellular distribution of a well-defined mucin carbohydrate epitope (sialylated Lewis A, as defined by the CA 19-9 monoclonal antibody) and the DU-PAN-2 epitope by Takasaki et al. (1987) reported a difference in cellular localization.

The DU-PAN-2 epitope was primarily present within the cytoplasm of pancreatic tumors, whereas the CA 19-9 antigen was predominantly present on the luminal surface and in the lumen of the tumor ducts of serial sections. In contrast, Satomura et al. (1991), in a comparative study of 6 sialylated carbohydrate antigens, found no significant differences in the cellular localization and frequency of DU-PAN-2 and on CA 19-9 antigen expression in pancreatic cancer tissues.

5. Relationship of DU-PAN-2 Mucin Expression to Staging and Grading of Pancreatic Adenocarcinomas

Several systems for staging pancreatic adenocarcinomas according to local disease, regional lymphatic involvement, and distant metastases have been proposed. Although survival times are influenced by staging, the difference between the mean survival time of stage I patients with local disease and stage III patients with distant metastases was only 9 mo (Kloppel and Fitzgerald, 1986). DU-PAN-2 can be expressed in primary pancreatic tumors and distant metastases, although there is considerable heterogeneity in the percentage of tumor cells stained upon immunohistological examination. Some of the heterogeneity is likely attributable to tumor grade. A system to grade exocrine pancreatic tumors into three categories of differentiation was primarily described (Kloppel and Fitzgerald, 1986) based on histological observations of glandular differentiation, nuclear size, anaplasia, and mitotic activity. The same grading system was applied by Kern et al. (1986) at the ultrastructural level. DU-PAN-2 antigen is expressed in pancreatic tumors of all three grades, although poorly differentiated and anaplastic tumors are noted to express a lower percentage of antigen-positive cells (Borowitz et al., 1984; Takasaki et al., 1987). The serum DU-PAN-2 levels of patients with tumors at different stages and grades of differentiation will be discussed in a subsequent section.

The relationship of mucin antigen expression to differentiation was clarified by in vitro studies of DU-PAN-2 antigen expression in several pancreatic tumor cell lines and clones (Kim et al., 1989; Metzgar et al., 1989). When a panel of these cell lines was tested with the DU-PAN-2 antibody by immunoperoxidase and immunofluorescence, some of the lines failed to express DU-PAN-2 and apomucin-peptide epitopes (Lan and Metzgar 1989; Lan et al., 1990a). The antigen-negative lines were derived from tumors that were originally classified as poorly differentiated and that formed undifferentiated or poorly differentiated xenografts in nude mice. Because there was also heterogeneity in DU-PAN-2 and mucin expression, as well as morphologic and ultrastructural heterogeneity in some of the moderately differentiated pancreatic tumor lines, such as HPAF, we cloned the HPAF line and studied some of the clones (Kim et al., 1989; Metzgar et al., 1989). This was the first reported cloning of a human pancreatic tumor cell line. Phenotypic analysis of the clones using a panel of murine monoclonal antibodies, some of which were reactive with mucin, demonstrated distinct profiles of antigen expression. Two clones, CD11 and CD18, which had distinct antigenic, morphologic, and ultrastructural characteristics, were selected for further study. CD11 cells demonstrated many of the characteristics of a well-differentiated state, including the formation of ductal structures with polarized, long, columnar-shaped cells; the presence of cytoplasmic secretory granules; and high levels of DU-PAN-2 antigen expression in nude-mouse xenografts. In contrast, CD18 cells exhibited characteristics of a poorly differentated state, including the formation of nests of isoprismatic cells without luminal spaces and lacking polarization. DU-PAN-2 antigen expression was absent or low in CD18 cells. Treatment of the poorly differentiated CD18 cells with sodium butyrate caused phenotypic, morphologic, and ultrastructural alterations that resulted in cells that resembled untreated well-differentiated CD11 cells. This included increased DU-PAN-2 mucin expression (Mullins et al., 1991). Recent unpublished studies of another poorly differentiated pancreatic tumor line, HS766T, not derived from HPAF cells, indicated that mucin mRNA was highly expressed after sodium butyrate treatment compared to pretreatment levels. These data indicate that mucin antigen and gene expression is absent or very low in poorly differentiated or undifferentiated cell types of pancreatic adenocarcinomas, but is highly expressed in well-differentiated cell types. However, there can be considerable heterogeneity in this expression within an individual tumor.

6. Clinical Studies on DU-PAN-2 Antigen Levels in Body Fluids of Patients with Benign and Malignant Disease

Because mucins are secreted and shed from many types of normal and malignant secretory epithelial cells, they have been intensively studied as serum tumor markers. Two methods have been employed, using the DU-PAN-2 monoclonal antibody to measure antigen in body fluids. A competition radioimmune assay (RIA) was developed by Metzgar et al. (1984) and a double determinant enzyme-linked immunoassay (ELISA) by Kyowa Medex, Ltd., Tokyo, Japan. Both assays gave remarkably similar results when standard antigen curves were compared, hence the arbitrary units in each assay were comparable and interchangeable. In the normal population the serum concentration of DU-PAN-2 antigen is <100 U/mL in >90% of the samples studied. When the population included a variety of benign disorders, a concentration of 100 U/mL was more frequently observed. Therefore, different arbitrary cutoff values between normal and abnormal levels have been used. A value of 300 or 400 U/mL has usually been selected, although 150 U/mL has been used for screening purposes.

DU-PAN-2 serum studies of patients with benign and malignant disease in the United States were summarized in a previous review (Hollingsworth and Metzgar, 1985). Independent serum DU-PAN-2 studies in Japan, correlated at Kanazawa University, using an ELISA assay and a 400 U/mL cutoff, gave similar results for patients with benign and malignant diseases (Figs. 2 and 3).

A different Japanese survey of serum DU-PAN-2 levels (Cho et al., 1986) applied the 400 U/mL cutoff and obtained the following results: 61% positive cases in 54 pancreatic cancer patients, 44% positive cases among 19 patients with cancer of the biliary

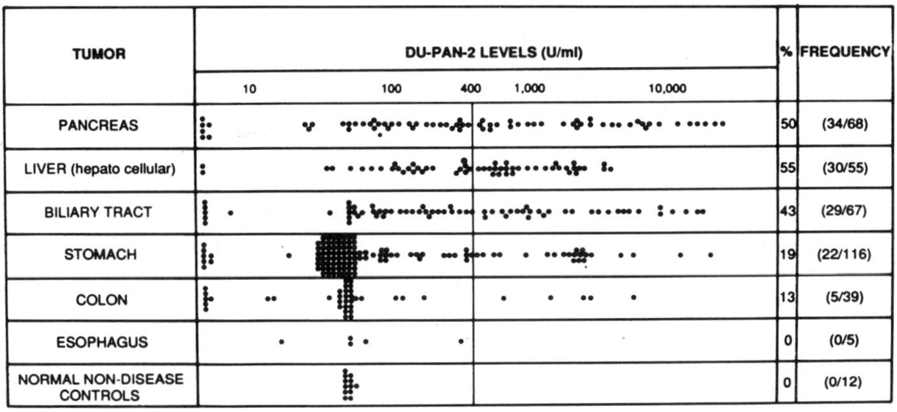

Fig. 2. Serum DU-PAN-2 levels of patients with malignant disease. Each solid dot represents the DU-PAN-2 level of a single sample, determined by a double-determinant EIA method with a 400 U/mL cutoff level, designated by a vertical line. Data provided by N. Sawabu from Takemori et al., 1987.

tract, and 44% positive cases in 23 patients with hepatocellular carcinoma. A cutoff level of 300 U/mL of DU-PAN-2 antigen was used by Ichihara et al., 1986a,b, who observed that serum from 54% of 65 pancreatic cancer patients, 47% of 15 patients with cancer of the biliary tract, and 44% of 32 patients with hepatocellular carcinoma had serum levels >300 U/mL.

When comparisons were made between serum levels of DU-PAN-2 and antigen expression in the tumor, some pancreatic cancer patients had significant DU-PAN-2 expression in the tumor, but had serum values <300 or 400 U/mL (Takasaki et al., 1988; Suzuki et al., 1988). When similar studies were carried out on hepatocellular carcinoma patients, a number of patients were identified that had elevated serum DU-PAN-2 levels but no antigen expression in tumor cells (Satomura et al., 1986; Haviland et al., 1988). These hepatocellular carcinoma patients with DU-PAN-2 antigen negative tumors often had numerous hyperplastic hepatic ductal cells in areas surrounding the tumor, which stained intensely for DU-PAN-

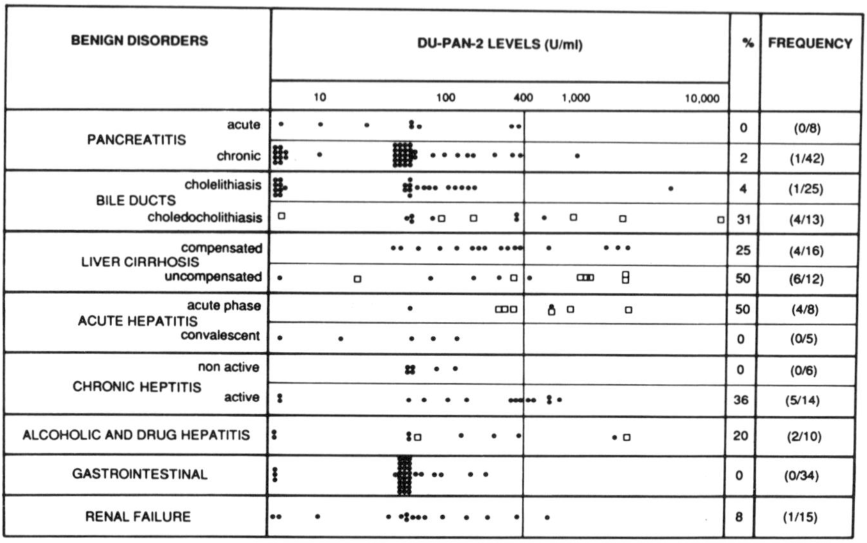

Fig. 3. Serum DU-PAN-2 levels of patients with various benign disorders. Each solid dot represents the DU-PAN-2 level of a sample of a patient without jaundice. Open squares represent samples from patients with jaundice. DU-PAN-2 units were determined by a double-determinant EIA method with a 400 U/mL cutoff level, designated by a vertical line. Data provided by N. Sawabu from Takemori et al., 1987.

2 by immunoperoxidase testing. Thus, these hyperplastic, nonmalignant DU-PAN-2-positive hepatic-duct cells may be contributing to the serum DU-PAN-2 antigen pool. Clearly, impaired liver function as a result of either malignant or benign disease could also increase serum DU-PAN-2 levels as a consequence of a generalized decreased catabolism of serum glycoproteins. Although there has been no direct examination of the mechanism by which tumor mucin and normal mucin reaches the circulation, there is indirect evidence that some mucin arrives from lymph. Immunohistological examination of DU-PAN-2 antigen expression in tumor-negative regional lymph nodes of pancreatic cancer patients and patients with benign hepatobiliary diseases indicated significant staining for the DU-PAN-2 mucin. This type of staining was not seen in normal

lymph nodes from these regional sites from patients with non-GI-tract diseases (unpublished data).

There have been a number of studies comparing serum and tissue DU-PAN-2 levels with another tumor mucin epitope, CA 19-9. Both of these epitopes can be expressed on the same mucin molecule. However, mucin from some donors may express one epitope and not the other. A comparative study by Ichihara et al. (1986a,b), examined the serum levels of CA 19-9 and DU-PAN-2 antigens in 61 pancreatic cancer patients and also studied expression of these epitopes in tumor tissue of 22 of these patients. DU-PAN-2 serum levels were elevated above a 150 U/mL cutoff level in 67% of the 61 samples studied, and CA 19-9 was elevated in 72% of these sera (Fig. 4). The six patients who were Lewis A negative all had elevated levels of DU-PAN-2. In a larger serum study of 168 cases of pancreatic cancer coordinated by the Kyowa Medex Company, similar results were obtained, with 75% of the patients having elevated DU-PAN-2 levels and 80% having elevated CA 19-9. The combination of the two serum assays increased the sensitivity to 91% with an *r* value of 0.0116. Other serum studies of pancreatic cancer patients comparing these two tumor markers gave *r* values between 0.01 and 0.2. In tumor tissue, CA 19-9 was expressed in 17 of 22 (77%) specimens. The five negative cases included three patients with Le(a–b–), one with Le(a+b–), and one with Le(a–b+) phenotypes. DU-PAN-2 antigen was expressed in 20 of 22 (91%) cancer tissues. The two DU-PAN-2-negative cases were CA 19-9-positive. In 19 of 21 (90%) cases, the serum CA 19-9 level correlated to the expression of the antigen in the cancer tissue. Discrepancy was seen in two cases: One patient had an elevated level of CA 19-9 in the serum, but lacked this antigen in the cancer cells. In the second patient, the situation was reversed. For DU-PAN-2, positive serum and tumor correlation was seen in 14 of 21 (67%) cases. Six of seven patients with low DU-PAN-2 levels expressed the antigen in their tumor cells, and one patient with DU-PAN-2-negative cancer tissue had an elevated level of this marker in the serum. The serum levels of these antigens, however, were likely the consequences of multiple factors, only one of which was

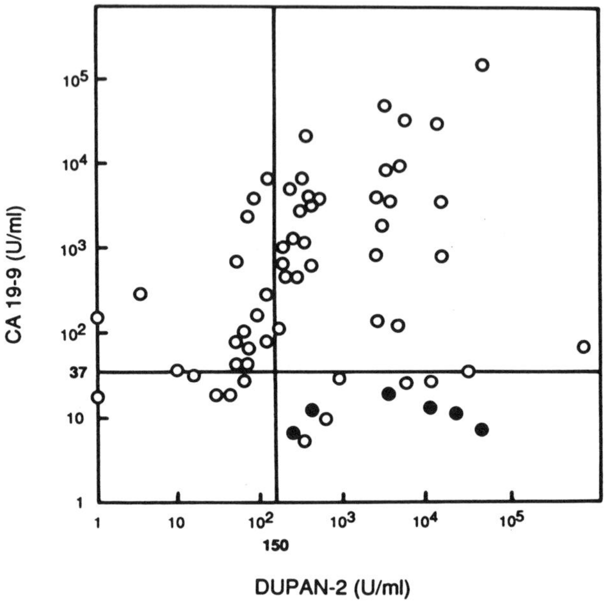

Fig. 4. Correlation of serum levels of DU-PAN-2 and CA 19-9 markers in pancreatic cancer patients. Open circles represent the serum DU-PAN-2 and CA 19-9 levels of a single sample from patients expressing the Lewis[a] antigen. Closed circles are values from patients that are Lewis[a] negative. The DU-PAN-2 and CA 19-9 levels were determined by double-determinant EIA methods with a 150 U/mL cutoff level for DU-PAN-2 and 37 U/mL cutoff level for CA 19-9. Data provided by N. Sawabu from Ichihara et al., 1987a.

the qualitative and quantitative expression of the antigens in tumors. The general conclusion from this and other combination tumor-marker studies is that whenever two or more parameters are used, the sensitivity of detection is usually improved, but the specificity is often decreased.

The use of serum DU-PAN-2 and other mucin epitopes has thus not markedly facilitated early tumor diagnosis because of a lack of tumor specificity of these epitopes, along with other factors related to their physiology. Nevertheless, DU-PAN-2 and other pancreatic mucin epitopes have been useful and accurate indicators of therapeutic effectiveness. Mahvi et al. (1985) reported serial studies of DU-PAN-2 serum antigen levels in six pancreatic cancer patients after surgical resection of their tumors. Elevated DU-PAN-2 levels in five of these patient's sera returned to a normal range within 1–3 wk postsurgery. This study also demonstrated that some pancreatic cancer patients receiving chemotherapy and radiation therapy exhibited posttreatment serum DU-PAN-2 levels in the normal range and that serum levels increased rapidly when progressive recurrent disease was noted. Takami et al. (1987) and Suzuki et al. (1988) also measured serial serum levels of DU-PAN-2 antigen before and after surgical treatment of pancreatic cancer. These investigators demonstrated that among those patients who were incorrectly thought to have curative resection, the serum DU-PAN-2 levels returned to normal levels, but again became elevated and predicted recurrence of the tumor several months before death. After most noncurative resections, the serum marker did not return to normal.

7. Future Clinical Perspectives on the Use of DU-PAN-2 and Other Mucin Markers

Efforts to improve specificity and thereby facilitate diagnosis by production of second-generation monoclonal antibodies to antigens purified with a primary murine monoclonal antibody have not as yet resulted in vastly improved reagents. When immunizations were done with native mucins, many of the new antibodies were directed to immunodominant terminal oligosaccharides that had already been defined by other antibodies. However, antibodies with other isotypes were sometimes obtained, and some had better binding characteristics than the original antibody. Currently, many laboratories are making and evaluating monoclonal and polyclonal antibodies to natural and synthetic tumor mucin peptides. Interest in mucin-peptide epitopes increased when an antibody, SM3, elicited to deglycosylated breast-tumor mucin reacted strongly with breast-tumor mucin and was weakly reactive or unreactive with normal breast mucin (Burchell et al., 1987). The explanation (with some confirmatory evidence) for the improved specificity of the SM3 antibody was that normal breast mucins are more heavily glycosylated than breast-tumor mucins. Therefore the SM3 epitope was probably masked by carbohydrates on the normal mucin. Thus far, other antibodies to deglycosylated mucin or to synthetic mucin peptides have not improved tumor diagnosis. However, most of these studies are still in progress, and comprehensive studies with different mucin peptides have not been fully evaluated.

Most clinical studies with antibodies to mucin-peptide epitopes to date have been immunohistological. Serological assays for mucin peptides in body fluids are currently being developed and evaluated with antibodies to different apomucin epitopes. Some tumors or benign secretory epithelial diseases of cells that are not high mucin secretors could still result in shed or released mucin precursors that have reactive peptide epitopes. In addition to serum, urine may be assayed and provide different information on the catabolism of these molecules.

Mucins and mucin peptides have recently been implicated as target antigens, for cytotoxic T cells with specificity for pancreatic tumors were generated by in vitro stimulation with pancreatic tumor cells (Barnd et al., 1989). Therefore, active immunotherapy is being considered as an alternative to passive antibody or cellular therapy to elicit *in situ* immune responses to tumor antigens in this and other malignant diseases. The tandem repeat segment of the pancreatic and breast mucin gene, which codes for >50% of the apomucin peptide, is highly immunogenic, both in the glycosylated and in the nonglycosylated state. The repeating oligosaccharide units of the native mucin apparently are good stimulators of allogeneic B-cell responses, whereas the repeating peptide units of the apomucin may activate autologous cytotoxic T cells.

References

Abe, M. and D. Kufe (1989), *Cancer Res.* **49,** 2834–2839.

Barnd, D., M. Lan, R. Metzgar, and O. Finn (1989), *Proc. Natl. Acad. Sci. USA* **86,** 7159–7163.

Borowitz, M., F. Tuck, W. Sindelar, P. Fernsten, and R. Metzgar (1984), *J. Natl. Cancer Inst.* **72,** 999–1005.

Burchell, J., S. Gendler, J. Taylor-Papadimitriou, A. Girling, A. Lewis, R. Millis, and D. Lamport (1987), *Cancer Res.* **47,** 5476–5482.

Cho, M., S. Watanabe, and T. Takeuchi (1986), *J. Jpn. Panc. Soc.* **1,** 69 (in Japanese).

Gendler, S., J. Taylor-Papadimitriou, T. Duhig, J. Rothbard, and J. Burchell (1988), *J. Biol. Chem.* **263,** 12820–12823.

Gendler, S., C. Lancaster, J. Taylor-Papadimitriou, T. Duhig, N. Peat, J. Burchell, L. Pemberton, E.M. Lelani, and D. Wilson (1990), *J. Biol. Chem.* **265,** 15286–15293.

Gum, J., J. Byrd, J. Hicks, N. Toribara, D. Lamport, and Y. Kim (1989), *J. Biol. Chem.* **264,** 6480–6487.

Haviland, A., M. Borowitz, P. Killenberg, M. Lan, and R. Metzgar (1988), *Int. J. Cancer* **41,** 789–793.

Hilkens, J. and F. Buijs (1988), *J. Biol. Chem.* **263,** 4215–4222.

Hollingsworth, M. and R. Metzgar (1985), in *Monoclonal Antibodies in Cancer,* Humana, Clifton, NJ, pp. 279–307.

Hollingsworth, M., M. Lan, S. Batra, W.N. Qi, T. Mullins, and R. Metzgar (1990), *Proc. Am. Assoc. Cancer Res.* **31,** 482–484.

Ichihara, T., A. Nakao, Y. Suzuki, N. Suzuki, T. Nonami, A. Harada, H. Takagi, and H. Nagura (1987a), *J. Jpn. Panc. Soc.* **2,** 439–449 (in Japanese).

Ichihara, T., A. Nakao, J. Sakamoto, Y. Suzuki, T. Nonami, A. Harada, T. Watanabe, H. Takagi, and H. Nagura (1987b), *J. Jpn. Panc. Soc.* **2,** 460–471 (in Japanese).

Kern, H., U. Rausch, and J. Mollenhauer (1986), in *The Exocrine Pancreas: Biology, Pathobiology and Diseases* (Go, V.L., ed.), Raven, New York, pp. 637–647.

Khorrami, A., M. Lan, R. Metzgar, and B. Kaufman (1989), *Glycoconjugate J.* **6,** 428 (Abstract).

Kim, Y., H. Kern, T. Mullins, M. Koriwchak, and R. Metzgar (1989), *Pancreas* **4,** 353–362.

Kloppel, G. and P. Fitzgerald (1986), in *The Exocrine Pancreas: Biology, Pathobiology and Diseases* (Go, V. L., ed.), Raven, NY, pp. 649–674.

Lan, M., M. Hollingsworth, and R. Metzgar (1990a), *Cancer Res.* **50,** 2997–3001.

Lan, M., S. Batra, W.N. Qi, R. Metzgar, and M. Hollingsworth (1990b), *J. Biol. Chem.* **265,** 15294–15299.

Lan, M., O. Finn, P. Fernsten, and R. Metzgar (1985), *Cancer Res.* **45,** 305–310.

Lan, M., A. Khorrami, B. Kaufman, and R. Metzgar (1987a), *J. Biol. Chem.* **262,** 12863–12870.

Lan, M., R. Bast, M. Colnaghi, R. Knapp, D. Colcher, and R. Metzgar (1987b), *Int. J. Cancer* **39,** 68–72.

Lan, M. and R. Metzgar (1989), in *Human Tumor Antigens and Specific Tumor Therapy,* Liss, New York, pp. 1–11.

Ligtenberg, M. J., H. Vos, A. M. Gennissen, and J. Hilkens (1990), *J. Biochem.* **265,** 5573–5578.

Mahvi, D., W. Meyers, R. Bast, H. Seigler, and R. Metzgar (1985), *Ann. Surgery* **202,** 440–445.

Metzgar, R., M. Lan, Y. Kim, M. Koriwchak, T. Mullins, and M. Hollingsworth (1989), in *Immunity to Cancer II* (Alan R. Liss, New York), pp. 53–61.

Metzgar, R., N. Rodriguez, O. Finn, M. Lan, V. Daasch, P. Fernsten, W. Meyers, W. Sindelar, R. Sandler, and H. Seigler (1984), *Proc. Natl. Acad. Sci. USA* **81,** 5242–5246.

Mullins, T., H. Kern, and R. Metzgar (1991), *Pancreas,* in press.

Nakamura, Y., M. Leppert, P. O'Connell, R. Wolff, T. Holm, M. Culver, C. Martin, E. Fujimoto, M. Hoff, E. Kumlin, and R. White (1987), *Science* **235,** 1616–1622.

Satomura, Y., H. Ohta, Y. Takemori, N. Sawabu, S. Minami, T. Kitamura, M. Mai, N. Hattori, T. Akiyama, and K. Watanabe (1986), *J. Clin. Exp. Med. (Igaku No Ayumi),* **137,** 143 (in Japanese).

Satomura, Y., N. Sawabu, Y. Takamori, H. Ohta, H. Watanabe, T. Okai, K. Watanabe, H. Matsuno, and F. Konishi (1991), *Pancreas* (in press).

Shimizu, M. and K. Yamauchi (1982), *J. Biochem.* **91,** 515–524.

Siddiqui, J., M. Abe, D. Hayes, E. Shami, E. Yumis, and D. Kufe (1988), *Proc. Natl. Acad. Sci. USA* **85,** 2320–2323.

Suzuki, Y., T. Ichihara, A. Nakao, J. Sakamoto, H. Takagi, and H. Nagura (1988), *Hepatogastroenterology* **35,** 128.

Swallow, D., S. Gendler, B. Griffiths, A. Kearney, S. Povey, D. Sheer, R. Palmer, and J. Taylor-Papadimitriou (1987), *Ann. Hum. Genet.* **51,** 289–294.

Takami, H., T. Furuchi, Y. Ogata, and O. Abe (1986), *Jpn. J. Cancer Chem.* **13,** 3207–3214 (in Japanese).

Takasaki, H., E. Uchida, M. Tempero, D. Burnett, R. Metzgar, and P. Pour (1987), *Int. J. Pancreatol.* **2,** 349–361.

Takasaki, H., E. Uchida, M. Tempero, D. Burnett, R. Metzgar, and P. Pour (1988), *Cancer Res.* **48,** 1435–1438.

Takemori, Y., N. Sawabu, Y. Satomura, H. Ohta, H. Watanabe, T. Okai, M. Mai, N. Hattori, T. Akiyama, and T. Hashimoto (1987), *Jpn. J. Cancer Chem.* **14,** 119–126 (in Japanese).

Tempero, M., H. Takasaki, E. Uchida, Y. Takiyama, D. Colcher, R. Metzgar, and P. Pour (1989), *Am. J. Surg. Pathol.* **13,** 89–95.

Wahab, Z., and R. Metzgar (1991), *Pancreas* **6,** 307–317.

Williams, C. S., D. H. Wieschner, A. Tanaka, I. Tsarfary, I. Keydar, and S. Pian (1990), *Biochem. Biophys. Res. Commun.* **170,** 1331–1338.

Chapter 17

CA 50

Caj Haglund, Pentti Kuusela, Peter J. Roberts, and Hannu Jalanko

1. Biochemistry and Biology

1.1. The CA 50 Epitope

The CA 50 antigen is defined by the monoclonal antibody C 50 (IgM) obtained by immunization of mice with the human colonic adenocarcinoma cell line COLO 205 (Lindholm et al., 1983). The C 50 antibody reacts with an epitope present on two carbohydrate moieties, sialosylfucosyllactotetraose (IV^3NeuAc,III^4Fuc-$LcOse_4$) (Månsson et al., 1985), corresponding to sialylated Lewis[a] blood group antigen, and sialosyllactotetraose (IV^3 NeuAc-$LcOse_4$), lacking the fucose molecule of the sialylated Lewis[a] structure (Nilsson et al., 1985). The CA 50 antigen occurs mainly on glycoproteins in serum and in tissues also as gangliosides (Nilsson et al., 1983,1985). Normally, sialylated Lewis[a] is the dominant CA 50 ganglioside in epithelial carcinomas (Månsson et al., 1985). Sialosyllactotetraose has been found in small amounts in various carcinomas (Nilsson et al., 1983, 1985), but, determined by a solid-phase assay, the reactivity of the C 50 antibody for sialosyllactotetraose is

From: *Serological Cancer Markers* Edited by Stewart Sell ©1992 The Humana Press, Totowa, NJ

one-tenth of that for sialylated Lewis[a] (Nilsson et al., 1985). Sialylated Lewis[a] is also the antigenic epitope in another tumor marker test, the CA 19-9 assay, based on the monoclonal antibody 1116 NS 19-9 (Koprowski et al., 1979; Magnani et al., 1982).

The metabolism and excretion of the CA 50 antigen have not been clarified in detail. Many tumor markers, including CA 50, appear in serum as glycoproteins. It is known that circulating glycoprotein levels are largely regulated by the liver (Ashwell and Harford, 1982). The elevated serum levels of CA 50 observed in many patients with extrahepatic cholestasis and benign liver diseases *(see* later discussion) suggest a clearance of CA 50 by the liver.

2. Tissue Expression of CA 50

2.1. Expression in Normal Tissues

The CA 50 antigen has been detected in tissue extracts from various gastrointestinal and nongastrointestinal epithelial tumors: pancreatic, colorectal, gastric, gallbladder, lung, urinary bladder, liver cell, breast, and cervical carcinomas. The antigen is also expressed in meconium and in normal adult pancreas, and probably in gallbladder and gastric mucosa, but has not been found in nonepithelial tumors (Nilsson et al., 1983).

The knowledge on the immunohistochemical expression of CA 50 is limited. In normal pancreatic tissue, the antigen is expressed in the apical border of ductal cells "predominantly of small terminal ducts," but focally also in large ducts, and in centroacinar cells (Haglund et al., 1986; Schwenk and Makovitzky, 1989). Acinar cells and Langerhans' islets are always negative. CA 50 is frequently expressed in normal colorectal mucosa (Ouyang et al., 1987; Enblad et al., 1988). In some specimens, more than half of the epithelial cells stain, whereas other specimens show positivity of only a few cells or are totally negative. The staining pattern is both cytoplasmic and luminal.

2.2. Tissue Expression in Benign Disorders

The staining pattern for CA 50 in chronic pancreatitis is similar to that of normal pancreas (Haglund et al., 1986; Schwenk and Makovitzky, 1989). In specimens of acute pancreatitis the staining is more intense than in normal pancreas (Haglund et al., 1986). Mucinous cystadenomas stain strongly for CA 50, whereas in serous cystadenomas only focal staining of some cells is seen. In most colonic adenomas, epithelial cells stain for CA 50 (Ouyang et al., 1987; Enblad et al., 1988). The staining pattern is heterogenous like in normal mucosa, but adenomas are more extensively stained (Enblad et al., 1988). An extensive staining of CA 50 is seen also in inflammatory bowel disease (Frykholm et al., 1987). There is no difference between ulcerative colitis and Crohn's disease. No correlation between disease duration and CA 50 expression has been found.

2.3. Tissue Expression in Malignant Lesions

Immunohistochemically, CA 50 is expressed in most pancreatic carcinomas, and the expression correlates with the degree of differentiation, being strongest in well-differentiated carcinomas (Haglund et al., 1986). In well-differentiated tumors, predominantly, the brush border and mucus is stained, whereas the staining pattern in moderately and poorly differentiated carcinomas is mainly cytoplasmic (Haglund et al., 1986; Schwenk and Makovitzky, 1989). There is no correlation between the histological expression and the serum levels of the CA 50 antigen, and many tissue-positive carcinomas are associated with a normal or only slightly elevated serum level (Haglund et al., 1986).

Most colorectal carcinomas express CA 50 (Enblad et al., 1987; Ouyang et al., 1987). A pronounced inter- and intratumoral heterogeneity has been described. The staining pattern does not correlate with Dukes' stage or degree of differentiation (Enblad et al., 1987).

CA 50 is expressed in normal pancreatic and colonic epithelium and in benign lesions of these organs, and there is no clear difference in staining pattern against carcinomas. Therefore, immunohistohemical staining for CA 50 cannot be used to distinguish between benign and malignant lesions.

3. Expression of CA 50 in Serum

3.1. The CA 50 Assay

The concentration of CA 50 can be determined in serum by immunological methods. Originally, an inhibition test was described (Holmgren et al., 1984). Later, immunoradiometric (IRMA) and DELFIA assays have been developed (Lindholm et al., 1985; Pharmacia, Gothenburg and Uppsala, Sweden). The correlation between the three tests is high (Kuusela et al., 1987; Masson et al., 1988). Cut-off values of 17 U/mL, 20 U/mL and 14 U/mL, respectively, have been recommended, by the manufacturer.

Masson et al. (1988) compared the three CA 50 methods in the differential diagnosis between pancreatic cancer and chronic pancreatitis. The inhibition test showed a slightly better discrimination, whereas the IRMA and DELFIA methods were easier to perform and had better analytic ranges. In our material, the IRMA method had better diagnostic accuracy than the inhibition test (Haglund et al., 1987).

3.2. CA 50 in Serum of Healthy Individuals

The CA 50 concentration is low in serum of healthy individuals (Holmgren et al., 1984; Paganuzzi et al., 1985; Chan et al., 1985; Habib et al., 1986). The abovementioned cut-off levels for the serum assays represent the mean +2 SD levels of healthy blood donors.

3.3. CA 50 in Serum of Patients with Benign Diseases

Using the recommended cut-off values, slightly to moderately increased serum concentrations of CA 50 have been found in patients with benign pancreatic (12–46%), biliary (35–38%), and liver diseases (22–59%) (Chan et al., 1985; Jalanko et al., 1985; Blind and Dahlgren, 1987; Haglund et al., 1987; Masson et al., 1988; Paganuzzi et al., 1988). In our material, the highest values in benign diseases were found in patients with extrahepatic cholestasis, half of which had elevated values. Particularly high levels are seen in patients with cholangitis (unpublished data). Elevated CA 50 values are less frequently seen in patients with hepatocellular jaundice, and the serum levels are usually lower (Haglund et al., 1987). The elevation of the CA 50 levels in extrahepatic cholestasis is probably due to impaired excretion in the bile (*see* earlier discussion). The elevation of the serum CA 50 level in patients with benign pancreatic diseases is usually slight and more often seen in acute than in chronic pancreatitis.

Increased serum CA 50 concentrations are more seldom seen in benign gastric (14%) or colorectal diseases (5–6%) (Kuusela et al., 1987; Persson et al., 1988). Elevated levels have also been reported in benign breast diseases, like fibrocystic disease (8–10%) (Paganuzzi et al., 1985; Habib et al., 1989), prostatic hyperplasia (15–17%) (Strømme et al., 1986; Lewenhaupt et al., 1990), benign lung diseases, like pneumonia (18–33%) (Paganuzzi et al., 1985; Marechal et al., 1988), and in some patients with benign gynaecological diseases.

3.4 CA 50 in Serum of Patients with Malignant Diseases

3.4.1. CA 50 in Pancreatic Cancer

The highest serum concentrations of CA 50 and the highest frequency of elevated values are seen in patients with pancreatic cancer. In several studies very high sensitivities of the CA 50 test for pancreatic cancer have been reported (81–97%). Many of these results have been based on small numbers of patients (Blind and Dahlgren, 1987; Benini et al., 1988; Masson et al., 1988; Paganuzzi et al., 1988; Habib et al. 1989), but Cooper et al. (1988) reported a 95% sensitivity in 58 patients (>14 U/mL), and Harmenberg et al. (1988) an 81% sensitivity, although in that study a cut-off value of 100 U/mL was used. In our own studies, lower sensitivities of the CA 50 assays have been obtained. Using the inhibition test, Jalanko et al. (1985) demonstrated elevated CA 50 levels in 58% of patients with pancreatic cancer. In a later study on 95 patients with pancreatic cancer, the serum CA 50 concentration was above 17 U/mL in 71% as quantitated by the IRMA assay (Haglund et al., 1987). High levels were particularly found in patients with advanced disease, but also half of the patients with a resectable pancreatic tumor had an elevated value. There was no difference in the proportion of elevated values between patients with well to moderately differentiated adenocarcinomas and those with poorly differentiated or anaplastic carcinomas (Haglund et al., 1987). In a few patients studied, the CA 50 concentration in serum predicted a recurrence after surgery for cure (Haglund et al., 1987).

As mentioned earlier, benign biliary diseases cause an increase of the CA 50 concentration in serum. In patients with pancreatic cancer, most of whom are jaundiced, obstruction of the common bile duct apparently contributes to the elevation of the CA 50 level. Patients with extrahepatic jaundice and a slightly or moderately elevated CA 50 level create a problem in differential diagnosis between benign and malignant diseases. In these patients, the clinicians have to use a higher cut-off level, when interpreting an elevated CA 50 value.

3.4.2. CA 50 in Colorectal Cancer

Elevated CA 50 serum levels are seen in 13–22% of primary Dukes A, in 19–43% of Dukes B, 30–59% of Dukes C, and 53–73% of Dukes D colorectal carcinomas (Kuusela et al., 1987; Persson et al., 1988; Ståhle et al., 1988a; Habib et al., 1989). Ståhle at al. (1988a) found no difference in mean serum levels between

Stages A, B, and C. Patients with metastazised disease had significantly higher serum levels of CA 50. Patients with a low preoperative serum concentration have a better prognosis than patients with an elevated CA 50 level (Ståhle et al., 1988b). An elevated CA 50 value predicted cancer mortality during the first two years postoperatively (Ståhle et al., 1989).

A rise in the CA 50 level may indicate recurrence many months prior to clinical signs or symptoms (Persson et al., 1988). By the time of clinical detection of the recurrence, 49–66% of the patients show an elevated CA 50 level (Kuusela et al., 1987; Persson et al., 1988). According to our experience, only a few patients with recurrent colorectal cancer had an elevated CA 50 level, but a normal CEA, at the time of detection of recurrence (Kuusela et al., 1987).

3.4.3. CA 50 in Other DigestiveTract Carcinomas

High frequencies of elevated CA 50 values have been reported also for other digestive tract carcinomas, e.g., esophageal (41–71%). gastric (41–78%), hepatocellular (14–78%), and biliary (58–70%) carcinomas (Bruhn et al., 1985; Chan et al., 1985; Kuusela et al., 1987; Cooper et al., 1988; Munck-Wikland et al., 1988; Habib et al., 1989). However, most studies have been based on small numbers of patients, including mainly patients with advanced disease. Chan et al. (1985) reported a large material of 153 hepatocellular carcinomas from Singapore, which is an area of high incidence. In this study, 78% of all patients had an elevated CA 50 level. CA 50 was equally often elevated in alpha-fetoprotein positive and negative patients. Elevated CA 50 values were associated with a poor prognosis of the patient. A possible utility of CA 50 as a complement to alpha-fetoprotein in the diagnosis of hepatocellular carcinoma needs to be further studied.

3.4.4. CA 50 in Other Malignancies

Elevated serum levels have also been found in some patients with breast (27–48%) (Rasmuson et al., 1987; Cooper et al., 1988, Habib et al., 1989), lung (34–47%) (Bruhn et al., 1985; Cooper et al., 1988, Marechal et al., 1988), renal (47%) (Habib et al., 1989), prostatic (19–28%) (Strømme et al., 1986; Lewenhaupt et al., 1990), bladder (62%) (Habib et al., 1989), and ovarian cancer (52%) (Pledger et al., 1988), mainly in patients with advanced disease. Useful clinical applications have not been shown in these studies.

3.5. Comparison with Other Tumor Markers

The CA 50 antigen is closely related to the CA 19-9 antigen. Both the C 50 and the 19-9 antibody react with the sialylated Lewis^{a} determinant. In addition, the C 50 antibody reacts with sialosyllactotetraose, but the reactivity is much weaker than for sialylated Lewis^{a}, and the expression of sialosyllactotetraose in various carcinomas is apparently rather weak. Originally, the broader reactivity of the C 50 antibody was thought to be an advantage in Lewis negative subjects, who normally do not express sialylated Lewis^{a}, but may synthesize sialosyllactotetraose (Nilsson et al., 1985). However, Masson et al. (1990) recently showed that there was no difference in the plasma levels of CA 50 and CA 19-9 between individuals with pancreatic cancer and blood cell phenotype Lewis (a–b–) and those with Lewis phenotypes Le (a+b–) and Le (a–b+).

It is evident that there is a strong correlation between the serum levels of CA 50 and CA 19-9 (Haglund et al., 1987; Harmenberg et al., 1988). To our experience, both markers are usually elevated in the same patients, although in some patients a clear difference in the serum levels may be seen. None of the studies comparing CA 50 and CA 19-9 have shown an advantage of the broader reactivity of the C 50 antibody. A combination of the CA 50 and CA 19-9 tests give no further benefit because of the similarity of the antigens (Haglund et al., 1987).

CA 50 and CA 19-9 have higher sensitivities for pancreatic cancer than CEA and CA 125 (Haglund et al., 1989). Using the recommended cut-off level for each tumor marker, CA 50 has a lower sensitivity for colorectal cancer than CEA, but higher than CA 19-9 (Table 1). However, using cut-off values representing the mean +2 SD of benign colorectal diseases the sensitivities of CA 50 and CA 19-9 are similar. Both markers have a higher sensitivity

Table 1
Comparison of CA 50, CA 19-9, and CEA
in Digestive Tract Diseases,
Using the Recommeded Cut-Off Levels[a]

		CA 50 >20 U/mL, %	CA 19-9 >37 U/mL, %	CEA >3 U/mL, %
Colorectal diseases				
(*N* = 53 primary, 24 recurrences; *n* = 24)				
Sensitivy	Dukes A–B	21	16	32
	Dukes C–D	47	44	71
	Total (A–D)	38	34	57
	Recurrences	38	46	83
Specificity		100	100	83
Gastric diseases				
(*N* = 27; *n* = 43)				
Sensitivity		48	48	41
Specificity		88	100	86
Liver diseases				
(*N* = 11; *n* = 33)				
Sensitivity		55	9	45
Specificity		67	85	67[b]
Pancreatic diseases				
(*N* = 95; *n* = 81)				
Sensitivity		69	77	54
Specificity		80	77	76
Biliary diseases				
(*N* = 17; *n* = 29)				
Sensitivity		88	88	50
Specificity		66	62	82

[a]The percentages are based on patient materials of the authors.
[b]12 patients.
N = number of patients with cancer.
n = number of patients with relevant benign disease.

for small tumors than CEA. Table 1 shows comparisons between CA 50, CA 19-9, and CEA in digestive tract malignancies.

The CA 50 levels correlate well with the serum concentrations of a novel tumor marker CA 242. The immunoassay for CA 242 uses the C 50 antibody as "catching" antibody and the C 242 antibody as "detecting" antibody. The structure of the CA 242 antigen is not yet defined. It is related, but not identical to CA 50 *(see* chapter on CA 242).

4. Summary

Elevated serum values of CA 50 have been found in association with most epithelial carcinomas. Like other available markers, CA 50 is neither organ- nor cancer-specific. Many benign diseases are associated with slightly or moderately elevated CA 50 levels in serum. In many cancers the serum concentration of CA 50 increases only in patients with advanced disease.

CA 50 is at its best in the diagnosis and monitoring of pancreatic cancer, the sensitivity and specificity being similar to those of CA 19-9. Further studies comparing CA 50 with CEA in monitoring patients with colorectal cancer will be needed to evaluate, whether a combination of these markers might be useful. Combinations of different markers improve the sensitivity only slightly compared to the use of CA 50 alone.

References

Ashwell, G. and J. Harford (1982), *Ann. Rev. Biochem.* **51,** 531.

Benini, L. G. Cavallini, D. Zordan. P. Rizzotti, L. Rigo, G. Brocco, L. Perobelli, M. Zanchetta, P. Pederzoli, and L. A. Scuro (1988), *Pancreas* **3,** 61.

Blind, P. J. and S. T. Dahlgren (1987), *Acta Chir. Scand.* **153,** 45.

Bruhn, H. D., A. Everding, B. Joos, and J. Hedderich (1985), in *Tumor Marker Antigens* (Holmgren J., ed.), Student litteratur, Lund, p. 94.

Chan, S. H., L. Lindholm, L. Wong, and C. J. Oon (1985), *in Tumor Marker Antigens* (Holmgren J., ed.), Studentlitteratur, Lund, p. 106.

Cooper, E. H., J. C. Knowles, D. Parker, and M. Taylor (1988), *Biomed. Pharmacother.* **42,** 189.

Enblad, P., B. Glimelius, C. Busch, J. Pontén, and L. Påhlman (1987), *Br. J. Cancer* **55,** 503.

Enblad, P., C. Busch, U. Carlsson, G. Ekelund, B. Glimelius, C. Lindström, J. Pontén, and L. Påhlman (1988), *Am. J. Clin. Pathol.* **89,** 121.

Frykholm, G., P. Enblad, L. Påhlman, and C. Busch (1987), *Dis. Colon Rectum* **30,** 545.

Habib, N. A., M. J. Hershman, F. Haberland, L. Papp, C. B. Wood, and R. C. N. Williamson (1986), *Br. J. Cancer* **53,** 697.

Habib, N. A., M. J. Hershman, S. B. Kelly, G. Taylor, R. C. N. Williamson, and C. B. Wood (1989), *Eur. J. Surg. Oncol.* **15,** 361

Haglund, C., J. Lindgren, P. J. Roberts, and S. Nordling (1986), *Int. J. Cancer* **38,** 841.

Haglund, C., P. Kuusela, H. Jalanko, and P. J. Roberts (1987), *Int. J. Cancer* **39,** 477.

Haglund, C., P. Kuusela, and P. J. Roberts (1989), *Ann. Chir. Gynaecol.* **78,** 41.

Harmenberg, U., B. Wahren, and K.-L. Wiechel (1988), *Cancer Res.* **48,** 1985.

Holmgren, J., L. Lindholm, B. Persson, T. Lagergård, O. Nilsson, L. Svennerholm, C.-M. Rudenstam, B. Unsgaard, F. Yngvason, S. Pettersson, and A.-F. Killander (1984), *Br. Med. J.* **288,** 1479.

Jalanko, H., C. Haglund, P. J. Roberts, and P. Kuusela (1985), in *Tumor Marker Antigen* (Holmgren J., ed.), Studentlitteratur, Lund, p. 114.

Koprowski, H., M. Herlyn, Z. Steplewski, M. Mitchell, M. Herlyn, D. Herlyn, and P. Fuhrer (1979), *Somat. Cell Genet.* **5,** 957.

Kuusela, P., C. Haglund, P. J. Roberts, and H. Jalanko (1987), *Br. J. Cancer* **55,** 673.

Lewenhaupt, A., P. Ekman, P. Eneroth, and A. Kallner (1990), *Eur. Urol.* **17,** 7.

Lindholm, L., J. Holmgren, L. Svennerholm, P. Fredman, O. Nilsson, B. Persson, H. Myrvold, and T. Lagergård (1983), *Int. Arch. Allergy Appl. Immun.* 71, 178.

Lindholm, L., C. Johansson, E.-L. Jansson, C. Hallberg, and O. Nilsson (1985), in *Tumor Marker Antigen* (Holmgren J., ed.), Studentlitteratur, Lund, p. 123.

Magnani, J. L., B. Nilsson, M. Brockhaus, D. Zopf, Z. Steplewski, H. Koprowski, and V. Ginsburg (1982), *J. Biol. Chem.* **257,** 14365.

Marechal, F., G. Berthiot, and G. Deltour (1988), *Anticancer Research* **8,** 677.

Masson, P., B. Pålsson, and Å. Andrén-Sandberg (1988), *Scand. J. Clin. Lab. Invest.* **48,** 751.

Masson, P., B. Pålsson, and Å. Andrén-Sandberg (1990), *Br. J. Cancer* **62,** 118.

Månsson, J. E., P. Fredman, O. Nilsson, L. Lindholm, J. Holmgren, and L. Svennerholm (1985), *Biochim. Biophys. Acta* **834,** 110.

Munck-Wikland, E., R. Kuylenstierna, B. Wahren, J. Lindholm, and S. Haglund (1988), *Cancer* **62,** 2281.

Nilsson, O., L. Lindholm, B. Persson, P. Fredman, J-E. Månsson, J. Holmgren, and L. Svennerholm (1983), in *Glycoconjugates, Proceedings of 7th International Symposium* (Chester M. A., D. Heinegård, A. Lundblad, and S. Svensson, eds.), Lund-Symposium Secretariat, Lund University, Lund, Sweden, p. 852.

Nilsson, O., J-E. Månsson, L. Lindholm, J. Holmgren, and L. Svennerholm (1985), *FEBS Lett.* **182,** 398.

Ouyang, Q., M. Vilien, B. Ravn Juhl, L. G. Larsen, and V. Binder (1987), *Acta Path. Microbiol. Immunol. Scand.* (Sect). A. **95,** 177.

Paganuzzi, M., P. Marroni, F. Boccordo, G. Valenti, G. B. Ferrara, E. Cerri, and G. B. Secco (1985), in *Tumor Marker Antigen* (Holmgren J., ed.), Studentlitteratur, Lund, p. 134.

Paganuzzi, M., M. Onetto, P. Marroni, D. Barone, M. Conio, H. Aste, V. Pugliese (1988), *Cancer* **61,** 2100.

Persson, B. E., E. Ståhle, L. Påhlman, B. Glimelius, O. Nilsson, L. Lindholm, B. Norrgård-Pedersen, and J. Holmgren (1988), *Med. Oncol. Tumor Pharmacother.* **5,** 165.

Pledger, D. R., A. Belfield, J. H. Kennedy, and S. B. Kaye (1988), *Eur. J. Cancer Clin. Oncol.* **24,** 219.

Rasmuson, T., G. R. Björk, L. Damber, L. Jacobsson, A. Jeppsson, T. Stigbrand, and G. Westman (1987), *Acta Oncol.* **26,** 261.

Schwenk, J. and J. Makovitzky (1989), *Int. J. Pancreatol.* **5,** 85.

Ståhle, E., B. Glimelius, R. Bergström, and L. Påhlman (1988a), *Eur. J. Surg. Oncol.* **14,** 277.

Ståhle, E., B. Glimelius, R. Bergström, and L. Påhlman (1988b), *Eur. J. Surg. Oncol.* **14,** 287.

Ståhle, E., B. Glimelius, R. Bergström, and L. Påhlman (1989), *Int. J. Colorect. Dis.* **4,** 182

Strømme, J. H., F. Haffner, N. B. Johannessen, T. Talseth, P. Frederichsen, and L. Theodorsen (1986), *Scand. J. Clin. Lab. Invest.* **46,** 443.

Chapter 18

TAG-72 as a Tumor Marker

Jeffrey Schlom, David Colcher, Diane E. Milenic, Patricia Horan Hand, John W. Greiner, Masahide Kuroki, Ann Thor, Alfredo Molinolo, and Noriaki Ohuchi

In 1981, the murine IgG monoclonal antibody (MAb) B72.3 was isolated. The immunogen employed was a membrane-enriched fraction of human mammary carcinoma metastasis (Colcher et al., 1981). The B72.3-reactive antigen has subsequently been purified and characterized and has been termed TAG-72, for tumor-associated glycoprotein (Johnson et al., 1986). As a result of the purification of TAG-72, a second generation of anti-TAG-72 MAbs has been generated and characterized (Muraro et al., 1988); because the TAG-72 was obtained from a human colon cancer xenograft (LS-174T), these second-generation MAbs have been given the designation CC (i.e., CC49 and so on).

In this chapter, the following topics will be reviewed and discussed:

1. The biochemical and serological characterization of TAG-72;
2. The range of expression of TAG-72 epitopes in human malignancies and normal tissues;

From: *Serological Cancer Markers* Edited by Stewart Sell ©1992 The Humana Press, Totowa, NJ

3. The preparation and characterization of the CC MAbs;
4. CA 72-4 as a serum marker for carcinoma; and
5. The use of radiolabeled B72.3 to detect tumor lesions in carcinoma patients.

Also discussed will be the construction of novel recombinant and chimeric forms of MAb B72.3 and their potential uses, and the modulation and upregulation of TAG-72 in carcinoma cells and the potential clinical consequences of this phenomenon.

1. Purification and Characterization of TAG-72

TAG-72 has been purified from the LS-174T human colon carcinoma xenograft (Johnson et al., 1986; Sheer et al., 1988) and serous effusions from human carcinoma patients (Katari et al., 1990). In the initial LS-174T studies (Johnson et al., 1986) the tumor homogenate was fractionated by Sepharose CL-4B chromatography. The high-mol-wt TAG-72 found in the exclusion volume was then subjected to two sequential passages through B72.3 antibody-affinity columns. At each step of the procedure, TAG-72 content was quantitated using a competition radioimmunoassay (RIA), and the degree of purification was expressed as the ratio of antigen in units to total protein. The three-step procedure produced a purification of TAG-72 with minimal contamination by other proteins, as shown by polyacrylamide gel electrophoresis, followed by staining with Coomassie blue or periodic acid/Schiff reagent. The density of affinity-purified TAG-72, as determined by cesium chloride gradient ultracentrifugation, was found to be 1.45 g/mL. This density determination, together with the high mol wt of TAG-72, its resistance to Chondroitinase digestion, the presence of blood-group-related oligosaccharides, and sensitivity to shearing into forms with low mol wt suggest that TAG-72 is a mucin-like molecule.

In subsequent studies (Sheer et al., 1988), a double-determinant liquid competition RIA for TAG-72 showed greater than a 1000-fold purification. Radiolabeled protein on sodium dodecyl sulfate-polyacrylamide gel electrophoresis (SDS-PAGE) demonstrated an apparently homogeneous high-mol-wt mucin. Chemical deglycosylation using trifluoromethanesulfonic acid yielded low-mol-wt proteins, which could be analyzed for amino acid sequence and also became susceptible to tryptic digestion. The amino acid composition of the purified TAG-72 mucin was similar to that of other purified mucins. The reactive epitope for B72.3 has been shown to be sialyl Tn (Kjeldsen et al., 1988). It is unclear, however, what role the protein backbone of the mucin plays in immunological reactivities, since it has been shown that disruption of the TAG-72 protein backbone will reduce B72.3-reactivity (Johnson et al., 1986; Kurosaka et al., 1988).

A recent study (Katari et al., 1990) demonstrated the isolation and characterization of TAG-72 secreted directly from effusions of patients with ovarian, colorectal, pancreatic, and endometrial carcinomas, and compared them with TAG-72 derived from the LS-174T colon carcinoma xenograft. A three-step purification procedure, utilizing heat extraction, antibody-affinity chromatography, and gel-filtration chromatography, resulted in 1000- to 4400-fold purifications of the TAG-72 derived from effusions, as analyzed using a double-determinant RIA. Radiolabeled TAG-72 from each of the effusions demonstrated similar high-mol-wt bands ($\geq 10^6$ dalton) on SDS-PAGE. Similar results from the various effusions were also obtained in Western blotting analyses. Analyses of TAG-72 from the different effusions in RIA using five different anti-TAG-72 MAbs revealed similar binding patterns. The results of these studies demonstrated that TAG-72 obtained directly from patients with ovarian, colorectal, endometrial, and pancreatic carcinomas and the LS-174T xenograft are highly similar in terms of immunochemical properties and antigenic profile.

2. Range of Reactivities of MAb B72.3

B72.3 has been shown to react equally well with both frozen sections and paraffin-embedded formalin-fixed tissue sections (Thor et al., 1986). Detailed analyses of the range of reactivity of MAb

Table 1
MAb B72.3 Reactivity with Human Neoplasia
Using Formalin-Fixed Tissues and Immunoperoxidase Methodology[a]

Organ	Histological tumor type	No. tested/ no. reactive	>20% reactive malignant cells
Ovary	Serous cystadenocarcinoma	30/30	14/30 (40)[b]
Ovary	Mucinous cystadenocarcinoma	10/10	6/10 (60)
Lung	Squamous cell carcinoma	3/3	1/3
Lung	Adenocarcinoma[c]	28/29	20/29 (69)
Lung	Large-cell carcinoma	1/1	0/1
Colon	Adenocarcinoma	51/54 (94)	23/54 (43)
Breast	Invasive ductal carcinoma	37/44 (84)	12/44 (27)
Esophagus	Squamous cell carcinoma	2/2	0/2
Stomach	Adenocarcinoma	3/4	1/4
Pancreas	Adenocarcinoma	3/3	0/3
Prostate	Adenocarcinoma	1/1	0/1
Bladder	Transitional cell carcinoma	0/1	0/1
Skin	Melanoma	0/2	0/2
Lymph nodes	Lymphoma	0/4	0/4
Bone marrow	Leukemia (chronic lymphocytic)	0/1	0/1
Bone	Thymoma	0/1	0/1
Bone	Osteogenic sarcoma	0/1	0/1
Brain	Glioblastoma multiform	0/1	0/1

[a]Taken from Thor et al., 1986.
[b]Numbers in parentheses are percentages.
[c]Tissue represents all primary tumors.

B72.3 have been undertaken by numerous groups. One of the more extensive studies is outlined in Tables 1 and 2. Adenocarcinomas demonstrated the most TAG-72 expression, with 100% of ovarian, 96% of lung, 94% of colon, 84% of breast, 100% of pancreatic, and 75% of stomach tumors reactive (Nuti et al., 1982; Stramignoni et al., 1983; Johnston et al., 1986a; Thor et al., 1986; Ohuchi et al.,

1987; Lyubsky et al., 1988). Of these, ovarian, colonic, lung, and breast adenocarcinomas demonstrated the highest average percentage of cellular reactivities. Squamous cell carcinomas demonstrated variable reactivity with MAb B72.3, and poorly differentiated squamous cell carcinomas often showed more TAG-72 antigen expression than well-differentiated keratin-producing tumors from the same primary organs (e.g., lung, esophagus). At least 5% of the malignant epithelial cells were positive in the majority of adenocarcinomas of the breast, colon, lung, pancreas, stomach, and ovary as well as esophageal squamous carcinomas (Thor et al., 1986).

Human neoplasias of nonepithelial origin failed to demonstrate reactivity with MAb B72.3 (Thor et al., 1986); these included melanomas, leukemia, lymphomas, a thymoma, sarcoma, and glioblastoma multiforme (high-grade astrocytoma). Heterogeneity of TAG-72 expression was observed between cells of primary tumors as well as between primary, regional, and distant colon carcinoma tumor metastases. Tumor metastases to a variety of tissues, including lymph nodes, omentum, liver, soft tissues, bladder, lung, and colon, also demonstrated a heterogeneity of TAG-72 expression. No correlation was observed between site of tumor metastasis and percentage of cellular reactivity. MAb B72.3 demonstrated greatly reduced reactivity with benign colon tissues.

Reactivity with breast epithelial cells demonstrating apocrine metaplasia has been noted (Thor et al., 1986; Castagna et al., 1987); however, this lesion has a characteristic histological appearance and can be easily differentiated from carcinomas. As summarized in Table 2, TAG-72 expression in normal tissues was noted in some cell types from 33 organ and tissue types evaluated (Thor et al., 1986; Molinolo et al., 1990). MAb B72.3 reactive cells were noted in secretory-phase endometrial glands (25% of cells), a major salivary-gland duct (15% of cells), the esophageal squamous epithelium (1% of cells), the gastric epithelium (1% of cells), respiratory epithelium from the bronchus of the lung (5% of cells), transitional epithelium lining renal pelvis (1% of cells), biliary duct epithelium from liver (1% of cells), and the endocervical glandular epithelium (1% of cells). Of particular interest were major organs, including

Table 2
MAb B72.3-Reactivity with Formalin-Fixed Normal Human Tissues[a]

Organ system	Positive cell types[b]	Negative cell types
Lymphoreticular		
Bone marrow	–	Myeloid and erythroid precursors, megakaryocytes, bone
Lymph node	–	Lymphocytes, histocytes
Spleen	–	Lymphocytes, reticuloendothelial cells, arteries, erythrocytes
Thymus	–	Lymphocytes
Gastrointestinal		
Esophagus	Squamous epithelium (<1)	Stroma, smooth muscle, submucosal glands
Stomach	Mucous epithelium (<1)	Mucin-secreting epithelium, chief cells, parietal cells
Small intestine	–	Epithelium, Brunner's glands, stroma, smooth muscle
Colon	–	Epithelial cells, stroma, smooth muscle
Other		
Heart	–	Cardiac muscle
Brain	–	Neural/glial cells
Peripheral nerve	–	Nerve fibers
Lung	Ciliated respiratory epithelium (5)	Type I and II pneumocytes, macrophages, stroma
Kidney	Transitional epithelium (1)	Tubular epithelium, glomerular epithelial cells, stroma, endothelial cells
Skeletal muscle	–	Skeletal muscle
Liver	Bile-duct epithelium (1)	Hepatocytes, stroma, Kupfer cells, bile-duct epithelium
Bladder	–	Transitional epithelium, stroma, smooth muscle

Salivary-gland ducts	Large striated duct epithelium (15)	Small intercalated duct epithelium
Salivary gland	–	Mucinous acinar cells, serous acinar cells
Smooth muscle	–	–
Uterus		
Proliferative	Uterine glandular epithelium (0)	Stroma, smooth muscle
Secretory	Uterine glandular epithelium (25)	–
Cervix		
Exo	–	Squamous epithelium, stroma
Endo	Columnar epithelium (1) (particularly with squamous metaplasia)	Stroma
Ovary	–	Follicular cells, stroma
Fallopian tube	–	Ciliated epithelium, smooth muscle, stroma
Prostate	–	Prostatic epithelium, stroma
Testes	–	Spermatogenic cells, sertoli cells, leydig cells, stroma
Endocrine/Exocrine		
Thyroid	–	Follicular cells, parafollicular cells (C-cells), stroma
Parathyroid	–	Oxyphil cells, chief cells
Adrenal	–	Cortical cells
Pancreas	–	Islet of Langerhans/acinar cells

[a]Taken from Thor et al., 1986.
[b]Numbers in parentheses are percentages.

bone marrow, lymph nodes, liver, spleen, heart, and pulmonary and kidney parenchyma, which were negative for immunoreactivity with MAb B72.3 (Thor et al., 1986; Molinolo et al., 1990).

B72.3 was also used to study the expression of the colorectal carcinoma associated antigen TAG-72 in premalignant colonic lesions with the immunoperoxidase technique. This antigen, which is rarely detectable in the normal colonic epithelium, was expressed in 13 of 19 adenomas with moderate to severe dysplasia and nine of nine cases of inflammatory bowel disease. The antibody reacted with the normal-appearing mucosa adjacent to a carcinoma in 10 of 12 cases, although only eight of the tumors expressed the antigen. The expression of the TAG-72 antigen in the colonic epithelium thus may be an early marker of malignant transformation (Wolf et al., 1989).

In another study (Xu et al., 1989), B72.3 reacted strongly with 21 of 21 transitional mucosas and with 17 of 21 adjacent colon cancers. Reactivity of B72.3 with transitional mucosa was strong and homogeneous, whereas reactivity with cancer tissue was weaker and more heterogeneous. Reactive mucosa adjacent to squamous carcinoma or lymphoma was also reactive with B72.3. In the colon, expression of TAG-72 antigen occurs during the process of epithelial cell transformation, but may also be regulated by factors unrelated to the process of carcinogenesis. TAG-72 has also been shown to be expressed in ulcerative colitis (Thor et al., 1989). The tendency for TAG-72 expression to correlate to disease duration in patients with quiescent disease and to increase with more severe degrees of dysplasia suggests that the expression of this gene product correlates to the dysplasia-to-carcinoma sequence (Thor et al., 1989).

B72.3 has also been extensively tested for reactivity to normal and malignant human endometrium (Thor et al., 1987). B72.3 reacted with normal postovulatory endometria; in contrast, proliferative-phase epithelia were nonreactive. Both immunohistochemical and RIA techniques were used to evaluate this phenomenon. TAG-72 expression was also detected in 100% of endometrial adenocarcinomas examined ($n = 32$). No MAb B72.3 reactivity was noted in resting, postmenopausal endometria; however, it was present in hyperplastic lesions and appeared to correlate to the severity of histologic abnormality (Thor et al., 1987).

MAb B72.3 demonstrated reactivity with selected fetal tissues (Thor et al., 1986; Stanick et al., 1988). Reactivity was observed only in tissues of the gastrointestinal tract, including the colon (10% of epithelial cells), esophagus (1% of epithelial cells), and stomach (1% of epithelial cells). No reactivity was noted with tissues from other organ systems, including the lymphoreticular, cardiovascular, hepatic, pulmonary, neural, muscular, skin, endocrine, and genitourinary tissues. Thus, TAG-72 can be characterized as a "pancarcinoma" antigen, an "oncofetal" antigen, and perhaps a "differentiation" antigen, as in the case of human endometrium.

MAb B72.3 has been used extensively by numerous institutions to aid in the detection of malignant cells in tissue sections and cytologic preparations of human effusions and for differential diagnoses between adenocarcinoma of the lung and malignant mesothelioma. These findings are listed in Table 3 with accompanying references.

3. Generation and Characterization of Second-Generation Anti-TAG-72 MAb

In studies culminating in 1988, TAG-72 was purified and used as immunogen to produce a second generation of anti-TAG-72 MAbs (Muraro et al., 1988). The MAbs were initially screened for reactivity with purified TAG-72. Via both RIA and immunohistochemical analyses, these MAbs have further shown differential reactivity to carcinoma relative to normal adult tissue biopsies. Nine CC MAbs (CC11, 15, 29, 30, 40, 46, 49, 83, and 92, all IgGs) were selected for further characterization. As a result of analyses using direct-binding RIA to a range of human carcinomas, Western blotting, live-cell surface binding assays, five liquid competition RIAs, and K_a measurements, all nine CC MAbs could be distinguished from each other and from B72.3. The K_a of B72.3 was determined to be $2.54 \times 10^9/M^{-1}$; most of the CC MAbs demonstrated higher

Table 3
MAb B72.3 as an Adjunct in the Immunohistochemical and Immunocytochemical Analyses of Human Carcinoma

Study Design	Reference
Detection of carcinoma in human effusions	Johnston et al., 1985
Detection of carcinoma in peritoneal washings	Szpak et al., 1989
Detection of adenocarcinoma in cytospin preparations	Martin et al., 1986
Cytological diagnosis of pancreatic carcinoma	Ness et al., 1988
Breast carcinoma in bronchoalveolar lavage	Radio et al., 1989
Diagnosis of adenocarcinoma in malignant effusions	Massod, 1989
Detection of carcinoma in FNAB (fine-needle aspiration biopsy)	Johnston et al., 1986b
Phenotypic characterization of lung cancers in FNAB	Johnston et al., 1986a
Evaluation of cytological specimens from the central nervous system	Vick et al., 1987
Fine-needle aspiration cytology of human breast tumors	Lundy et al., 1986; Nuti et al., 1986; Massod, 1990; Kline et al., 1989; Bergeron et al., 1989; Natali et al., 1990
An adjunct in cytological diagnosis of adenocarcinoma of the pancreas	Lyubsky et al., 1988
Study of breast apocrine metaplasia	Castagna et al., 1987
Distinction between malignant mesothelioma of the pleura and adenocarcinoma	Szpak et al., 1986; Nance and Silverman, 1990
Differentiation of adenocarcinoma of the lung from mesothelioma	Warnock et al., 1988
Differential diagnosis of mesothelioma	Ordonez, 1989

Table 4
Comparison of Affinity Constant of B72.3
and Second-Generation (CC) Anti-TAG-72 MAbs[a]

MAb	Affinity Constant, $10^9/M^{-1}$
B72.3	2.54
CC46	3.64
CC30	8.15
CC15	9.13
CC29	9.49
CC11	12.60
CC92	14.26
CC49	16.18
CC83	27.72

[a]Taken from Muraro et al., 1988.

K_a values (Table 4). These studies thus demonstrated that one or more of the anti-TAG-72 CC MAbs may be more efficient than B72.3, or useful in combination with B72.3, toward the further study of human carcinoma cell populations and in the diagnostic and therapeutic procedures presently utilizing MAb B72.3.

Studies were then conducted (Kuroki et al., 1990) employing B72.3 and 18 of the second-generation CC MAbs to construct a serological map of the TAG-72 molecule. MAbs produced immune precipitate lines against purified TAG-72 in double immunodiffusion, indicating that each epitope recognized by a single MAb is present at least twice on the TAG-72 molecule. Immunodepletion analyses utilizing 11 of the anti-TAG-72 MAbs indicated that each recognizes the same molecule or population of molecules. Nineteen competition RIAs were developed, and 19 purified competitor immunoglobulins were employed in each assay (Fig. 1). The patterns of cross-competition indicated the presence of a complex array of tumor-associated epitopes on the TAG-72 molecule (Kuroki et al., 1990). Some of the MAbs recognized epitopes that were structurally or spatially related to one another, but none appeared to recognize identical epitopes. The spectrum of inhibitory reactivities

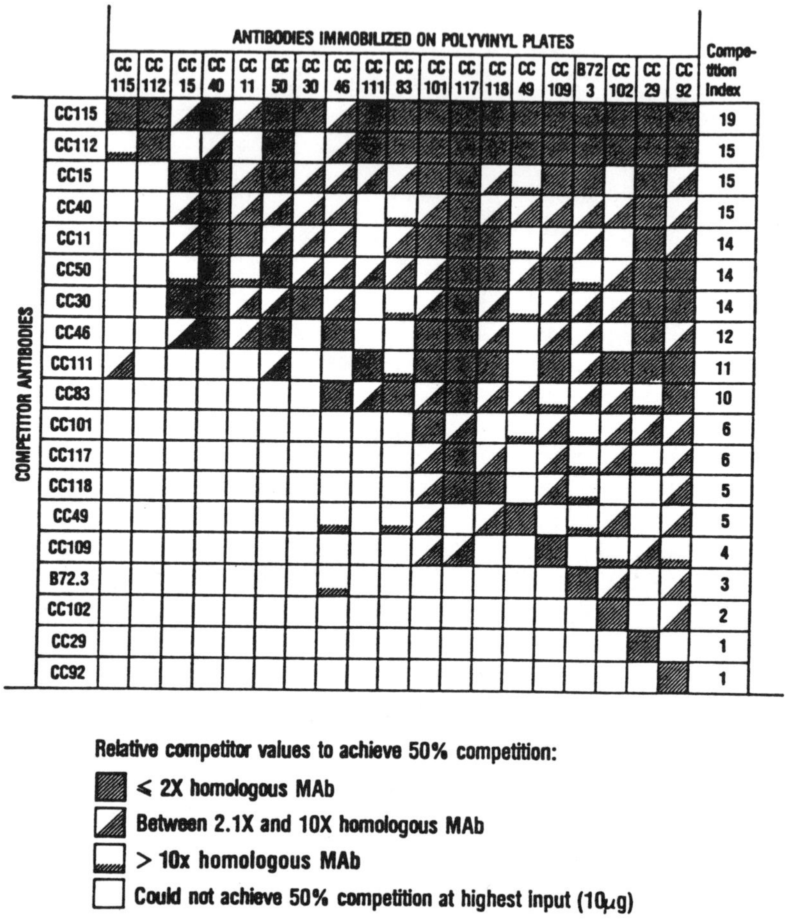

Fig. 1. Graphic representation of relative competitions among anti-TAG-72 MAbs. The relative competition values derived from the amounts of competitor antibodies required to obtain 50% inhibition in cross-competition assays among MAbs were classified into four groups as indicated. Competition index refers to the relative ability of a given MAb to compete in its own and other anti-TAG-72 competition assays. The order of MAbs listed was reorganized according to the competition index. Taken from Kuroki et al., 1990.

of these MAbs for TAG-72 binding varied from extremely restricted to broader inhibition. The serological mapping studies provided information as to the range and nature of the epitopes expressed on the TAG-72 molecule and helped to form the basis for selecting alternative anti-TAG-72 MAbs to define further the nature of this pancarcinoma and oncofetal antigen.

Some of the second-generation CC MAbs were also compared with B72.3 for reactivity to normal and malignant tissues using immunohistochemical assays (Molinolo et al., 1990). Two of these MAbs, CC49 (an IgG) and CC112 (an IgM), were selected for extensive immunohistochemical characterization. These MAbs were tested against a spectrum of normal, benign, and malignant human adult tissues using the avidin–biotin–peroxidase technique, and their reactivity was compared with B72.3. Both CC MAbs were more reactive than B72.3 against a range of tumors. Extensive testing with MAbs CC49 and B72.3 using serial tissue sections demonstrated that both MAbs reacted similarly to most normal adult tissues, with MAb CC49 reacting more strongly to inflammatory colonic tissue. In 35 of 48 (72%) carcinoma biopsies of the gastrointestinal tract, ovary, breast, and lung, in which one of the MAbs reacted to at least 20% of the cells, CC49 reacted to a greater percentage of carcinoma cells and/or tumor-associated mucin than B72.3 (Table 5). The reciprocal was observed in only 2% of the carcinomas. This study thus provides evidence that these second-generation anti-TAG-72 MAbs may be more efficient than B72.3 in the further study of human carcinoma cell populations and in the diagnostic and therapeutic procedures presently being pursued with MAb B72.3.

4. The CA 72-4 Radioimmunoassay for the Detection of TAG-72 in the Serum of Carcinoma Patients

In previous studies (Paterson et al., 1986; Klug et al., 1986) MAb B72.3 has been used to detect the presence of TAG-72 in the serum of carcinoma patients. In recent studies (Gero et al., 1989),

Table 5
Differences Between CC49 and B72.3 Staining of Carcinomas that Showed at Least 20% Reactive Cells

Organ	Total	CC49 = B72.3	CC49 > B72.3	CC49 < B72.3
Colon	9	2	7	0
Breast	13	2	11	0
Ovary	5	1	4	0
Pancreas	11	3	8	0
Stomach	4	2	2	0
Lung	6	2	3	1
Totals	48	12 (25)[b]	35 (73)	1 (2)

[a]Taken from Molinolo et al., 1990.
[b]Numbers in parentheses are percentages.

second-generation MAb CC49 was used as the "catcher" MAb with ^{125}I-B72.3 as the detecting antibody in a double-determinant immunoradiometric assay. This combination enabled the development of a sequential assay (designated CA 72-4) that showed optimal qualitative properties, as demonstrated by such parameters as linear dose response, high reproducibility, and lack of serum-matrix and "hook-back" effects (Gero et al., 1989).

Using the CA 72-4 assay, only 3.5% of 744 normal sera and 6.7% of 134 sera from patients with benign gastrointestinal diseases had TAG-72 levels of >6 U/mL (Table 6). Approximately 40% of 303 patients with gastrointestinal malignancies had serum TAG-72 levels of >6 U/mL (55% of the patients with advanced disease). Thirty-six percent of patients with adenocarcinomas of the lung and 24% of patients with ovarian cancer (53% stage IV patients) also had elevated serum TAG-72 levels (Gero et al., 1989).

A poor correlation was found between the carcinoembryonic antigen (CEA) and TAG-72 values of sera obtained from patients with gastric cancer (Fig. 2); 34% of CEA-negative cases were scored positive in the CA 72-4 assay, suggesting the complementarity of the CA 72-4 assay to CEA assays in the analysis of sera from

Table 6
The Use of the CA 72-4 Serum Assay to Detect TAG-72 in Carcinoma Patients[a,b]

Disease type	No. of cases	Percentage of patients >6 U/mL	Percentage of patients >10 U/mL
Gastric carcinoma	199	42	34
Stage IV	77	55	47
Colorectal carcinoma	104	38	29
Stage IV	41	54	39
Lung carcinoma	165	16	12
Adenocarcinoma	28	36	25
Squamous cell CA	60	17	10
Small-cell CA	61	11	7
Non-small-cell CA	16	19	19
Ovarian carcinoma	92	24	20
Stage IV	15	53	40
Breast carcinoma	66	12	11
Prostatic carcinoma	50	20	10
Squamous carcinoma	25	4	0
Sarcoma	29	3	3
Benign stomach disease	75	5	1
Benign colorectal disease	59	8	3
Misc. benign diseases	17	0	0
Normal (disease-free)	744	3.5	0.5

[a]Taken from Gero et al., 1989.

[b]The percentage of patients with positive TAG-72 values in the CA 72-4 radioimmunoassay are shown using two reference levels, 6 and 10 U/mL.

patients with certain malignancies. Thus, the utility of the CA 72-4 assay to measure TAG-72 levels is clearly demonstrated in the case of patients with gastric cancer. As shown in Fig. 2, 37% of patients with stage III and stage IV disease were scored as positive in the CEA assay. The RIA for TAG-72 was positive in 48% of the sera tested. There is no correlation between the positivity in the CEA assay and the CA 72-4 assay. Thirty-four percent of CEA-negative

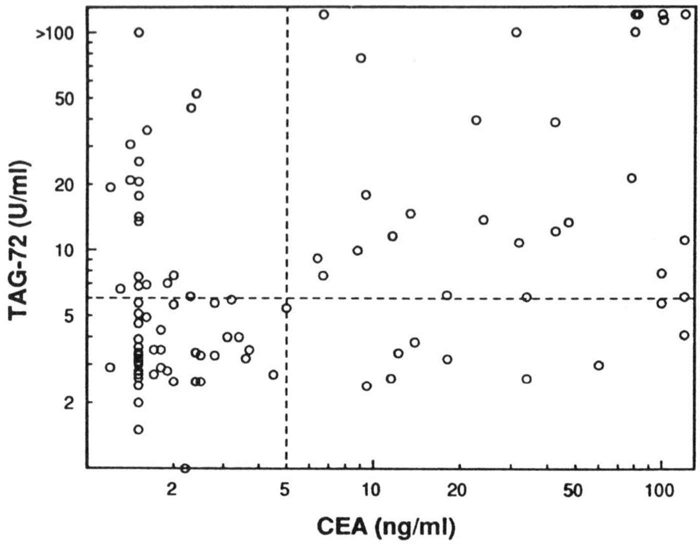

Fig. 2. Complementarity of CEA and TAG-72 values in the sera (n = 99) of patients with gastric carcinoma (stages III and IV). Taken from Gero et al., 1989.

cases showed elevated TAG-72 levels, suggesting the complementary value of the CA 72-4 assay when employed with the widely used CEA assay. Other advantages in the use of multiple assays have been demonstrated when the use of CA 72-4 and/or CA 15-3 assays can improve the specificity of using the CA 125 assay to discriminate between benign and malignant pelvic masses. Similarly, the use of the CA 72-4 assay with the CA 15-3, CA 19-9, and/or DuPAN-2 assays may improve the utility of serum RIAs for analysis of the disease state of patients with malignancies. Studies have also shown that the CA 72-4 assay can also be used in conjunction with the CA 125 assay to help discriminate between malignant and nonmalignant diseases of the ovary (Einhorn et al., 1989; Soper et al., 1990).

In studies conducted in Japan (Ohuchi et al., 1990), serum levels of TAG-72 in patients with carcinoma were investigated by the CA 72-4 assay, utilizing MAbs CC49 and B72.3. The cutoff value for CA 72-4 was determined as 4 U/mL according to the mean ± 2 SD (3.9 U/mL), and only 3% of healthy individuals ($n = 514$) demonstrated elevated levels of TAG-72. The average concentration of TAG-72 in patients with carcinoma ($n = 265$) was 37.9 U/mL, much higher than that (2.6 U/mL) in patients with benign diseases ($n = 212$). Elevated TAG-72 was found in 48% of patients with gastric carcinoma, 55% with colorectal carcinoma, 38% with pancreatic carcinoma, 37% with breast carcinoma, and 60% with ovarian carcinoma (Table 7). Serum TAG-72 in patients with primary carcinoma was measured serially to determine plasma clearance, and the mean decrease period to the cutoff value was 23.2 d after removal of the tumors (Fig. 3). These results indicate (Gero et al., 1989; Ohuchi et al., 1989, 1990) that the CA 72-4 immunoradiometric assay may be useful for detecting serum TAG-72 antigen in patients with gastrointestinal, breast, ovarian, and other epithelial malignancies.

5. Targeting of Human Carcinoma Lesions with Radiolabeled MAb B72.3

In addition to the use of radiolabeled MAbs to detect occult carcinoma and to aid in staging, this modality also has therapeutic implications: the use of a given MAb–radionuclide conjugate in low doses (for diagnostic gamma scanning), may provide a "therapeutic index" for that particular MAb, whether the MAb is given coupled to a high-energy killer isotope or drug, or used unconjugated. Thus, these types of trials are now referred to as "pre Phase I" trials.

Preclinical studies in mice using ^{125}I-radiolabeled B72.3 have demonstrated good tumor localization (several pre Phase I trials have subsequently been conducted with MAb B72.3 [Colcher et al., 1984]). Radiolabeled MAb B72.3 was administered to colorectal

Table 7
Positive Rates and Average Values of Serum TAG-72 Antigen Defined by CA 72-4 Immunoradiometric Assay in Patients with Carcinoma or Benign Disease, and Controls[a]

		Fraction of TAG-72-positive sera			
	No. tested	≥4.0[b]	≥6.5[b]	≥8.0[b]	Mean TAG-72, U/mL
Carcinomas	265	0.47	0.37	0.31	37.92
Esophagus	12	0.25	0.25	0.25	7.08
Stomach	92	0.48	0.36	0.30	27.82
Primary	71	0.35	0.25	0.21	25.14
Stage I	38	0.18	0.08	0.05	4.92
Stage II	7	0.29	0.29	0.14	11.26
Stage III	10	0.30	0.20	0.20	5.21
Stage IV	16	0.81	0.69	0.63	19.71
Recurrent	21	0.90	0.71	0.62	32.13
Colorectum	73	0.55	0.49	0.40	62.04
Primary	64	0.50	0.45	0.36	57.20
Stage I	20	0.10	0.05	0.05	2.66
Stage II	7	0.43	0.29	0.14	4.27
Stage III	4	0.75	0.75	0.75	6.45
Stage IV	5	0.80	0.80	0.60	14.98
Stage V	28	0.71	0.64	0.57	116.24
Recurrent	9	0.89	0.78	0.67	81.30
Pancreas	13	0.38	0.31	0.23	13.32
Gallbladder	4	0.50	0.50	0.50	14.53
Choledochus	7	0.57	0.57	0.43	6.31
Breast	52	0.37	0.21	0.19	18.89
Primary	34	0.29	0.15	0.12	3.49
Recurrent	18	0.50	0.33	0.33	47.99
Ovary	5	0.60	0.60	0.60	190.12
Others	7	0.71	0.42	0.28	6.70
Benign diseases	212	0.10	0.05	0.03	2.57
Controls	514	0.03	0.01	0.003	1.90

[a]Taken from Ohuchi et al., 1990.
[b]Cutoff values in TAG-72 U/mL (Paterson et al., 1986).

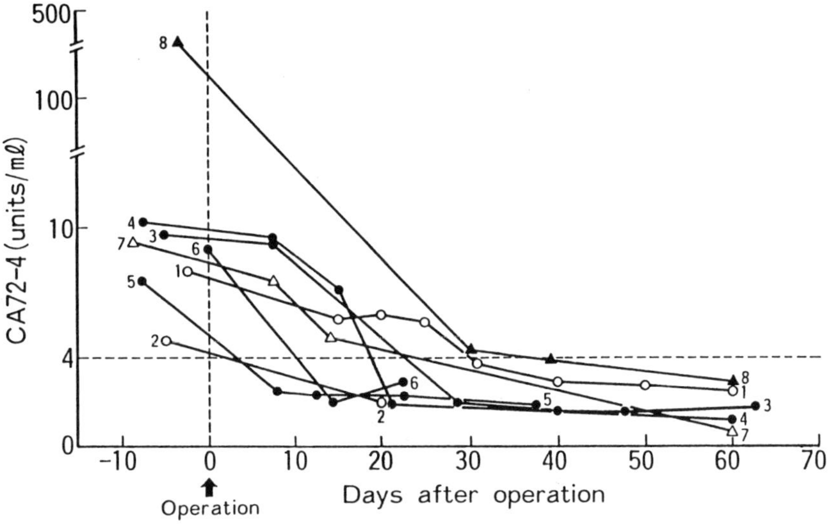

Fig. 3. Serial determination of TAG-72 antigen concentration in sera from patients with gastric cancer (○; 1 and 2), colorectal cancer (●; 3, 4, 5, and 6), breast cancer (Δ;7), and ovarian cancer (▲;8). The values were determined before and after radical curative surgeries for respective primary cancer. The reference value of 4 U/mL is indicated by the dotted horizontal line. Taken from Ohuchi et al., 1990.

cancer patients for a quantitative evaluation of its reactivity with tumor lesions vs a wide range of normal tissues (Esteban et al., 1987; Colcher et al., 1987a; Carrasquillo et al., 1988). These studies included patients with metastatic colorectal carcinoma that involved the surgical resection of metastatic colorectal cancer lesions plus adjacent "normal" tissues for staging and therapeutic purposes. Thus, gamma scanning followed by a comprehensive direct examination of the tumor and a variety of normal tissues could be achieved. Approximately 7 d before surgery, patients received ^{131}I-labeled MAb B72.3 IgG. Patients were scanned with a gamma camera at various times until surgery. At surgery, suspected carcinoma lesions and selected normal tissues were removed. Specimens from all biopsies were immediately weighed and placed in a gamma counter to determine cpm/g; biopsy specimens were subsequently analyzed for the percentage of tumor cells of total cells present and the percentage of TAG-72 antigen-positive cells.

In the initial study (Esteban et al., 1987), 27 patients received ^{131}I-labeled B72.3 IgG. Positive gamma scans (confirmed at surgery) were observed in 14 of 27 patients and in 10 of 20 patients for whom direct examination of tissues were available. There was no effect of IgG dose, milliCurie amount, or specific activity on whether a gamma scan was positive or negative. Gamma scans identified tumor lesions accurately in the liver, bone, orbit, rectum, colon, cecum, and pelvis, and diffusely in the peritoneal cavity (Carrasquillo et al., 1988). No toxicity was observed. Perhaps the most important part of these studies, however, revolved around analysis of a radiolocalization index (RI). The RI value is defined as the ratio of the uptake of ^{131}I-labeled MAb in tumor to that in histologically confirmed normal tissue on a per gram basis; average values (cpm/g) from biopsy of normal liver and/or intestinal tissue of each patient were normalized to 1.0. RI values of ≥3.0 were arbitrarily considered "positive" for these studies. At least one tumor lesion in 17 of 20 of the patients studied had an RI of ≥3.0. In eight of these patients, all 50 tumor lesions biopsied had RI values of ≥3.0. Five of the patients studied displayed 26 lesions with RI values of ≥10.0. In total, 99 of 142 (70%) carcinoma lesions biopsied displayed RI values of ≥3.0. Of 210 histologically confirmed normal tissues biopsied, 198 showed negative RI values, that is, values <3.0. In 12 patients, all apparently normal tissues biopsied had a negative RI. Twelve biopsy specimens from eight patients showed RI values of ≥3.0. In all but two cases, these tissues were immediately adjacent to carcinoma or draining carcinoma; in two cases, positive RI values were seen in spleen biopsies. These values apparently were caused by the presence of antigen–antibody immune complexes.

B72.3 was also labeled with approx 5 mCi of ^{111}In after site-specific conjugation to the antibody oligosaccharide moiety with the linker-chelator glycyltyrosyl-(*N*, ε-diethylenetriaminepentaacetic acid)-lysine (GYK-DTPA). Single iv infusions (0.2, 1, 2, or 20 mg) of the radiolabeled B72.3 conjugate, designated ^{111}In-CYT-103, were administered to 127 presurgical cancer patients (Maguire et al., 1989). Six patients (4.7%) had adverse effects related to the antibody conjugate. In all cases, these effects resolved either spontaneously or with appropriate countermeasures. A positive human antimouse antibody (HAMA) response was detected in 23% of patients. Of the 64 patients in this study with suspected colorectal adenocarcinoma, 55 underwent surgery, of whom 50 were found to have tumor at surgery. Antibody images were positive for 37 of the 50 patients (74.0%). Of the 78 lesions confirmed at the time of surgery, 57 (73.1%) were detected by the antibody scans. The gamma-camera scans detected six biopsy-confirmed false positive lesions. When compared with the results of CT scans, the antibody scans showed greater sensitivity (73 vs 52%) for tumor lesions. ^{111}In-CYT-103 affected the management of 26% (16/62) of the patients evaluated (Maguire et al., 1989). These results indicate that radiolabeled B72.3 (^{111}In-CYT-103) is safe and shows promise as a radioimmunoscintigraphic agent for the presurgical staging of patients with colorectal adenocarcinoma.

Twenty patients with known ovarian cancer were investigated (Lastoria et al., 1988) to define the clinical usefulness of radioimaging using MAb B72.3 labeled with ^{131}I. No adverse reactions occurred after intravenous injection. The radioimaging results were compared with those obtained with other diagnostic methods, including computed X-ray tomography and ultrasound. A sensitivity of 85% in the detection of primary ovarian cancers and collections of ascites, and of 84% in the detection of abdominal and extraperitoneal metastases, was demonstrated. No false localization occurred. Negligible uptake of radiolabeled MAb B72.3 was seen in the unaffected ovary.

An alternative approach in the use of MAbs for diagnostic or therapeutic purposes involves intracavitary administration. MAbs administered directly into a cavity or body site may localize tumors in that cavity more efficiently than systematically administered MAb. Studies have been conducted with B72.3 to (a) determine the feasibility of intraperitoneal administration of radiolabeled MAb for tumor localization or therapy, (b) determine the specificity of tumor localization by the concomitant ip administration of ^{131}I-MAb and an isotype-matched control ^{125}I-labeled MAb, (c) compare tumor localization of iv- vs ip-administered MAb by the simultaneous administration of ^{125}I-MAb iv and the same ^{131}I-MAb ip, and (d) define the pharmacokinetics of plasma clearance of both ip- and iv-administered radiolabeled MAb.

Patients were administered ^{131}I-labeled MAb B72.3 murine IgG ip and scanned with a gamma camera at various time-points prior to surgery (Colcher et al., 1987b; Carrasquillo et al., 1988). Gamma scans of seven of 10 patients showed clearly discernible concentrations of radiolabeled MAb in tumor. A representative positive gamma scan is shown in Fig. 4. Three of the initial 10 patients studied that were positive for MAb localization via gamma scanning (areas confirmed as tumor at surgery) were negative for tumor via CT scanning and X-ray studies. Lesions as small as approx 1.5 cm in diameter were clearly defined via gamma scans. The RI values of biopsy specimens were determined. Using RI ≥3, arbitrarily chosen, as a "positive" radiolabeled uptake, 83 of 112 (74%) of carcinoma lesions showed positive values. Of the 95 histologically confirmed normal tissues biopsied, all but one demonstrated RI values <3. Phase I trials using ^{131}I-B72.3 (Raubitschek et al., 1988) and ^{90}Y-B72.3 (Kavanagh et al., 1990) administered ip are now in progress.

6. Intraoperative Probe MAb-Directed Surgery

A novel use of MAbs involves their use in conjunction with a hand-held gamma-detecting probe used at surgery to detect occult tumor. This probe has now been used in several hundred patients at numerous centers with ^{125}I-labeled MAb B72.3. In studies involving colorectal carcinoma patients, the intraoperative probe local-

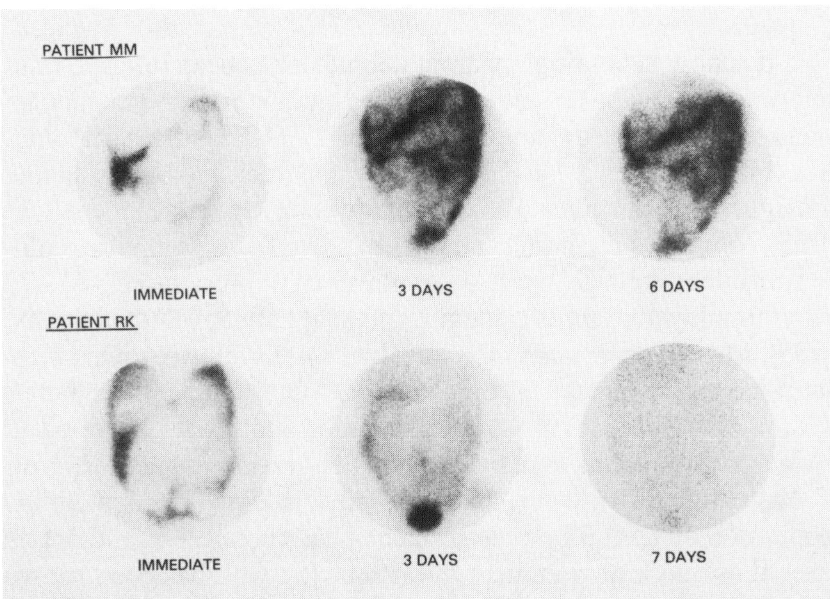

Fig. 4. Radioimmunoscintigraphy in patients with metastatic colorectal cancer after ip administration of ^{131}I-B72.3 IgG. Two patients were injected ip with radiolabeled B72.3 IgG. Patients RK and MM were scanned immediately after antibody administration and at various times, as indicated in the Fig. Patient RK, with no peritoneal tumor, was negative for B72.3 localization, whereas the peritoneal tumor was visualized by B72.3 in patient MM. Taken from Colcher et al., 1987b.

ized the ^{125}I-B72.3 in 83% of sites and altered the surgical approach in 26% of patients with recurrent colorectal cancer (Sickle-Santanello et al., 1987; Martin et al., 1988; Tuttle et al., 1988). In a more recent study (Nieroda et al., 1989) 14 patients with carcinoma of the breast confirmed at biopsy received ^{125}I-labeled MAb iv prior to further exploration; the gamma-detecting probe, used externally for this application, was able to identify residual, subclinical, and multicentric carcinoma of the breast in some cases.

7. Future Studies

It is now becoming apparent that what has been referred to as heterogeneity of TAG-72 expression in carcinoma lesions may actually be the more dynamic process of TAG-72-antigen modulation. For example, it has been shown that such factors as spatial configuration can alter TAG-72 expression (Horan Hand et al., 1985). Very few carcinoma cell lines express TAG-72 in vitro; colonies of tumor cells grown in agar, however, express more TAG-72 than monolayer cultures (Horan Hand et al., 1985; Friedman et al., 1985). Moreover, when tumor cells like LS-174T are grown as xenografts, they express 100 times more TAG-72 than cultured cells (Horan Hand et al., 1985). These studies and others have led to investigations that have demonstrated that recombinant interferons (IFNs) α (clone A), β-ser, and γ can all selectively upregulate the expression of TAG-72 on the surface of carcinoma cells and not on normal cells (Greiner et al., 1984, 1986, 1987). It has been shown that the concentrations of IFN required to induce this phenomenon are well below cytostatic and cytotoxic doses. The mechanism for this phenomenon is not clearly understood at this time, but it has recently been shown that TAG-72 can be upregulated on approx 80% of fresh biopsy specimens of effusions of a variety of carcinomas and not upregulated on benign effusions and a variety of normal cell lines (Guadagni et al., 1989) (Fig. 5). Recent studies (Greiner et al., 1990) of ovarian and gastrointestinal cancer patients have demonstrated that relatively low doses of ip-administered recombinant IFNγ can increase the expression of the TAG-72 antigen on carcinoma cells in effusions within 24 h after administration (Fig. 6). These findings thus may ultimately prove extremely important in enhancing both diagnostic and therapeutic modalities of anti-TAG-72-based therapies.

Finally, recombinant and chimeric forms of MAb B72.3 have now been constructed, both with a human γ4 (Whittle et al., 1987; Colcher et al., 1989) and a human γ1 (Primus et al., 1990; Hutzell et al., 1991) backbone. These constructs should be of use in clinical studies in reducing HAMA responses, thus enabling multiple-

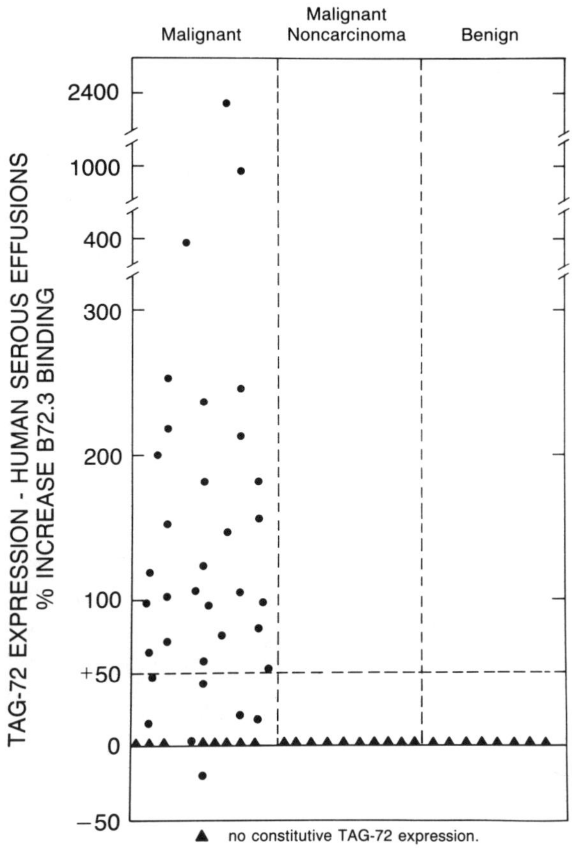

Fig. 5. Effect of recombinant IFN on the cell-surface expression of fresh human effusions. Effusions from patients with carcinoma; patients with malignant noncarcinoma, i.e., melanoma, lymphoma (which do not constitutively express TAG-72); and patients with benign diseases were incubated with and without IFN and then reacted with ^{125}I-B72.3 to detect surface TAG-72 expression. *See* Guadagni et al., 1989 for details.

dose therapeutic regimens. Furthermore, modified recombinant constructs, such as aglycosylated or domain-deleted forms, may alter pharmacokinetic properties and thus enable an individual B72.3 or other anti-TAG-72 recombinant constructs to better fit a designated diagnostic or therapeutic modality.

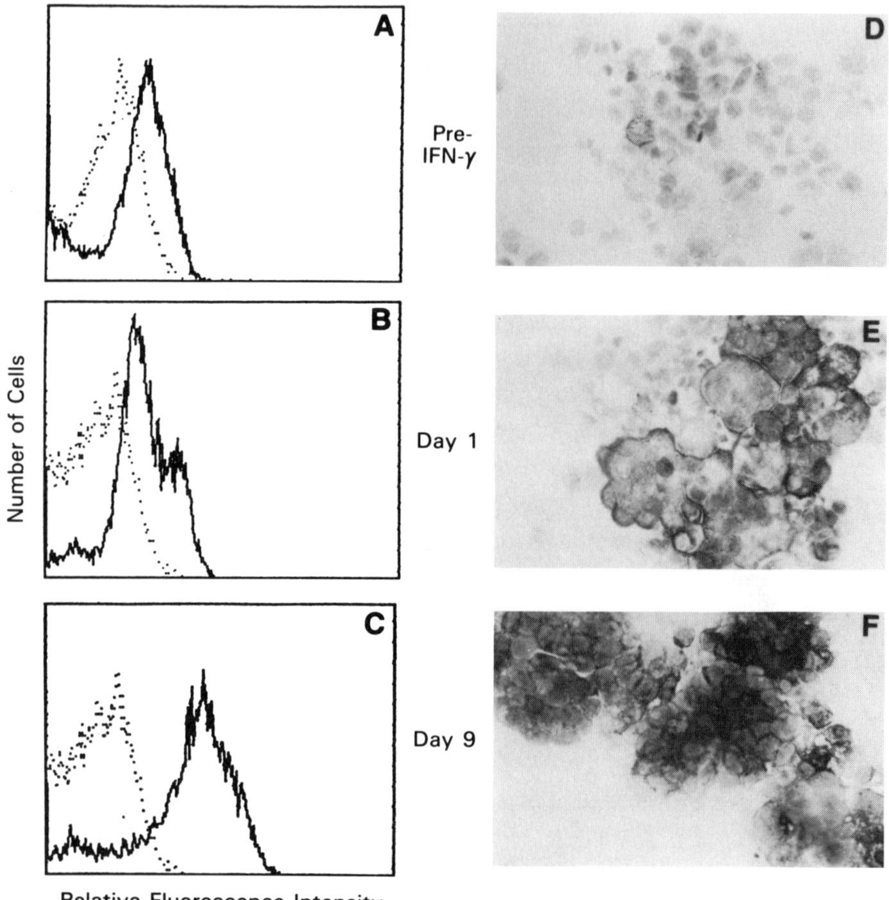

Fig. 6. The use of recombinant IFN to upregulate tumor antigen expression (Greiner et al., 1990). Changes induced in B72.3 binding to human ovarian carcinoma cells isolated from adenocarcinomatous ascites before and after the patient received two successive weekly ip administrations of IFNγ (0.1 mU). Prior to the initial ip treatment with 0.1 mU IFNγ, ascites was removed, and the constitutive TAG-72 expression was measured by B72.3 binding using flow cytometry (**A**) and immunocytochemistry (**D**). Panels **B** and **E** illustrate the alterations in B72.3 reactivity to carcinoma cells isolated 24 h after ip IFNγ treatment. The patient was given a second ip treatment with 0.1 mU IFNγ, and B72.3 binding was analyzed by flow cytometry (**C**) and immunocytochemical staining (**F**) 48 h later (i.e., day 9).

References

Bergeron, C., P. Shatz, R. Margolese, P. Major, and A. Ferenczy (1989), *Anal. Quant. Cytol. Histol.* **11,** 33–42.

Carrasquillo, J. A., P. Sugarbaker, D. Colcher, J. C. Reynolds, J. Esteban, G. Bryant, A. M. Keenan, P. Perentesis, K. Yokoyama, D. E. Simpson, P. Ferroni, R. Farkas, J. Schlom, and S. M. Larson (1988), *J. Nucl. Med.* **29,** 1022–1030.

Castagna, M., M. Nuti, and F. Squartini (1987), *Cancer Res.* **47,** 902–906.

Colcher, D., P. Horan Hand, M. Nuti, and J. Schlom (1981), *Proc. Natl. Acad. Sci. USA*, **78,** 3199–3203.

Colcher, D., A. M. Keenan, S. M. Larson, and J. Schlom (1984), *Cancer Res.* **44,** 5744–5751.

Colcher, D., J. M. Esteban, J. A. Carrasquillo, P. Sugarbaker, J. C. Reynolds, G. Bryant, S. M. Larson, and J. Schlom (1987a), *Cancer Res.* **47,** 1185–1189.

Colcher, D., J. Esteban, J. A. Carrasquillo, P. Sugarbaker, J. C. Reynolds, G. Bryant, S. M. Larson, and J. Schlom (1987b), *Cancer Res.* **47,** 4218–4224.

Colcher, D., D. Milenic, M. Roselli, A. Raubitschek, G. Yarranton, D. King, J. Adair, N. Whittle, M. Bodmer, and J. Schlom (1989), *Cancer Res.* **49,** 1738–1745.

Einhorn, N., R. C. Knapp, R. C. Bast, and V. R. Zurawski, Jr. (1989), *Acta Oncol.* (Madr.) **28,** 655–657.

Esteban, J. M., D. Colcher, P. Sugarbaker, J. A. Carrasquillo, G. Bryant, A. Thor, J. C. Reynolds, S. M. Larson, and J. Schlom (1987), *Int. J. Cancer* **39,** 50–59.

Friedman, E., A. Thor, P. Horan Hand, and J. Schlom (1985), *Cancer Res.* **45,** 5648–5655.

Gero, E. J., D. Colcher, P. Ferroni, R. Melsheimer, S. Giani, J. Schlom, and P. Kaplan (1989), *J. Clin. Lab. Anal.* **3,** 360–369.

Greiner, J. W., P. B. Fisher, S. Pestka, and J. Schlom (1986), *Cancer Res.* **46,** 4984–4990.

Greiner, J. W., F. Guadagni, R. V. Smalley, D. Goldstein, E. C. Borden and J. Schlom (1990), *AACR Proceedings*, **31,** 1672 (Abstract).

Greiner, J. W., P. Horan Hand, P. Noguchi, P. Fisher, S. Pestka, and J. Schlom(1984), *Cancer Res.* **44,** 3208–3214.

Greiner, J. W., F. Guadagni, P. Noguchi, S. Pestka, D. Colcher, P. B. Fisher, and J. Schlom (1987), *Science* **235,** 895–898.

Guadagni, F., J. Schlom, W. W. Johnston, C. A. Szpak, D. Goldstein, R. Smalley, J. Simpson, E. C. Borden, S. Pestka, and J. W. Greiner (1989), *J. Natl. Cancer Inst.* **81,** 502–512.

Horan Hand, P., D. Colcher, D. Salomon, J. Ridge, P. Noguchi, and J. Schlom (1985), *Cancer Res.* **45,** 833–840.

Hutzell, P., S. Kashmiri, D. Colcher, J. Primus, P. Horan Hand, M. Roselli, G. Yarranton, M. Bodmer, N. Whittle, D. King, C. C. Loullis, D. W. McCoy, R. Callahan, and J. Schlom (1991), *Cancer Res.* **51,** 181–189.

Johnson, V. G., J. Schlom, A. J. Paterson, J. Bennett, J. L. Magnani, and D. Colcher (1986), *Cancer Res.* **46,** 850–857.

Johnston, W. W., C. A. Szpak, S. C. Lottich, A. Thor, and J. Schlom (1985), *Cancer Res.* **45,** 1894–1900.

Johnston, W. W., C. A. Szpak, A. Thor, and J. Schlom (1986a), *Cancer Res.* **46,** 6462–6470.

Johnston, W. W., C. A. Szpak, S. C. Lottich, A. Thor, and J. Schlom (1986b), *Hum. Pathol.* **17,** 501–513.

Katari, R. S., P. D. Fernsten, and J. Schlom (1990), *Cancer Res.* **50,** 4885–4890.

Kavanagh, J. J., M. Rosenblum, T. Burke, L. Lamki, L. Murrary, J. Shanken, L. Thompson, and J. T. Wharton (1990), *AACR Proceedings*, **31,** 1116 (Abstract).

Kjeldsen, T., H. Clausen, S. Hirohashi, T. Ogawa, H. Iijima, and S. Hakomori (1988), *Cancer Res.* **48,** 2114–2120.

Kline, T. S., J. Lundy, and M. Lozowski (1989), *Cancer* **63,** 2253–2256.

Klug, T. L., M. A. Sattler, D. Colcher, and J. Schlom (1986), *Int. J. Cancer* **38,** 661–669.

Kuroki, A., P. Fernsten, D. Wunderlich, D. Colcher, J. F. Simpson, D. J. Poole, T. G. Ooley, and J. Schlom (1990), *Cancer Res.* (in press).

Kurosaka, A., H. Kitagawa, S. Fukui, Y. Numata, H. Nakada, I. Funakoshi, T. Kawasaki, T. Ogawa, H. Iijama, and I. Yamashina (1988), *J. Biol. Chem.* **263,** 8724–8726.

Lastoria, S., P. D'Amico, L. Mansi, G. G. Giordano, R. Rossiello, J. Schlom, E. Pace, N. Panza, G. Pacilio, and M. Salvatore (1988), *Nucl. Med. Comm.* **9,** 347–356.

Lundy, J., M. Lozowski, Y. Mishriki (1986), *Ann. Surg.* **203,** 399–402.

Lyubsky, S., J. Madariaga, M. Lozowski, Y. Mishriki, A. Schuss, S. Chao, and J. Lundy (1988), *Am. J. Clin. Pathol.* **89,** 160–167.

Maguire, R. T., R. F. Schmelter, V. L. Pascucci, and J. J. Conklin (1989), *Antibody Immunoconjugates Radiopharm.* **2,** 257–269.

Martin, E. W., C. M. Mojzisik, G. H. Hinkle, J. Sampsel, M. A. Siddiqi, S. E. Tuttle, B. Sickle-Santanello, D. Colcher, M. O. Thurston, J. G. Bell, W. B. Farrar, and J. Schlom (1988), *Am. J. Surg.* **156,** 386–392.

Martin, S. E., S. Moshiri, A. Thor, V. Vilasi, E. W. Chu, and J. Schlom (1986), *Am. J. Clin. Pathol.* **86,** 10–18.

Massod, S. (1989), American Society of Clinical Pathologists and the College of American Pathologists (Abstract).

Massod, S. (1990), American Society of Clinical Pathologists and the College of American Pathologists **438,** 14 (Abstract).

Molinolo, A., J. F. Simpson, A. Thor, and J. Schlom (1990), *Cancer Res.* **50,** 1291–1298.

Muraro, R., M. Kuroki, D. Wunderlich, D. J. Poole, D. Colcher, A. Thor, J. W. Greiner, J. F. Simpson, A. Molinolo, P. Noguchi, and J. Schlom (1988), *Cancer Res.* **48,** 4588–4596.

Nance, K. V. and J. F. Silverman (1990), American Society of Clinical Pathologists and the College of American Pathologists, **436,** 4 (Abstract).

Natali, P. G., M. Mottolese, R. Perrone Donnorso, R. Buffa, G. Bussolati, G. Coggi, G. Corradi, L. Coascia-Porrazzi, M. Ferretti, E. Rondanelli, M. Castagna, A. Vecchione, and G. A. Siccardi (1990), *Int. J. Cancer* **45,** 12–15.

Ness, M. J., P. M. Pour, M. A. Tempero, and J. Linder (1988), *Mod. Pathol.* **1,** 279–283.

Nieroda, C., C. Mojzisik, A. Sardi, W. Farrar, G. Hinkle, A. Siddiqi, P. J. Ferra, A. James, J. Schlom, M. Thurston, and E. Martin (1989), *Surg. Gynecol. Obstetr.* **169,** 35–40.

Nuti, M., M. Mottolese, M. Viola, R. Perrone Donnorso, J. Schlom, and P. G. Natali (1986), *Int. J. Cancer* **37,** 493–498.

Nuti, M., Y. A. Teramoto, R. Mariani-Costantini, P. Horan Hand, D. Colcher, and J. Schlom (1982), *Int. J. Cancer* **29,** 539–545.

Ohuchi, N., J. Simpson, D. Colcher, and J. Schlom (1987), *Int. J. Cancer* **40,** 726–733.

Ohuchi, N., K. Takahashi, N. Matoba, T. Sato, Y. Taira, N. Sakai, M. Masuda, and S. Mori (1989), *Jpn. J. Clin. Oncol.* **19,** 242–248.

Ohuchi, N., E. Gero, S. Mori, M. Akimoto, N. Matoba, T. Nishihira, K. Nirayama, D. Colcher, and J. Schlom (1990), *J. Tumor Marker Oncol.* **5,** 1–10.

Ordonez, N. G. (1989), *Am. J. Surg. Pathol.* **13,** 276–291.

Paterson, A. J., J. Schlom, H. F. Sears, J. Bennett, and D. Colcher (1986), *Int. J. Cancer* **37,** 659–666.

Primus, F. J., T. K. Pendurthi, P. Hutzell, S. Kashmiri, D. Slavin, R. Callahan, and J. Schlom (1990), *Cancer Immunol. Immunother.* **31,** 349–357.

Radio, S. J., S. I. Rennard, A. Kessinger, W. P. Vaughan, and J. Linder (1989), *Arch. Path. Lab. Med.* **113,** 333–336.

Raubitschek, A., D. Colcher, S. Lastoria, P. Perentesis, R. Neumann, S. Larson, J. Reynolds, P. Sugarbaker, J. Schlom, and J. Carrasquillo (1988, September), *Second Conference on Radioimmunodetection and Radioimmunotherapy of Cancer,* Princeton, NJ (Abstract).

Sheer, D. G., J. Schlom, and H. L. Cooper (1988), *Cancer Res.* **48,** 6811–6818.

Sickle-Santanello, B. J., P. J. O'Dwyer, C. Mojzisik, S. E. Tuttle, G. H. Hinkle, M. Rouseau, J. Schlom, D. Colcher, M. O. Thurston, C. Nieroda, A. Sardi, J. P. Minton, and E. W. Martin (1987), *Dis. Colon Rectum* **30,** 761–764.

Soper, J. T., V. J. Hunter, L. Daly, M. Tanner, W. T. Creasman, and R. C. Bast, Jr. (1990), *Obstet. Gynecol.* **75,** 249–254.

Stanick, D., A. Schuss, Y. Mishriki, S. Chao, A. Thor, and J. Lundy (1988), *Cancer Invest.* **6,** 279–287.

Stramignoni, D., R. Bowen, B. Atkinson, and J. Schlom (1983), *Int. J. Cancer* **31,** 543–552.

Szpak, C. A., W. W. Johnston, V. Roggli, J. Kolbeck, C. Lottich, R. Vollmer, A. Thor, and J. Schlom (1986), *Am. J. Pathol.* **122,** 252–260.

Szpak, C. A., J. T. Soper, A. Thor, J. Schlom, and W. W. Johnston (1989), *Acta Cytol.* **33,** 205–214.

Thor, A., N. Ohuchi, C. A. Szpak, W. W. Johnston, and J. Schlom (1986), *Cancer Res.* **46,** 3118–3124.

Thor, A., M. J. Viglione, R. Muraro, N. Ohuchi, J. Schlom, and F. Gorstein (1987), *Int. J. Gynecol. Pathol.* **6,** 235–247.

Thor, A., S. H. Itzkowitz, J. Schlom, Y. S. Kim, and S. Hanauer (1989), *Int. J. Cancer* **43,** 810–815.

Tuttle, S. E., S. D. Jewell, C. Mojzisik, G. H. Hinkle, D. Colcher, J. Schlom, and E. W. Martin (1988), *Int. J. Cancer* **42,** 352–358.

Vick, W. W., C. J. Wikstrand, D. E. Bullard, J. Kemshead, H. B. Coakham, J. Schlom, W. W. Johnston, D. D. Bigner, and S. H. Bigner (1987), *Acta Cytol.* **31,** 815–824.

Warnock, M. L., A. Stoloff, and A. Thor (1988), *Am. J. Pathol.* **133,** 30–38.

Whittle, N., J. Adair, C. Lloyd, L. Jenkins, J. Schlom, A Raubitschek, D. Colcher, and M. Bodmer (1987), *Protein Eng.* **1,** 499–505.

Wolf, B. C., J. C. D'Emilia, R. R. Salem, D. DeCoste, H. F. Sears, L. S. Gottlieb, and G. D. Steele, Jr. (1989), *J. Natl. Cancer Inst.* **81,** 1913–1917.

Xu, M., F. X. Real, S. Welt, M. H. Schussler, H. F. Oettgen, and L. J. Old (1989), *Int. J. Cancer* **44,** 985–989.

Chapter 19

CA 125

Fredrick J. Montz

1. Introduction

In the decade following Bast and associates' initial reports on the usefulness of CA 125 in the management of epithelial adenocarcinomas of the ovary (Bast et al., 1981), there has been extensive investigation of the potential clinical value of CA 125 determination. In this chapter we will review the present status of CA 125 determination for screening and management of gynecologic malignancies and will as summarize the biochemistry of CA 125 and the assay utilized to determine levels of the antigen in human fluids.

2. Biochemistry of CA 125 and Assay Techniques

CA 125 is an antigenic determinant defined by a monoclonal IgG immunoglobulin (OC 125) that was developed by somatic hybridization of spleen cells from mice immunized with an epithelial ovarian carcinoma cell line (OVCA433) (Bast et al., 1981). CA 125 is associated with a high-mol-wt glycoprotein that is expressed

From: *Serological Cancer Markers* Edited by Stewart Sell

in coelomic epithelium during embryonic development (Kabawat et al., 1983). The antigen is expressed in a wide range of benign, inflamed, and malignant tissues in the adult female (de Bruijn et al., 1986; Einhorn et al., 1986; Vasilev et al., 1988; Marechal et al., 1989; Duk et al., 1990a). There is a fluctuation of CA 125 serum levels in normal ovulatory women that appears to parallel the growth of the dominant follicle (Jager et al., 1988).

The assay for CA 125 is an immunoradiometric assay that uses polystyrene beads (6.4 mm) coated with OC 125 antibody. Bound antigen is detected by simultaneous incubation of the bead and the serum sample with ^{125}I-labeled OC 125, incubated at room temperature for 20 h and washed and measured in a gamma counter.

3. Clinical Application of CA 125 Assay

3.1. Ovarian Malignancies

The vast majority of the available data covering the clinical usefulness of CA 125 focuses on patients with ovarian epithelial malignancies or patients that are felt to be at high risk for this disease and are being screened for it.

3.1.1. Screening of the Population at Risk

Realizing that between 28 (Vasilev et al., 1988) and 78% (Einhorn et al., 1986) of patients who have palpable pelvic masses and a serum CA 125 level of >35 U/mL will have an ongoing malignant disease process, it had been proposed that random screening of patients at risk for gynecologic, and particularly ovarian, malignancies would diagnose these diseases at early stages, prior to their becoming clinically apparent. Unfortunately, published literature does not demonstrate that such screening has lived up to the clinician's expectations.

In a large study of 915 high-risk patients, (Zurawski et al., 1987), CA 125 determinations were useful in <1% of the patients screened. Of seven elevated CA 125 values >65 U/mL, six patients had benign conditions, none had a gynecologic malignancy, and one patient had a colonic malignancy. However, Skates and associates (1990), using a computer-based simulation approach to model the potential impact of screening for ovarian malignancies, claim that random CA 125 determination is an effective tool. Their model predicted that yearly screening would detect approx 60% of cases, with 50% of cases having some years of life saved. In the subgroup of women between 50 and 74 yr of age, an average of 4 yr of life would be saved by the screening. The investigators theorized that each year of life saved would cost between $10,000 and $30,000, with the actual amount being dependent on the false positive rate.

A recent collaborative follow-up study from Sweden (Einhorn et al., 1990) reports the results of annual serum CA 125 determinations in a cohort of women over the age of 40 yr. Of 5550 women evaluated with annual CA 125 determinations, those with initial-screening CA 125 levels ≥30–35 U/mL were followed every 3 mo with serum CA 125 determinations and every 6 mo with physical examinations and transabdominal ultrasound evaluations. An age-matched cohort of women with CA 125 <30–35 U/mL was similarly followed. Elevated CA 125 was noted in 175 women. Six of these women had ovarian malignancies (3.4%). Two patients were in stage IA, two in stage IIB, and two in stage III. In each of these patients, CA 125 had doubled or reached 95 U/mL during a median follow-up of 32 mo. When patients were stratified by age ≤50 or >50, it was evident that this screening protocol failed to diagnose any of the younger patients, but detected malignancies in six of nine patients over the age of 50. Future controlled trials will need to be completed to confirm these findings as well as to determine the impact, if any, on reducing mortality.

3.1.2. Evaluation of Patients with a Pelvic Mass

Though CA 125 has not definitively demonstrated its worth in screening the asymptomatic population at risk, serum determinations are valuable tools when evaluating the patient with a pelvic mass.

Elevated serum CA 125 levels are associated with a variety of benign and malignant causes for pelvic masses. These include endometriosis with endometriomas, salpingo-oophoritis with tubo-ovarian abscess, leiomyomata uteri, adenomyosis, and benign epithelial ovarian neoplasms (Bast et al., 1983; Niloff et al., 1984a; Einhorn et al., 1986b; Malkasian et al., 1986; Pittway and Fayez, 1986; Vasilev et al., 1988; Azziz, 1989), as well as the acknowledged gynecologic malignancies (nonmucinous ovarian epithelial, fallopian tube, metastatic endometrial, primary papillary serous carcinoma arising from the peritoneum, and adenocarcinoma of the endocervix [Niloff et al., 1984; Azziz, 1989; Wik et al., 1989]).

As noted previously, in patients with a palpable pelvic mass, a CA 125 level >35 U/mL may be predictive of a malignant disease process in up to three-fourths of the patients and in as few as slightly more than a quarter. This wide range of positivity is a function of the type of patient population studied. For instance, in a younger population, which is more likely to have nonmalignant causes of elevated CA 125 levels, there is a lower chance that an elevated CA 125 is a true positive.

Malkasian et al. (1988) reported their experience with CA 125 levels used to discriminate benign from malignant disease. They enrolled 158 patients with pelvic masses who were to undergo exploratory celiotomies. When the 68 patients found to have cancer were compared with the 90 patients with benign disease, those with malignancies were significantly older, were more frequently menopausal, and had significantly higher values of serum CA 125. Of patients with benign pelvic masses, 8% had CA 125 levels >65 U/mL, whereas 75% of patients with malignant disease had CA 125 levels >65 U/mL. If only those patients who had frankly malignant, primary, nonmucinous epithelial ovarian carcinomas were considered, CA 125 levels >65 U/mL predicted malignancy with a sensitivity of 91% for all patients. Greater sensitivity and specificity were observed in the postmenopausal subgroup than in the premenopausal subgroup. In the postmenopausal group with a 63% prevalence of ovarian cancer, the positive predictive value was 98% and the negative predictive value was 72%. In a premenopausal population with a 15% prevalence of ovarian cancer, the predictive value for a positive test was 49%, whereas the predictive value for a negative test was 93%. Other authors have demonstrated similar predictive capacities of the test in these different patient groups (O'Connell et al., 1987; Chen et al., 1988; Jacobs et al., 1988).

Finkler et al. (1988) attempted to compare serum CA 125, clinical impression, and ultrasound for accuracy in preoperative diagnosis, i.e., whether a pelvic mass was benign or malignant. When these tests were used individually, the sensitivity and specificity of CA 125 levels were equal to those of a "review" ultrasound. Overall, the sensitivity of clinical impression and original ultrasound were poor. Sensitivity and specificity were highest for CA 125 assays in postmenopausal patients, especially when these were used as the second diagnostic tool. Positive and negative predictive values significantly increased among postmenopausal patients when CA 125 was added to any of the other diagnostic tests evaluated. In conjunction with these tests, measurement of serum CA 125 significantly increased the diagnostic accuracy and thus may have an important role in the preoperative evaluation of women with ovarian masses. Gadducci and associates (1988) have substantiated these impressions.

Several authors have proposed that a "bank" of biochemical tumor markers should be used, rather than a single marker. In theory, utilizing a bank of markers should increase both the sensitivity and specificity of preoperative serum determination by a single tumor marker. This theory, however, has not been fully substantiated (Bast et al., 1984; LaHousen et al., 1987; Schwartz et al., 1987; Stratton et al., 1988).

Patsner et al. (1988a) reported on their investigation comparing lipid-associated sialic acid with CA 125. In their small series (27 patients), serum lipid-associated sialic acid levels correlated well to CA 125 levels during all phases of treatment. There was no significant difference in predictive value of elevated or normal levels, and no added diagnostic worth. Of note is that lipid-associated sialic acid was less expensive than CA 125 and therefore offered an affordable alternative.

3.1.3. Patients with Epithelial Malignancies

In patients who have histologically confirmed ovarian malignancies and an associated CA 125 elevation, serum CA 125 determination has become a standard tool in monitoring clinical course and disease status (Lavin et al., 1987). Elevated CA 125 is an excellent predictor of a positive disease status at the time of second-look laparotomy, whereas negative CA 125 at a second look does not exclude disease (Niloff et al., 1985; Berek et al., 1986).

The rate of fall of CA 125 in patients with a confirmed malignancy and an initially elevated CA 125 level may be predictive of response to chemotherapy. Van Der Burg et al. (1988) followed 85 patients with epithelial ovarian cancer and assessed the prognostic value of the pretreatment serum concentration of CA 125 and its half-life during induction chemotherapy. The focal point of their analysis was time to initial progression and subsequent progression rate. The prechemotherapy CA 125 level had no prognostic value if the patients were stratified by size of tumor. The half-life of CA 125, however, was an independent prognostic variable ($p = 0.01$). Patients with a CA 125 half-life of ≥20 d had a progression rate 3.2 times higher and a significantly shorter median time to progression of only 11 mo, as compared with 43 mo for patients with a CA 125 half-life of <20 d.

Similarly, in patients undergoing second-line therapy, Ng and associates (1989) demonstrated a significant association between clinical response and what they described as CA 125 trend, with a trend being described as a change in CA 125 of ≥26% from baseline value to last value prior to demonstration of clinical response. In eight of 11 patients (73%), increasing CA 125 levels were predictive of progressive disease, whereas in six of eight patients (86%), decreasing values predicted clinical regression. They noted that even in patients with baseline levels <35 U/mL, CA 125 appeared to have some predictive value of disease response.

Efforts have been made to correlate volume of disease to serum CA 125 concentration. To date, these studies have demonstrated little correlation. Goldhirsch et al. (1988), attempting to correlate the serum values of potential markers (such as CA 125, galactosyltransferase, and total sialic acid) with residual tumor mass after initial surgery, studied 43 patients with International Federation of Obstetrics and Gynecology stage IIB, IIIC, and IV ovarian cancer. The sensitivity of galactosyltransferase and sialic acid levels were sufficient to correlate their serum values to the corresponding residual tumor mass. A similar correlation for CA 125 was not demonstrated. Furthermore, 28 patients were histopathologically evaluated for their response to chemotherapy. Determination of these tumor markers did not permit discrimination between small residual disease (<1 cm) and "no evidence of disease." Conversely, progression of disease has been associated with a sensitive increase in the levels of all three markers. CA 125 has been found to be the most useful of the three for distinguishing between responding and nonresponding patients.

3.2. Endometrial Malignancies

Ca 125 is elevated above normal in between 30 and 50% of all patients with endometrial adenocarcinomas. Patients with higher-FIGO-stage malignancies are more likely to have an elevated CA 125 than those with lower-stage malignancies. Panici and associates (1988) noted CA 125 levels >35 U/mL in 30% of patients with stage I disease, 44% of stage II, and 87% of stage III patients, confirming the findings of earlier investigators (Niloff et al., 1984b; Duk et al., 1986). In general, investigators have failed to demonstrate definitively that level of CA 125 elevation is related to tumor differentiation or depth of invasion, though in Duk and associates' small study (1986) that was the case. Preoperative elevated levels do, however, appear to predict those patients that are at increased risk for developing recurrent disease postoperatively or for having occult extrauterine spread of the disease preoperatively (Patsner et al., 1988b). Recent reviews have noted that serum CA 125 levels may reflect the clinical course of the disease and the response to therapy in patients with advanced or recurrent adenocarcinoma of the endometrium (Lootsma-Miklosova et al., 1987; Patsner et al., 1989). Patsner et al. noted that CA 125 levels were more likely to accurately predict disease status in patients with either intraperitoneal disease or pulmonary metastasis. Of the three patients in this review that had recurrence of disease isolated to the vaginal vault, only one had an elevated CA 125 >35 U/mL. Changes in CA 125 levels did not appear to mirror the disease status in this latter group of patients. As is true in patients with epithelial ovarian malignancies, diminishing CA 125 levels predicted resolution of disease in only 40% of patients, whereas rising or persistently elevated levels accurately predicted clinical disease status in 70% of patients. This study suffered severely from the lack of definitive (surgical) documentation of disease status. In a further review of these patients, Patsner reported that all of his patients who suffered from radiation enteritis had elevated CA 125 levels (between 74 and 493 U/mL). At time of exploration, no evidence of recurrent disease was found and CA 125 levels subsequently either returned to normal or significantly declined postoperatively (Patsner et al., 1990).

The absolute value, specificity, and sensitivity of serial monitoring of serum CA 125 levels in patients with endometrial malignancies is yet to be determined and will require a thorough study, including surgical reexploration and/or documentation of disease status.

3.3. Cervical Adenocarcinoma

In his initial review, Niloff (1984a) reported elevated levels of CA 125 in five of six patients with adenocarcinoma of the endocervix. Subsequent investigations have confirmed this finding and demonstrated that elevated serum CA 125 levels prior to treatment correlate well to both the clinical stage of the disease (Duk et al., 1989), and surgically documented extracervical spread (Duk et al., 1990a), and are more likely to be elevated in patients with an adenosquamous cell type. CA 125 levels were noted to be more likely elevated in patients who had abdominal recurrence (15 of 15) than in patients with their recurrence localized to the vaginal vault (4 of 7). A major difficulty with these studies is that Duk uses varying levels of CA 125 as being the upper limits of normal (10 U/mL in some patients and 16 U/mL in others) and uses levels that many investigators would argue are too low to have acceptable specificity. These preliminary studies suggest that there may be some value in serial determinations of serum CA 125 in patients with adenocarcinoma of the cervix, since levels may be able to predict recurrence and clinical course. These observations as yet are unsubstantiated.

3.4. Other Gynecologic Malignancies

Case reports have indicated that CA 125 may be elevated in patients with adenocarcinoma of the fallopian tube (Niloff et al., 1984b; Lootsma-Miklosova et al., 1987) and uterine sarcomas (Patsner and Mann, 1988). Patient numbers are too small to make any definitive comment about the usefulness of this tumor marker in the management of diseases in patients with these malignancies.

References

Azziz, R. (1989), *Obstet. Gynecol. Clin. North Am.* **16,** 221.

Bast, R. C., M. Feeney, H. Lazarus, L. M., Nadler, R. B. Colvin, and R. C. Knapp (1981), *J. Clin. Invest.* **68,** 1331–1337.

Bast, R. C., T. L. Klug, E. Schaetzl, P. Lavin, J. M. Niloff, T. F. Greber, V. R. Zurawski, and R. C. Knapp (1984), *Am. J. Obstet. Gynecol.* **149,** 553–559.

Bast, R. C., T. L. Klug, E. St. John, E. Jenison, J. M. Niloff, H. Lazarus, R. S. Berkowitz, T. Leavitt, C. T. Griffiths, L. Parker, V. R. Zurawski, and R. C. Knapp (1983), *N. Engl. J. Med.* **309,** 883–887.

Berek, J. S., R. C. Knapp, G. D. Malkasian, P. T. Lavin, C. Whitney, J. M. Niloff, and R. C. Bast (1986), *Obstet. Gynecol.* **67,** 685–688.

Chen, D., P. E. Schwartz, L. Xinguo, and Y. Zhan (1988), *Obstet. Gynecol.* **72,** 23–27.

De Bruijn, H. W. A., S. Jager, J. M. Duk, and et al. (1986), *Am. J. Obstet. Gynecol.* **154,** 1088–1091.

Duk, J. M., J. G. Aalders, G. J. Flueren, and H. W. A. de Bruijn (1986), *Am. J. Obstet. Gynecol.* **155,** 1097–1102.

Duk, J. M., J. G. Aalders, M. Krans, and H. W. A. de Bruijn (1989), *Obstet. Gynecol.* **73,** 661–668.

Duk, J. M., H. W. A. de Bruijn, K. H. Groenier, G. J. Fleuren, and J. G. Aalders (1990a), *Cancer* **65,** 1830–1837.

Einhorn, N., K. Sjovall, D. A. Schoenfeld, G. Eklund, R. C. Knapp, R. C. Bast, and V. R. Zurawski (1990), *Program Proc. Am. Soc. Clin. Oncol.* **9,** 157 (abstract 607).

Einhorn, N., R. C. Bast, R. C., Knapp, B. Tjernberg, and V. R. Zurawski (1986b), *Obstet. Gynecol.* **67,** 414–416.

Finkler, N. J., B. Benacerraft, P. T. Lavin, C. Wojciechowski, and R. C. Knapp (1988), *Obstet. Gynecol.* **72,** 659–664.

Gadducci, A., P. Capriello, T. Bartolini, E. Barale E, and et al. (1988), *Eur. J. Gynaecol. Oncol.* **9,** 373–376.

Goldhirsch, A., E. Berger, O. Muller, R. Maibach, S. Misteli, K. Buster, H. Roesler, and K. Brunner (1988), *Oncology* **45,** 281–286.

Jacobs, I., I. Stabile, J. Bridges, P. Kemsley, and et al. (1988), *Lancet* **1**(8580), 268–271.

Jager, W., C. Meier, L. Wildt, W. Sauerbrei, and N. Lang (1988), *Fertil. Steril.* **50(2),** 223–227.

Kabawat, S. E., R. C. Bast, Jr., A. K. Chan, W. R. Welch, R. C. Knapp, R. B. Colvin (1983), *Int. J. Gynecol. Pathol.* **2,** 275–285.

LaHousen, M., H. Stettner, H. Pickel, W. Urdl, and P. Purstner (1987), *Cancer* **60,** 2228–2232.

Lavin, P. T., R. C. Knapp, G. Malkasian, C. W. Whitney, J. S. Berek, and R. C. Bast (1987), *Obstet. Gynecol.* **69,** 223–227.

Lootsma-Miklosova, E., J. B. Aalders, P. H. B. Willemse, and H. W. A. de Bruijn (1987), *Eur. J. Obstet. Gynecol. Reprod. Biol.* **124,** 231–235.

Malkasian, R. D., R. C. Knapp, P. T. Lavin, V. R. Zurawski, K. C. Podratz, C. R. Stanhope, R. Morel, J. S. Berek, R. C. Bast, and R. E. Ritts (1988), *Am. J. Obstet. Gynecol.* **159,** 341–346.

Malkasian, G. D., K. C. Podratz, C. R. Stanhope, R. E. Ritts, V. R. Zurawski (1986), *Am. J. Obstet. Gynecol.* **155,** 515–518.

Marechal, F, G. Berthiot, T. Kritly, M. G. Legrand, and G. Deltour (1989), *Anticancer Res.* **9,** 593–599.

Ng, L. W., H. D. Homesley, R. J. Barrett, C. E. Welander, and L. D. Case (1989), *Am. J. Clin. Oncol.* **12,** 106–109.

Niloff, J. M., R. C. Bast, E. M. Schaetzl, and R. C. Knapp (1985), *Am. J. Obstet. Gynecol.* **151,** 981–986.

Niloff, J. M,., R. C. Knapp, E. Schaetzl, and R. C. Bast (1984a), *Obstet. Gynecol.* **64,** 703–706.

Niloff, J. M., T. L. Klug, E. Schaetzl, V. R. Zurawski, R. C. Knapp, and R. C. Bast (1984), *Am. J. Obstet. Gynecol.* **148,** 1057–1061.

O'Connell, G. J., E. Ryan, K. J. Murphy, and M. Prefontaine (1987), *Obstet. Gynecol.* **70,** 930–932.

Panici, P. B., G. Scambia, G. Baiocchi, L. Perrone, S. Greggi, F. Battaglia, and S. Mancuso (1988), *Gynecol. Obstet. Invest.* **27,** 208–212.

Patsner, B. and W. J. Mann (1988), *Cancer* **62,** 1355–1358.

Patsner, B., J. W. Orr, and W. J. Mann (1990), *Am. J. Obstet. Gynecol.* **162,** 427–429.

Patsner, B., D. J. Tenhoppen, and W. J. Mann (1989), *Eur. J. Gynecol. Oncol.* **10,** 322–325.

Patsner, B., H. Mann, H. Cohen, and M. Loesch (1988b), *Am. J. Obstet. Gynecol.* **158,** 399–402.

Patsner, B., W. J. Mann, M. Vissicchoi, and M. Loesch (1988a), *Gynecol. Oncol.* **30,** 98–103.

Pittway, D. E. and J. A. Fayez (1986), *Fertil. Steril.* **46,** 790–794.

Schwartz, P. E., S. K. Chambers, J. T. Chambers, J. Gutmann, N. Katopodis, and R. Foemmel (1987), *Cancer* **60,** 353–361.

Skates, S. and D. Singer (1990), *Program Proc. Am. Soc. Clin. Oncol.* **9,** 162, (abstract 628).

Stratton, J. A., M. A. Rettenmaier, H. B. Phillips, S. Herabutya, and P. J. DiSaia (1988), *Obstet. Gynecol.* **71,** 20–26.

Van Der Burg, M. E. L., F. B. Lammes, W. L. J. Van Putten, and G. Stoter (1988), *Gynecol. Oncol.* **30,** 307–312.

Vasilev, S. A., J. B. Schlaerth, J. Campeau, and C. P. Morrow (1988), *Obstet. Gynecol.* **71,** 751–756.

Wik, M. R., S. E. Mills, L. P. Dehner, D. J. Bollinger, and R. E. Fechner (1989), *Int. J. Gynecol. Pathol.* **8,** 179–188.

Zurawski, V. R., S. F. Broderick, P. Pickens, R. C. Knapp, and R. C. Bast (1987), *Obstet. Gynecol.* **69,** 606–611.

Chapter 20

CA 242

Pentti Kuusela, Caj Haglund,
Hannu Jalanko, and Peter J. Roberts

1. Biochemistry and Biology

1.1. The CA 242 Epitope

The tumor marker CA 242 is defined by a monoclonal antibody, C-242, which was obtained by immunizing mice with a human colorectal carcinoma cell line, COLO 205 (Lindholm et al., 1985). The chemical structure of the antigenic determinant, which is still largely unresolved, is a sialylated carbohydrate, possibly a type-I chain (Johansson et al., 1991b). The CA 242 is related, but not identical, to the epitopes of well-characterized tumor markers CA 19-9 and CA 50.

1.2. The CA 242 Assay

In serum, CA 242 is found on the same macromolecular mucin complex as CA 19-9 and CA 50. Thereby, it has been possible to set up an immunoassay for CA 242, using antibodies against CA 50 and CA 242 epitopes as "catching" and "detecting" antibodies, respectively (Johansson et al., 1991a). At present, the only com-

From: *Serological Cancer Markers* Edited by Stewart Sell ©1992 The Humana Press, Totowa, NJ

mercially available assay kit is based on a dissociation-enhanced lanthanide fluoroimmunoassay (DELFIA; Pharmacia Diagnostic, Uppsala, Sweden). An upper limit for normal of 20 U/mL, corresponding to the 99.4th percentile of healthy blood donors, has been recommended for the assay (Nilsson et al., 1988). For comparisons between CA 242 and other markers, cutoff values representing the mean concentration + 2 SD found in patients with relevant benign diseases have been used (Kuusela et al., 1991).

2. Immunohistochemical Expression of CA 242

2.1. Expression in Normal Tissues

Knowledge of the tissue expression of CA 242 is still limited. In normal human pancreas CA 242 is typically found in the apical border of some ductal cells (Haglund et al., 1989). Large ducts are more often positive and show stronger staining than the small ducts. Acinar cells and Langerhans' islets do not express CA 242 (Haglund et al., 1989).

Ouyang et al. (1987) demonstrated expression of CA 242 in normal colonic mucosa in about half of the sections studied. Usually columnar epithelial cells and goblet cells are positive without cytoplasmic staining.

2.2. Tissue Expression in Benign Disorders

In chronic pancreatitis more than 90% of the specimens stain for CA 242. The staining pattern resembles that of normal pancreatic tissue, but the intensity is stronger. The extracellular mucus shows intense staining for CA 242.

The CA 242 staining pattern in acute pancreatitis clearly differs from that found in chronic pancreatitis: Mainly small ductal cells and centroacinar cells are positive for CA 242; only a few large ducts show a positive staining reaction. In both forms of pancreatitis, acinar cells and Langerhans' islets are negative for CA 242 (Haglund et al., 1989).

In the colon, dysplastic polyps and mucosa express CA 242 more frequently than normal colonic mucosa, although the differences are not significant (Ouyang et al., 1987).

2.3. Tissue Expression of CA 242 in Pancreatic and Colorectal Cancer

In pancreatic carcinomas, the expression of CA 242 seems to be dependent on the degree of differentiation of the tumor. Haglund et al. (1989) demonstrated that, altogether, 93% of well to moderately differentiated pancreatic adenocarcinomas and all cystadenomas express positive CA 242 staining. The strongest staining is found in the apical border of the cells and in the intraluminal mucus. In areas with very intense expression, diffuse staining is seen in adjacent tissues. Importantly, carcinoma tissue always shows a more intense staining than the surrounding normal tissue.

In less-differentiated tumors the frequency of CA 242 positive specimens is lower (Haglund et al.,1989) The staining is less intense and fewer cells are stained.

There was no clear-cut correlation between histological expression and serum levels of CA 242 (Haglund et al., 1989). High serum values may be found in patients with weak or moderate tissue staining of the tumor. On the other hand, a strong tissue staining may be associated with only slightly elevated or normal serum CA 242 values. In this respect CA 242 seems to behave similarly to CA 50 and CA 19-9 (Haglund et al., 1986; Nishida et al., 1988).

CA 242 is expressed in a majority of colorectal carcinomas. In opposition to the findings on pancreatic tissue, no correlation could be found between the marker expression and tumor classification or staging (Ouyang et al., 1987).

3. Clinical Data

3.1. CA 242 in Serum of Patients with Benign Diseases

As stated by the inventor of the CA 242 assay, 95% of normal healthy blood donors have a serum CA 242 level below 20 U/mL

(Nilsson et al., 1988). Slightly elevated serum levels (up to 125 U/mL) are also found in 5–33% of patients with benign colonic, gastric, hepatic, pancreatic, or biliary tract diseases (Kuusela et al., 1991). Characteristic to CA 242 is the finding that its concentration seldom increases in conjunction with benign pancreatic and biliary tract diseases (Johansson et al., 1991a). Only 5% of the patients with those diseases had an elevated CA 242 level, whereas the corresponding percentages for CA 19-9 and CA 50 were 26 and 33%, respectively (Kuusela et al., 1991).

3.2. Serum CA 242 in Malignant Diseases

The highest percentage of elevated CA 242 serum levels is found in colorectal and pancreatic carcinomas. In a study by Kuusela et al. (1991), patients with colorectal and pancreatic cancer had CA 242 levels above 20 U/mL in 55 and 68%, respectively (Table 1). In these patients the highest marker values (up to 22,100 and 84,000 U/mL, respectively) were usually associated with advanced disease. Johansson et al. (1991a) found higher frequencies of elevated values, i.e., 85% in colorectal cancer and 79% in pancreatic cancer. The differences in colorectal cancer are difficult to explain. In the report of Kuusela et al. (1991), the percentage of elevated values in patients with Dukes C–D carcinomas was not higher than 59%. Johansson et al. (1991a) do not report the stages of patients with colorectal cancer. A large number of patients with advanced disease might partly explain the difference. The difference found in pancreatic cancer is probably explained by differences in the patient material.

Almost half (44%) of the patients with gastric cancer show CA 242 values above the recommended cutoff value (Kuusela et al., 1991). This percentage decreases to 30% when the cutoff value is determined on the basis of benign gastric diseases.

Liver cancers were not associated with elevation of CA 242 (Kuusela et al., 1991). Johansson et al. (1991a) have found elevated CA 242 levels in some patients with ovarian, urinary bladder, and small-cell lung carcinoma.

Table 1
Assay Parameters For CA 242, CA 19-9, CA 5O, and CEA in Patients with Colorectal, Pancreatic and Biliary Diseases*

	CA242 %	CA 19-9 %	CASO %	CEA %
Colorectal diseases: $N = 53$; $n = 29$[a]	>20 U/mL[b]	>37 U/mL	>17 U/mL	>3 ng/mL
Sensitivity				
Dukes A–B	47	16	26	32
Dukes C–D	59	44	47	71
Total	55	34	40	57
Specificity	90	100	97	83
	>29 U/mL[c]	>21 U/mL	>13 U/mL	>9 ng/mL
Sensitivity[d]				
Dukes A–B	31	38	43	11
Dukes C–D	53	47	47	56
Total	45	43	45	40
Pancreatic and billary diseases: $N = 66$; $n = 42$[a]	>20 U/mL[b]	>37 U/mL	>17 U/mL	>3 ng/mL
Sensitivity	68	76	73	59
Specificity	95	74	67	79
	>20 U/mL[c]	>155 U/mL	>145 U/mL	>24 U/mL
Sensitivity[d]	68	61	46	17

*Determined at the recommended and "corrected" cutoff levels.

[a]N = Number of patients with cancer; n = Number of patients with relevant benign disease.

[b]Recommended cutoff levels.

[c]"Corrected" cutoff values determined as the mean + 2SD of levels found in patients with relevant benign diseases.

[d]Sensitivity of the "corrected" cutoff levels representing specificity of 95% for all the assays.

3.3. Comparison of Serum CA 242 with CA 19-9, CA 50, and CEA

In general, the serum CA 242 levels correlate very well to corresponding CA 19-9 and CA 50 levels. The correlation coefficients (r^2 values; linear regression) vary from 0.81 to 0.95 in colorectal, liver, pancreatic, and biliary tract diseases (Kuusela et al., 1991). In gastric diseases the corresponding coefficients were somewhat lower: 0.69 and 0.78, respectively. There was no correlation between CA 242 and CEA, except in gastric diseases, for which an r^2 value of 0.89 was observed between CA 242 and CEA.

CA 242 and CEA are equally often elevated in patients with colorectal cancer. The sensitivities of the markers are reported to be 55 and 57%, respectively, whereas CA 19-9 and CA 50 levels are elevated in 34 and 40%, respectively (Kuusela et al., 1991). Interestingly, CA 242 is more often elevated in Dukes A and B carcinomas (47%) than CEA (32%), CA 19-9 (16%), and CA 50 (26%). When cutoff values based on benign colorectal diseases are used, CA 242, CA 19-9, and CA 50 are elevated in 31–43% and CEA in only 11% of these patients.

CA 242 seems to be slightly less efficient than CA 19-9 and CA 50 in detecting pancreatic cancer when the recommended cutoff values are used. In these patients the high sensitivities of CA 19-9 and CA 50 are hampered by lower specifities, resulting from elevated marker values associated with obstructive biliary tract diseases (Jalanko et al., 1984; Paganuzzi et al., 1985; Haglund et al., 1986, 1987; Habib et al., 1986; Steinberg et al., 1986; Kuusela et al., 1987). Therefore, the use of cutoff values based on benign pancreatic and biliaty tract diseases make the applicability of the test more reliable. Using the "corrected" cutoff values, the CA 242 and CA 19-9 tests showed similar sensitivities (68 and 61%, respectively) whereas the sensitivity of the CA 50 assay was somewhat lower (46%) (Kuusela et al., 1991).

4. Conclusions

CA 242 is a new tumor marker of a carbohydrate nature. It has an expression rather similar to that of CA 19-9 and CA 50, both in tissues and in serum. However, there are certain differences. CA 242 shows a low frequency of elevated values associated with benign pancreatic and biliary tract diseases. This may be an advantage in the diagnosis of pancreatic cancers. To assess the value of CA 242 in patients with colorectal cancer, further studies will be needed.

References

Habib, N. A., M. J. Hersman, F. Haberland, L. Papp, C. B. Wood, and R. N. C. Williamson (1986), *Br. J. Cancer* **53,** 697–699.

Haglund, C., P. Kuusela, H. Jalanko, and P. J. Roberts (1987), *Int. J. Cancer* **39,** 477–481.

Haglund, C., J. Lindgren, P. J. Roberts, P. Kuusela, and S. Nordling (1989), *Br. J. Cancer* **60,** 845–851.

Haglund C., P. J. Roberts, P. Kuusela, T. M. Scheinin, O. Mäkelä, and H. Jalanko (1986), *Br. J. Cancer* **53,** 197–202.

Jalanko, H., P. Kuusela, P. Roberts, P. Sipponen, C. Haglund, and O. Mäkelä (1984), *J. Clin. Pathol.* **37,** 218–222.

Johansson, C., O. Nilsson, and L. Lindholm (1991a), *Int. J. Cancer,* in press.

Johansson, C., O. Nilsson, D. Baeckström, E.-L. Jansson, and A. Lindholm (1991b), *Tumor Biol.,* in press.

Kuusela, P., C. Haglund, and P. J. Roberts (1991), *Br. J. Cancer* **63,** 636–640.

Kuusela, P., C. Haglund, P. J. Roberts, and H. Jalanko (1987), *Br. J. Cancer* **55,** 673–676.

Lindholm, L., C. Johansson, E.-L. Jansson, C. Hallberg, and O. Nilsson (1985), in *Tumor Marker Antigens* (Holmgren, J., ed.), Studentlitteratur, Lund, Sweden, pp. 122–133.

Nilsson, O., E.-L. Jansson, C. Johansson, and L. Lindholm (1988), *J. Tumor Marker Oncol.* **3,** 314.

Nishida, K., H. Miyagawa, T. Yoshikawa, and M. Kondo (1988), *Oncology* **45,** 166–171.

Ouyang, Q., M. Vilen, B. Ravn Juhl, L. Grupe Larsen, and V. Binder (1987), *Acta Pathol. Microbiol. Imrnunol. Scand. Sect. A,* **95,** 177–183.

Paganuzzi, M., M. Onetto, P. Marroni, D. Barone, M. Conio, H. Aste, and V. Pugliesi (1988) *Cancer* **61,** 2100–2108.

Steinberg, W. M., R. Gelfand, K. K. Anderson, J. Glenn, S. H. Kurzman, W. F. Sindelar, and P. P. Toskes (1986), *Gastroenterology* **90,** 343–349.

Chapter 21

Squamous Cell Carcinoma Antigen

Hiroshi Kato

1. Introduction

Squamous cell carcinoma (SCC) antigen, formerly referred to as TA-4, was originally purified from SCC of the uterine cervix (Kato and Torigoe, 1977). Since very few tumor markers have been prepared especially for squamous cell carcinoma, a radioimmunoassay of SCC antigen has become a promising aid for the management of squamous cell carcinoma in a variety of sites. Also, SCC antigen has provided new information regarding the biological nature of squamous cells. Recent reports indicated that the expression of SCC antigen was closely related to the grade of differentiation of squamous cells (Ueda et al., 1984; Suehiro et al., 1986; Hoshina et al., 1986; Kimura et al., 1987; Gion et al., 1987; Cromback et al., 1989) and also to some environmental factors (Kobayashi, 1989). Thus, SCC antigen is an interesting marker not only for detecting malignant lesions, but also for understanding biological behaviors of squamous cells. This chapter will review the clinical features of SCC antigen and discuss current understanding regarding the expression of SCC antigen in squamous cells.

From: *Serological Cancer Markers* Edited by Stewart Sell ©1992 The Humana Press, Totowa, NJ

1.1. Nature of SCC Antigen

Squamous cell carcinoma antigen is a protein, which shows a single peak on SDS polyacrylamide gel electrophoresis. However, extensive charge heterogeneity was found by isoelectric focusing (Kato et al., 1984a). These subfractions of SCC antigen had almost the same molecular weight, ranging from 42,000 to 48,000 Da, and showed at least several epitopes in common. These subfractions are grouped roughly into the acidic fraction and the neutral fraction. Generally, the neutral fraction is present in both the malignant and nonmalignant squamous cells, whereas the acidic fraction is increased mainly in malignant cells. It is also interesting to note that the neutral fraction remains inside the cells, whereas the acidic fraction is released easily outside the cells and appears in the blood circulation (*see* Fig. 1). Little information is available regarding the molecular differences between the acidic and neutral fractions. The epitope analyses using monoclonal antibodies indicated that there was at least one epitope specific for the acidic fraction, whereas more than seven epitopes were present in common in both the acidic and neutral fractions. A preliminary study of DNA sequencing suggested that the gene for these subfractions might be the same. Also, our data with a lectin (PHE-A) affinity column chromatography indicated that some of the acidic fractions would contain sugar chains, suggesting the involvement of sugar chains in heterogeneous expression of this marker (Kato, 1987). Molecular structure of these subfractions is an topic of intense investigation.

2. Factors that Influence the Expression of SCC Antigen

2.1. Differentiation of Squamous Cells

Immunohistochemical studies indicated that SCC antigen was present in the cytoplasm of squamous cells (Kato et al., 1977; Matsuta et al., 1987). This antigen is particularly increased in the keratinizing or large-cell nonkeratinizing types of squamous cell carcinoma (Ueda et al., 1984; Hoshina et al., 1986; Kimura et al., 1987; Gion

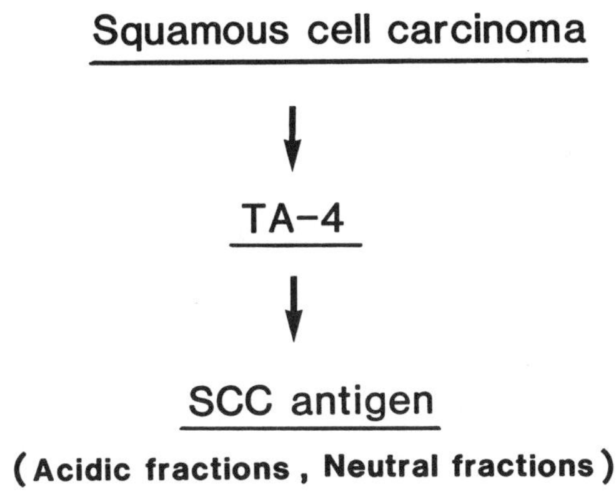

Fig. 1. Preparation of SCC antigen.

et al., 1987). Squamous cell carcinoma antigen is generally negative in the small-cell type of SCC, but the positive rate of serum SCC antigen was almost the same in three types of squamous cell malignancies, with appearance rates of 75% in the keratinizing type, 64.5% in the large-cell nonkeratinizing type, and 70.0% in the small-cell type (Kato, unpublished findings). Thus, the intracellular content and the release of SCC antigen do not necessarily correlate. Since it has been demonstrated that the dominant form of SCC antigen in the circulation is the acidic fraction, the small-cell type of cancer may produce mainly the acidic fraction, but not much neutral fraction, and the amounts of the acidic fraction in these cells would not be enough to be visualized by the ordinary immunostaining method. This hypothesis was supported by a recent study in our laboratory using a cultured cell line, which showed greater production and release of the acidic fraction, but negative staining of SCC antigen by immunohistochemistry (Tsuyama et al., 1991).

Squamous cell carcinoma antigen is also present at the intermediate layer of the nonmalignant squamous epithelium. The basal or parabasal cells are usually negative. It is interesting to note that, in patients with squamous cell carcinoma, SCC antigen of the normal epithelium is increased in the area adjacent to the malignant cells. There is no clear evidence that these normal cells with increased

SCC antigen will change to the malignant in the future, but these results may indicate the influence of some environmental changes related to the appearance of malignant cells. These aspects will be discussed further in the following section.

2.2. Environmental Factors

It was found that mononuclear cells release factors that stimulate the production of acidic fraction in an SCC cell line (Kobayashi, 1989). Immunohistochemical studies using a specific monoclonal antibody showed that the acidic fraction appeared mainly at the periphery of the tumor nest. Recent data also suggested the stimulatory effects of tumor necrosis factor (TNF) on the production of acidic fraction in both malignant and nonmalignant squamous epithelium (Nakamura and Kato, unpublished findings). These findings strongly indicate that the production of acidic fraction is influenced by environmental factors.

It may be surprising that even normal cells produce the acidic fraction of SCC antigen. However, since both the malignant and nonmalignant cells originate from a single cell during embryogenesis, they do carry the same genetic information. Therefore, any types of cell may be able to produce SCC antigen, once they receive proper signals necessary for activating the gene. Tumor necrosis factor may be one such signal. Knowledge of the effects of host environment on the production of SCC antigen would be helpful for understanding the appearance of false positive data in the circulation and also should be taken into consideration for evaluating the values of circulating tumor markers.

3. Clinical Value of SCC Antigen

3.1. Serum SCC Antigen in Healthy Women

In the initial studies using a double-antibody radioimmunoassay, the cutoff of serum SCC antigen was 2.0 ng/mL (Kato et al., 1987c). The present immunoradiometric assay can detect 0.3 ng/mL of serum SCC antigen, and the new cutoff is 1.5 ng/mL. Recently, the sensitive enzyme immunoassay (IMx assay) has been em-

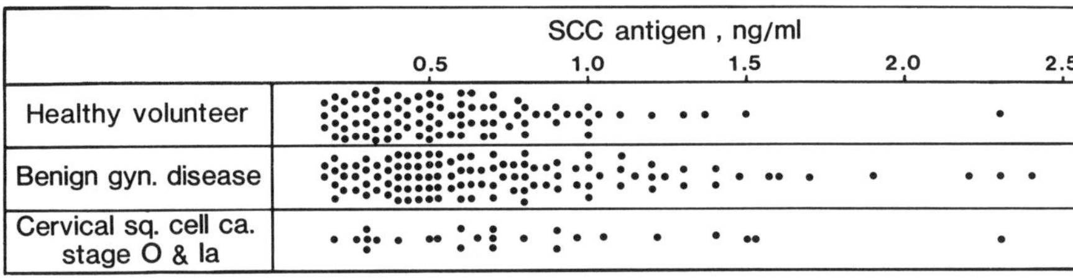

Fig. 2. Serum SCC antigen values in healthy women and in patients with benign gynecological diseases and early stages of cervical squamous cell carcinoma.

ployed (Takeshima et al., 1990). The IMx assay is fully automated and can detect 0.05 ng/mL of serum SCC antigen. Figure 2 shows serum SCC antigen values in healthy women and in patients with benign gynecological diseases. Mean serum SCC antigen levels were 0.57 + 0.04 ng/mL in healthy women and 0.73 + 0.45 ng/mL in benign gynecological diseases, respectively. It has been expected that the sensitive assay can lower the cutoff and make it easier to detect early cancer. However, approx 5% of healthy women still showed values >1.5 ng/mL. Also, the distribution patterns of serum SCC antigen in the controls were essentially the same as that in patients with early cervical cancer, which indicates that SCC antigen is not very useful in the detection of early cancer. On the other hand, each individual case shows relatively constant serum antigen values with a mean daily variation of approx 24%. Individualizing the cutoff may be helpful to identify an early rise of serum SCC antigen, particularly while monitoring recurrent disease.

3.2. False Positive in Benign Disease

It is now clear that SCC antigen is present in the normal squamous epithelium, and its production is further stimulated by environmental factors. Circulating SCC antigen is thus elevated in several benign lesions of squamous cells, including pulmonary disease (severe infections) or skin disease (pemphigus, eczema, or psoriasis) (Kudo et al., 1988; Alajaji et al., 1988; Numahara et al., 1989) (Table 1). Renal or hepatic dysfunctions also influence the metabolism

Table 1
Some Benign Diseases
that Show False Positive Serum SCC Antigen[a]

	Positive rates, range
Benign gynecological disease ovarian tumor, submucus myoma	4.7%, 0.1–5.0 ng/mL
Pulmonary disease pneumonia, bronchitis	12.2%, 0.5–5.0 ng/mL
Skin disease (psoriasis, pemphygus, eczema	85.0%, 1.0–90 ng/mL

[a]Data derived from Kato and Torigoe, 1977; Kudo et al., 1988; Alajaji et al., 1988; Numahara et al., 1989; Duk et al., 1989b.

of SCC antigen, resulting in an increase in circulating levels. In fact, serum SCC antigen was elevated in some patients on hemodialysis (Kato, unpublished findings). On the other hand, cachexia in advanced stage of malignancies, which is usually associated with renal dysfunction, is not always associated with a rise of serum SCC antigen. It should also be noted that the false positive results may often be caused by contamination with saliva or sweat during the assay procedure. Large amounts of SCC antigen are present in the saliva, sweat, or respiratory secretion as a result of destructon of normal squamous cells. In practice, technicians in laboratories should therefore be required to mask during the assay of SCC antigen.

3.3. SCC Antigen in Malignant Diseases

3.31. Cervical Cancer

A number of reports have appeared regarding serum SCC antigen in cervical cancer (Kato et al., 1987c; de Bruijn et al., 1987; Cazin et al., 1987; Magdelenat et al., 1987; Torre et al., 1987; Fruith and Daxenbichler, 1988). The positive rates of serum SCC antigen are increased according to the clinical stage, showing 12.3% in stage 0, 32.9% in stage I, 65.6% in stage II, 86.5% in stage III, 92.2% in stage IV, and 87.0% in recurrent diseases (Table 2). In general, high pretreatment values of serum SCC antigen indicated the presence

Table 2
Positive Rates of Serum SCC Antigen in Patients with Squamous Cell Carcinoma

	Clinical stage					
	0	I	II	III	IV	Recurrence
Cervix	40/226 (12.3%)	113/343 (32.9%)	214/326 (65.6%)	166/192 (86.5%)	47/51 (92.2%)	100/115 (87.0%)
Lung	– –	28/88 (31.8%)	41/95 (43.2%)	101/160 (63.1%)	55/97 (56.7%)	9/12 (75.0%)
Esophagus	– –	0/11 –	8/40 (20.0%)	13/30 (43.3%)	23/46 (50.0%)	14/17 (82.4%)
Head and neck	– –	8/49 (16.3%)	18/64 (28.1%)	43/107 (40.2%)	61/112 (54.5%)	12/15 (80.0%)

Data derived from Kato et al., 1987c; de Bruijn et al., 1987; Senekjian et al., 1987; Cazin et al., 1987; Magdelenat et al., 1987; Torre et al., 1987; Bugiardini et al., 1987; Ebert et al., 1987; Johnson et al., 1987; Mino et al., 1988; Fruith and Daxenbichler, 1988.

of unresectable tumor (Kato et al., 1982) and were often associated with poor prognosis (Kato et al., 1983). Furthermore, since the metabolic clearance of circulating SCC antigen is rapid, this marker is useful for monitoring disease progress (Kato et al., 1979; Maruo et al., 1985). Serum SCC antigen decreases, usually under the cutoff value, within 2 d after complete tumor resection, and a rapid decrease in antigen value during the radiotherapy or chemotherapy indicated the regression of tumor. Interestingly, Maruo et al. reported that serum SCC antigen values were increased transiently during radiotherapy, probably reflecting the biological response of tumor cells (Maruo et al., 1985). Yabushita et al. (1988) also demonstrated that the production of SCC antigen was stimulated by anticancer drug. These effects of therapy may be seen in clinical practice.

In recurrent disease of cervical cancer, approx 87% of patients showed elevations in serum SCC antigen levels (Kato et al., 1984b). The clinical implication is particularly clear for distant recurrences, which are often difficult to detect by conventional screening methods. The lead time of serum SCC antigen to other clinical signs of recurrence was 3.1 mo for distant recurrence (Fig. 3). Since a positive cytological smear test is usually the first indicaiton of vaginal recurrence, a combination of SCC antigen and vaginal-smear testing would be promising for monitoring recurrent cervical cancer.

Cervical adenocarcinoma showed a positive rate of 17–33% in serum SCC antigen, but endometrial carcinoma is usually negative for serum SCC antigen (Senekjian et al., 1987; Duk et al., 1989a).

In an attempt to use SCC antigen for detecting early cancer, Suehiro et al. applied flow cytometric analysis of cervical exfoliated cells (Suehiro et al., 1986). The cell specimens from patients with cervical cancer were immunostained by an antibody against SCC antigen and applied to flow cytometry. Approximately 82% of patients with cervical squamous cell carcinoma showed abnormal patterns on histogram. Nozawa et al. also reported the usefulness of immunostaining of SCC antigen in cervical smear (Nozawa et al., 1986). These approachs would be useful for detecting early cancer.

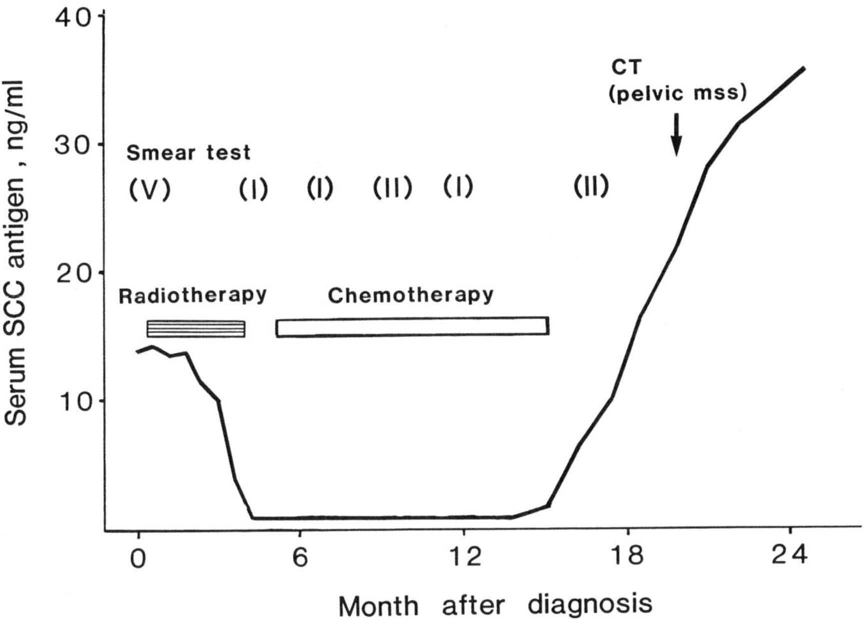

Fig. 3. Serum SCC antigen values in a patient with cervical squamous cell carcinoma.

3.3.2. Lung Cancer

Serum SCC antigen is a useful marker in squamous cell carcinoma of the lung, with a positive rate of 54%. The positive rate is increased in advanced stages of disease, and serial determinations of serum SCC antigen is correlated to the progress of the disease (Johnson et al., 1987; Ebert et al., 1987; Bugiardini et al., 1987; Mino et al., 1988; Body et al., 1990). Regarding the detection of recurrent disease, Mino et al. demonstrated that serum SCC antigen was abnormal in 14 of 16 patients (88%) with recurrent carcinoma (Mino et al., 1988). On the other hand, the positive rate of serum SCC antigen is low in other histological types of lung cancer, e.g., 14.8% in adenocarcinoma, 14.3% in small-cell carcinoma, and 15.2% in large-cell carcinoma. The limited diagnostic value of SCC antigen for these malignancies may be increased by the use of other tumor markers, such as CEA for adenocarcinoma and neuron-specific enolase (NSE) for small-cell carcinoma. Several benign diseases that showed positive serum SCC antigen included severe pneumonia and bronchitis.

3.3.3. Skin Cancer

In 1986, Maruguchi et al. presented a case report on a patient with squamous cell carcinoma of the skin who had an elevation of serum SCC antigen. Yagi et al. (1987) also reported that serum SCC antigen was a useful marker in patients with squamous cell carcinoma of the skin. Squamous cell carcinoma antigen thus has been applied to testing for skin cancer. On the other hand, serum SCC antigen is often elevated in nonmalignant skin lesions. The positive rates were 86.1% in patients with psoriasis, 83.3% in cases with eczema, and 80.0% in those with pemphigus. The values of serum SCC antigen were surprisingly high in these benign diseases, and sometimes reached nearly 100 ng/mL. Duk et al. demonstrated the correlation of serum SCC antigen values and the percentage of involvement of the body surface in psoriasis (Duk et al., 1989b). Interestingly, serum SCC antigen is usually negative in bullous pemphigoid, which will provide an interesting question about the production or secretion of this marker in the epidermal cells (Kudo et al., 1988). Recently, Numa et al. found that TNF stimulated the production of SCC antigen in the normal squamous epithelium (Numa and Kato, unpublished findings). Studies regarding the production of SCC antigen in benign skin lesions may be a useful model to investigate the false positive appearance of this marker in the circulation.

3.3.4. Head and Neck

Most head and neck cancers are squamous cell carcinoma and express SCC antigen (Mino et al., 1988; Yamanaka et al., 1988; Yoshimura et al., 1988; Fischback et al., 1990). The positive rates of serum SCC antigen were 34.9% in laryngeal cancer, 22.2% in hypopharyngeal cancer, 28.6% in nasopharyngeal cancer, and 38.5% in maxillary carcinoma (Mino et al., 1988; Yamanaka et al., 1988; Yoshimura et al., 1988). Yoshimura et al. (1988) demonstrated the correlation of serum SCC antigen values and tumor extension in the maxillary sinus cancer, showing the positive rates of 0% in stage 0, 20% in stage I, 14.3% in stage II, 42.9% in stage III, and 77.8% in stage IV disease. SCC antigen was also useful for detection of recur-rence of head and neck cancer.

3.3.5. Cancer of the Digestive Tract

Several reports indicated that serum SCC antigen could be a useful marker in oesophageal cancer (Kitamura et al., 1985; Gion et al., 1987; Burtin et al., 1987). The detection rate of serum SCC antigen is usually low in early stages of disease, but 40–50% in stage III and IV disease. Also, Petrelli et al. (1988) reported the elevation of serum SCC antigen in 11 of 14 patients with anal cancer.

3.3.6. Ovarian and Urogenital Cancer

Some of the ovarian squamous cell carcinoma showed positive values of serum SCC antigen, but the incidence rate is low. Recently Kimura et al. (1989) reported that serum SCC antigen was elevated with the malignant transformation of mature cystic teratoma of the ovary. The ovarian mature teratoma is generally screened by ultrasonography or X-ray examination, but differential diagnosis of malignant change is often difficult before surgical biopsy. Serum SCC antigen would, therefore, be a useful aid in clinical practice.

Few reports are available regarding the use of SCC antigen in urogenital cancer. Wishnow et al. demonstrated the positive values of serum SCC antigen in five of 11 patients with penile cancer and one of three patients with urethral cancer (Wishnow et al., 1989). Tsukamoto et al. also reported that serum SCC antigen was positive in patients with pure transitional cell carcinoma of uroepithelial carcinoma (personal communication).

4. Future of SCC Antigen

Discovery of the molecular heterogeneity of SCC antigen has extended our interest to the biological role of this marker in squamous cells. The neutral fraction is present in both the malignant and nonmalignant cells and appears to reflect some biological events related to the differentiation or multiplication of squamous cells. The acidic fraction is of particular interest. It is not only related to the grade of differentiation, but is influenced by host environmental factors. It is not fully understood what the expression of acidic fraction means in the pathogenesis of squamous cells. However, it is at least clear that SCC antigen is a useful aid not only as a tumor marker for malignant lesions, but also as a cell marker for nonmalignant changes of squamous cells. More attention should be focused on the mechanism for the expression of SCC antigen, e.g., determination of DNA sequence, which will provide useful information for understanding the biological behavior of squamous cells, perhaps different from the traditional information based on the morphological evaluation.

Acknowledgment

The experimental work from this laboratory was supported in part by a Grant-in-Aid for Cancer Research (56-17, 58-22) from the Ministry of Health and Welfare and by a Grant-in-Aid for Scientific Research (548286, 60480369, 63570782) from the Ministry of Education, Science, and Culture, Japan.

References

Alajaji, J. T., M. H. Courey, H. A. Azar, K. M. Ries, P. M. Skipper, and J. N. Endicott (1988),*Cancer* **62,** 2291–2296.

Body, J. J., J. P. Sculier, N. Raymakers, M. Paesmans, P. Ravez, P. Libert, M. Richez, G. Dabouis, H. Lacroix, G. Bureau, J. Thiriaux, J. Lecomte, D. Brohee, P. Mommen, J. Fruhling, and J. Klastersky (1990), *Cancer* **65,** 1552–1556.

de Bruijn, H. W. A., J. Bouma, M. Krans, H. Boonstra, R. von der Seijde, and J. G. Aalder (1987), in *SCC Antigen in the Management of Squamous Cell Carcinoma* (H. Kato, H. W. A. de Bruijn, W. Ebert, R. B. Herberman, and J. T. Johnson, eds.), Excerpta Medica, Princeton, NJ, pp. 18–33.

Bugiardini, G., M. Capelli, L. Plate, D. Bianchi, F. Falcone, M. Faraca, and P. Lagatta (1987), in *SCC Antigen in the Management of Squamous Cell*

Carcinoma (H. Kato, H. W. A. de Bruijn, W. Ebert, R. B. Herberman, and J. T. Johnson, eds.), Excerpta Medica, Princeton, NJ, p. 175.

Burtin, P., A. K. Ben Bouali, J. Boyer, A. Daver, F. Larra, and J. Ronceray (1987), in *SCC Antigen in the Management of Squamous Cell Carcinoma* (H. Kato, H. W. A. de Bruijn, W. Ebert, R. B. Herberman, and J. T. Johnson, eds.), Excerpta Medica, Princeton, NJ, pp. 142–148.

Cazin, J.-L., P. Gosselin, M.-C. Demaille, C. Sulman, and J.-P. Dehaut (1987), in *SCC Antigen in the Management of Squamous Cell Carcinoma* (H. Kato, H. W. A. de Bruijn, W. Ebert, R. B. Herberman, and J. T. Johnson, eds.), Excerpta Medica, Princeton, NJ, pp. 64–69.

Cromback C., A. Scharl, M. Vierbuchen, H. Wurz, and A. Bolte (1989), *Cancer* **63,** 1337–1342.

Duk, J. M., J. D. Aalders, G. J. Fleuren, M. Krans, and H. W. A. de Bruijn (1989a), *Obstet. Gynecol.* **73,** 661–667.

Duk, J. M., P. C. van Voorst Vader, K. A. ven Hoor, H. Hollema, H. M. G. Doeglas, and H. W. A. de Bruijn (1989b), *Cancer* **64,** 1652–1656.

Ebert, W., K. W. Kayse, and H. Bulzebruck (1987), in *SCC Antigen in the Management of Squamous Cell Carcinoma* (H. Kato, H. W. A. de Bruijn, W. Ebert, R. B. Herberman, and J. T. Johnson, eds.), Excerpta Medica, Princeton, NJ, pp. 154–161.

Fischback, W., T. Meyer, and K. Barthel (1990), *Cancer* **65,** 1321–1324.

Fruith, L. C. and G. Daxenbichler (1988), *Gynecol. Obstet. Invest.* **26,** 77–82.

Gion, M., R. Mione, R. Dittadi, G. Bruscagnin, C. Tremolada, C. Zari, and D. Palma (1987), in *Antigen in the Management of Squamous Cell Carcinoma* (Kato, H., H. W. A. de Bruijn, W. Ebert, R. B. Heberman, and J. T. Johnson, eds.), Excerpta Medica, Princeton, NJ, pp. 130–141.

Hoshina M., A. Kimura, K. Shibata, T. Maruo, and M. Mochizuki (1986), *Asia Oceania J. Obstet. Gynaecol.* **12,** 119–126.

Johnson, J. T., R. L. Wagner, D. E. Eibling, and S. Su (1987), in *SCC Antigen in the Management of Squamous Cell Carcinoma* (H. Kato, H. W. A. de Bruijn, W. Ebert, R. B. Herberman, and J. T. Johnson, eds.), Excerpta Medica, Princeton, NJ, pp. 112–123.

Kato, H. (1987), *Acta Obstet. Gynaecol.* **39,** 1204–1212.

Kato, H. and T. Torigoe (1977), *Cancer* **40,** 1621–1626.

Kato H., T. Nagaya, and T. Torigoe (1984a), *Gann* **75**, 433–435.

Kato, H., F. Miyauchi, H. Morioka, T. Fujino, and T. Torigoe (1979), *Cancer* **43,** 585–590.

Kato, H., H. Morioka, H. Tsutsui, S. Aramaki, and T. Torigoe (1982), *Cancer* **50,** 1294–1296.

Kato, H., H. Morioka, S. Aramaki, K. Tamai, and T. Torigoe (1983), *Am. J. Obstet. Gynecol.* **145,** 350–354.

Kato, H., K. Tamai, H. Morioka, M. Nagai, T. Nagaya, and T. Torigoe (1984b), *Cancer* **54,** 1544–1546.

Kato, H., H. Morioka, K. Hashimoto, Y. Suehiro, K. Hayashi, M. Kobayashi, and T. Torigoe (1987a), in *SCC Antigen in the Management of Squamous Cell Carcinoma* (H. Kato, H. W. A. de Bruijn, W. Ebert, R. B. Herberman, and J. T. Johnson, eds.), Excerpta Medica, Princeton, NJ, pp. 1–15.

Kato, H., Y. Suehiro, H. Morioka, T. Torigoe, A. Myoga, K. Sekiguchi, and I. Ikeda (1987b), *Jpn. J. Cancer Res. (Gann)* **78,** 1246–1250.

Kimura, A., T. Maruo, M. Hoshima, and M. Mochizuki (1987), *J. Jpn. Soc. Cancer Ther.* **22,** 1159–1162.

Kimura, T., M. Inoue, A. Miyake, O. Tanizawa, Y. Oka, K. Amemiya, H. Mineta, R. Neki, H. Nishino, K. Horishige, and T. Yanagida, (1989), *Cancer* **64,** 480–483.

Kitamura, M., H. Matuda, H. Matsuura, H., Kai, H., Kamio, and K. Sugimachi (1985), *J. Jpn. Surg. Soc.* **86,** 1561.

Kobayashi, M. (1989), *Acta Obstet. Gynecol. Jpn.* **41,** 412–418.

Kudo, H., M. Yamamoto, Y. Miyachi, K. Danno, and S. Imamura (1988), *Br. J. Dermatol.* **118,** 471–474.

Magdelenat, H., J. Fenton, and A. Ouhajjou (1987), in *SCC Antigen in the Management of Squamous Cell Carcinoma* (H. Kato, H. W. A. de Bruijn, W. Ebert, R. B. Herberman, and J. T. Johnson, eds.), Excerpta Medica, Princeton, NJ, pp. 70–74.

Maruguchi, Y., H. Yagi, T. Mitani, K. Danno, and S. Imamura (1986), *Hifu Rinsho* **28,** 783–786.

Maruo, T., K. Shibata, A. Kimura, M. Hoshina, and M. Mochizuki (1985), *Cancer* **56,** 302–308.

Matsuta M., T. Kababu, and I. Nishiya (1987), *Acta Histochem. Cytochem.* **20,** 75–85.

Mino, N., A. Iio, and K. Hamamoto (1988), *Cancer* **62,** 730–734.

Nozawa, S., M. Okada, D. Tsai, K. Sekiguchi, S. Kurihara, H. Kato, and T. Torigoe (1986), *J. Jpn. Soc. Clin. Cytol.* **25,** 402–411.

Numahara, T., K. Nakashima, S. Yamamoto, and M. Nishimoto (1989), *Dermatologica* **178,** 73,74.

Petrelli, N., N. Shaw, A. Bhargava, L. Herrera, B. Sischy, J. Daufelet, and A. Mittelman (1988), *Proc. Am. Assoc. Cancer Res.* **48,** 182.

Senekjian, E. K., J. M. Young, P. A. Weiser, C. E. Spencer, S. E. Magic, and A. Herbst (1987), *Am. J. Obstet. Gynecol.* **157,** 433–439.

Suehiro, Y., H. Kato, M. Nagai, and T. Torigoe (1986), *Cancer* **57,** 1380.

Takeshima, N., K. Nakamura, O. Takeda, H. Morioka, H. Tamura, N. Takasugi, and H. Kato (1990), *Tumor Biol.* **11,** 167–172.

Torre, G. C., E. Chisale, V. Barbetti, R. Rembado, D. Bianchi, G. Bugiardini, M. Capelli, L. Plate, A. Marabini, C. Orlandi, E. Cortesi, and A. Vecchione (1987), in *SCC Antigen in the Management of Squamous Cell Carcinoma* (H. Kato, H. W. A. de Bruijn, W. Ebert, R. B. Herberman, and J. T. Johnson, eds.), Excerpta Medica, Princeton, NJ, pp. 78–85.

Tsuyama, S., K. Hashimoto, K. Nakamura, H. Tamura, K. Sasaki, and H. Kato (1991), *Tumor Biol.* **12,** 28–34.
Ueda, G., T. Inoue, M. Yamasaki, M., Inoue, Y. Tanaka, K. Hiramatsu, J. Saito, T. Nishino, T., and Y. Abe (1984), *Int. J. Gynecol. Pathol.* **3,** 291–298.
Wishnow, K. I., D. E. Johnson, and H. A. Fritsche (1989), *Int. J. Biol. Markers* **4,** 226–228.
Yabushita, H., Y. Nakagawa, K. Sawaguchi, M. Noguchi, and M. Ishihara (1988), *Asia Oceania J. Obstet. Gynaecol.* **14,** 493–500.
Yagi, H., K. Danno, and Y. Maruguchi (1987), *Arch. Dermatol.* **123,** 902–906.
Yamanaka, N., T. Himi, Y. Harabuchi, K. Hoki, and A. Kataura (1988), *Cancer* **62,** 1932–1939.
Yoshimura, Y., T. Harada, M. Oka, T. Sugihara, T., and H. Kishimoto (1988), *Int. J. Oral Maxillofac. Surg.* **17,** 49–53.

Chapter 22

Tumor-Marker Detection by Isotachophoresis in Porous Membranes

Bence Jones Protein in Chronic Lymphocytic Leukemia and Non-Hodgkin's Lymphoma

Garri I. Abelev and Eleonora R. Karamova

1. Introduction

Isotachophoresis (ITP) is a very powerful electrophoretic method for separation of native macromolecules as well as substances of low molecular weight (Haglund, 1970; Chrambach, 1980). ITP combines very effective concentration of the substances with their sharp separation according to electrophoretic mobility of each component. Since ITP is hardly compatible with electroosmosis, it is usually carried out in free medium, as in capillary electrophoresis, or in gels lacking electroosmotic properties. We have modified ITP using highly "electroosmotic" cellulose acetate (CAM) as a supporting medium (Abelev and

From: *Serological Cancer Markers* Edited by Stewart Sell ©1992 The Humana Press, Totowa, NJ

Karamova, 1982, 1984). This modification (ITP-CAM) has two major advantages over "standard" ITP:

1. ITP-CAM exploits electroosmotic flow in CAM to create very effective counterflow, which completely equilibrates the electrophoretic migration of the separated components. This permits the use for analysis of highly diluted solutions of proteins or other macromolecules, which are transferred by counterflow to the ITP area, concentrated, and separated in this area.
2. The concentrated and separated bands of macromolecules on CAM can be easily detected by different immunochemical methods: immunodiffusion, immunoelectrophoresis, immunofixation, or immunoblotting. Hence, ITP-CAM is an extremely useful technique for analysis of low-protein biological fluids, such as urine, cerebrospinal and amniotic fluids, tears, saliva, and so on.

New possibilities were created by using nitrocellulose membranes (NCM) for ITP. The very strong electroosmotic counterflow created by ITP in NCM was used for the consecutive transfer of different immunoreagents to proteins (antigens or antibodies) fixed on NCM. This permits the performance of multistep immunochemical reactions, including immunoblotting or ELISA, in a semiautomatic way (Abelev and Karamova, 1989; Abelev et al., 1989). We have used ITP-CAM in combination with different kinds of immunodevelopment for detecting monoclonal Ig light chains (Bence Jones protein, BJP) produced by neoplastic B-cells in vitro or in vivo (Abelev et al., 1983, 1990; Abelev and Karamova, 1987). It was possible to develop a very simple immunoassay for detection of BJP in chronic lymphocytic leukemia (CLL) and non-Hodgkin's lymphoma (NHL), which was used for diagnosis, monitoring, and detection of residual disease in clinical remission of these conditions.

This chapter will consider

1. The principle of ITP-CAM and ITP-NCM;
2. Their application for BJP detection in CLL and NHL; and
3. Some further perspectives on ITP-CAM and ITP-NCM in tumor-marker studies.

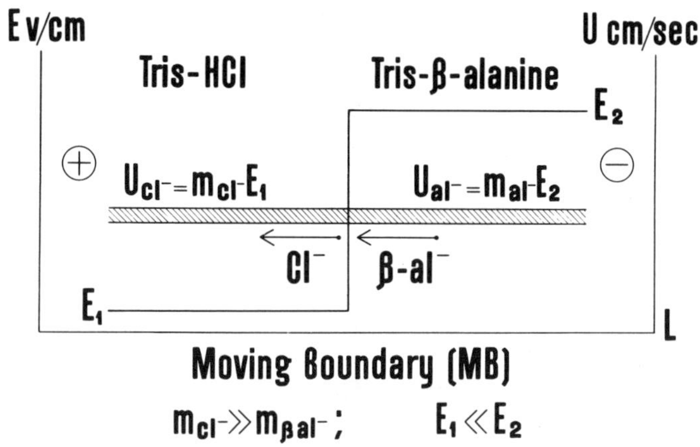

Fig. 1. Main parameters of isotachophoresis (explanations in the text).

2. Principle

Isotachophoresis (ITP)* is discontinuous electrophoresis that uses two buffer solutions, including a common cation (for instance, $Tris^+$) but different anions: a fast-moving, leading anion (L^-), e.g., Cl^-, and a slow-migrating, terminating one (T^-), e.g., β-alanine$^-$ (Fig. 1). In this case, to provide the requirement of constant current, the leap of potential is formed on the moving boundary (MB) between L^- and T^- (Fig. 1A), so that $E_1 \cdot m_{Cl} = E_2 \cdot m_{\beta al}$, where E_1 and E_2 represent the potential gradient in the area of L^- and T^-, and m_{Cl} and $m_{\beta al}$ represent the electrophoretic mobilities of Cl^- and β-alanine$^-$, respectively. Since $m_{Cl} >> m_{\beta al}$, $E_1 << E_2$. If protein, p, is present in terminating buffer and $m_p > m_{\beta al}$, but $< m_{Cl}$, the protein will migrate faster than β-alanine$^-$, but will not cross the MB, because it is slower than Cl^-, forming the front of MB. This means that p is expected to be separated from terminating buffer and condensed on the MB as a distinct band (Fig. 2) when $E_1 \cdot m_{Cl} = E_p \cdot m_p = E_2 \cdot m_{\beta al}$, where E_p is a potential gradient in p area. Since mE is the velocity (U) of the

*Anionic ITP, commonly used in the work with anionic biological macromolecules, is discussed here.

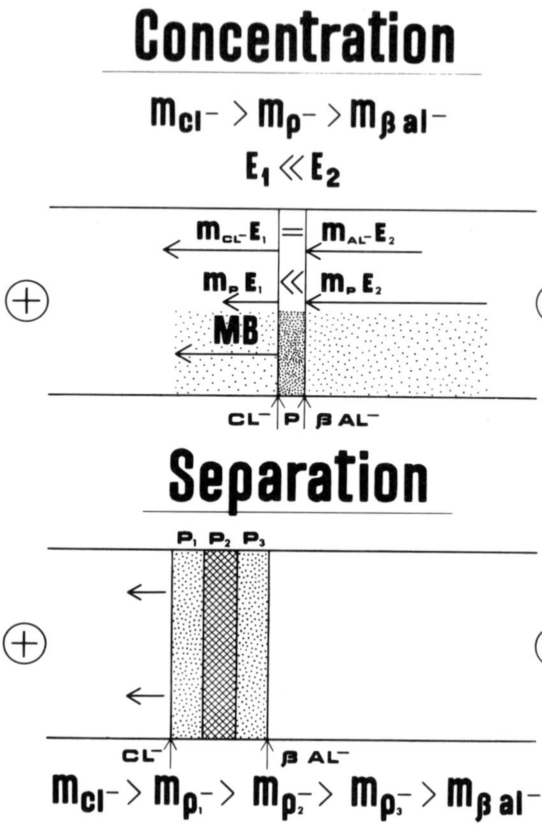

Fig. 2. Protein concentration and separation during isotachophoresis (explanation in the text).

given anion, and it is the same for each of three anions, they will migrate with the same velocity, creating isotachophoresis.

In the case in which terminating buffer contains several kinds of p anions, but each of them has $m_{\mathrm{Cl}}>m_p>m_{\beta\mathrm{al}}$, each component at equilibrium will form its own band, according to the rule $m_{\mathrm{Cl}}{\cdot}E_1 = m_p{\cdot}E_p = m_{\beta\mathrm{al}}{\cdot}E_2$ (Fig. 2). Thus, ITP concentrates protein bands from the diluted solutions and separates them from each other at the same time. The final results are not dependent on the initial presence of

p in terminating or leading buffer, or on the initial concentration of p in solution.

2.1. Counterflow ITP

Let one carry out ITP in porous membranes possessing electroosmotic properties (EO), such as CAM or NCM. Then the fluid incorporated into the membrane should move in the electric field from the anode to the cathode (opposite to MB during ITP), and the rate of this migration (U_{EO}) is proportional to E in the given area of the membrane ($U_{EO} = kE$). Since in ITP $E_{Cl}<E_p<E_{\beta al}$, then $U_{EO \cdot Cl}<U_{EO \cdot p}<U_{EO \cdot \beta al}$, which means that the inflow of the fluid to Cl^-/p^- and $p^-/\beta al^-$ boundaries will not compensate for the outflow from them. That is incompatible with ITP. However, this "incompatibility" is overcome by the fact that the liquid in the membrane creates an inseparable layer, which cannot be interrupted on the L/p or p/T boundaries. Therefore, the average U_{EO} should be established and will be roughly proportional to the average potential on the membrane ($U_{EO}=kE_{av}$). If ITP is carried out at constant voltage, E_{av} is not changing, so as U_{EO}. At the same time the rate of MB migration is progressively dropping when it migrates along the membrane, since the resistance of the membrane is rising. At a certain point U_{MB} will be completely counterbalanced by the electroosmotic flow. When this state is reached and the MB is stopped relative to the supporting membrane, all the anions participating in ITP are stopped on the membrane. Therefore, $m_L \cdot E_L = m_p \cdot E_p = m_T \cdot E_T = {}^-U_{EO}$. Thus, any protein with $m_p > m_T$ present in the T area will migrate electrophoretically to MB, and the same protein present in the L area will be transferred by EO counterflow to MB. Hence, if the sample containing trace amounts of several proteins is placed on the membrane in the L area, in front of MB, it will be soaked into membrane and "pumped" through MB by EO, whereas the proteins will be stopped on MB, condensed into narrow bands, and separated from each other according to their electrophoretic mobilities. Addition to the sample of ampholytes with intermediate mobilities will create spacers between the bands. The described

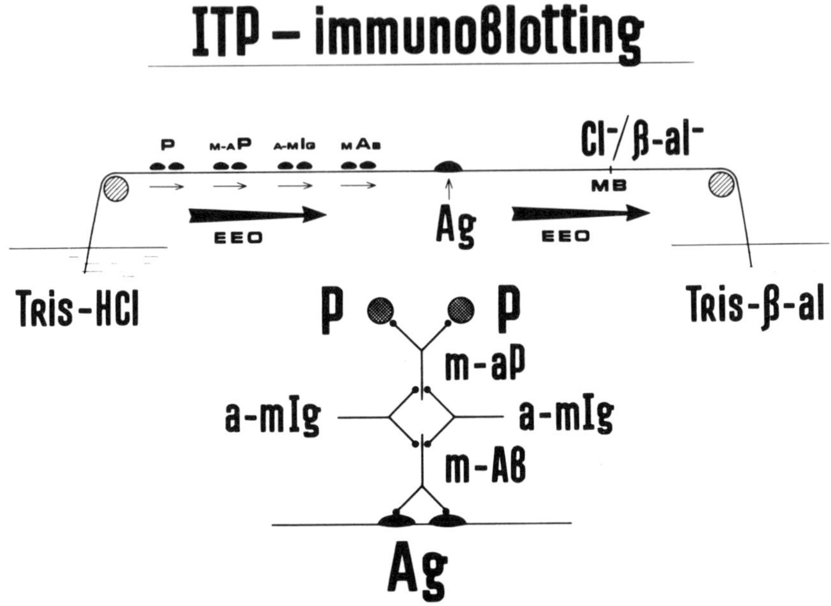

Fig. 3. Counterflow ITP on nitrocellulose membrane. Immunoenzymatic detection of antigens and antibodies. Ag, antigen; m-AB, mouse monoclonal antibody; a-mIg, rabbit or goat antimouse; IgG; m-aP, mouse monoclonal antiperoxidase; P, horseradish peroxidase; MB, moving boundary in stationary position; EEO, electroosmotic flow.

events exactly take place during ITP on CAM, i.e., on the protein nonabsorbing membrane. When Cl^- and β-alanine$^-$ anions are used as leading and terminating ions, respectively, the ITP acts effectively for separating proteins with mobilities of serum albumin–immunoglobulin ranks (Abelev and Karamova, 1982, 1984, 1987).

ITP opens quite different possibilities when carried out on a protein-absorbing support, such as NCM. In this case, the formation of MB, its migration along membrane with deceleration, and reaching a steady state is the same as in CAM. Moreover, because EO in NCM is higher than in CAM, the steady state of MB is displaced more to cathode than in CAM, so a greater part of NCM remains in the area of high counterflow (Fig. 3). NCM possesses the capacity to firmly fix different proteins. Thus, if the protein antigen was fixed somewhere in the area of counter-flow and the membrane was completely blocked with unrelated protein, the counter-flow could be used as a "conveyer belt," consecutively transferring immunoreagents to the antigen and then washing out its unbound fraction (Fig. 3). The same could be done with antibodies fixed on NCM and reacting with antigen and immunodeveloping reagents. This created a new principle for semiautomatic performance of multistep immunochemical reactions, such as, for instance, immunoblotting (Abelev and Karamova, 1989; Abelev et al., 1989).

3. General Techniques

3.1. ITP-CAM

The technique of ITP-CAM is described in detail by Abelev and Karamova (1984, 1987). Briefly, ITP was performed on strips of cellogel (Chemotron, Milan, Italy) 17 cm in length and width, depending on the purpose of the analysis. Each strip had two folds, "cathodic" and "anodic," which served as reservoirs for the liquid (Fig. 4A). The strip saturated with leading buffer, 0.06*M* Tris-HCl, pH 6.7, was inserted into an electrophoretic chamber of Gelman type (Gelman, USA) or "Biophyspribor" (Moscow, USSR), so that its anode end was bridged with leading buffer, which filled the anode section, and the cathode end was connected (by filter-paper bridge) with terminating buffer (0.012*M* Tris-β-alanine, pH 8.6) in the cathode section of the chamber. Both folds of the membrane were filled with leading buffer containing traces of bromphenol blue (BPB). After constant tension was applied the MB started to form, which was easily marked by BPB concentration. When MB was clearly formed and straightened, the liquid from the "cathodic" fold was evacuated and the sample was introduced instead. The sample contained 30 μL of 2.5% ampholine, pH 3.5–10 (LKB, Bromma, Sweden). Its volume ranged from 50 to 200 μL/cm of width. It should be dialyzed prior to electrophoresis. During ITP the sample was soaked into CAM, concentrated, and separated on the MB. The final separation took place when the "cathodic" fold was empty and the second steady state relative to the "anodic" fold was established.

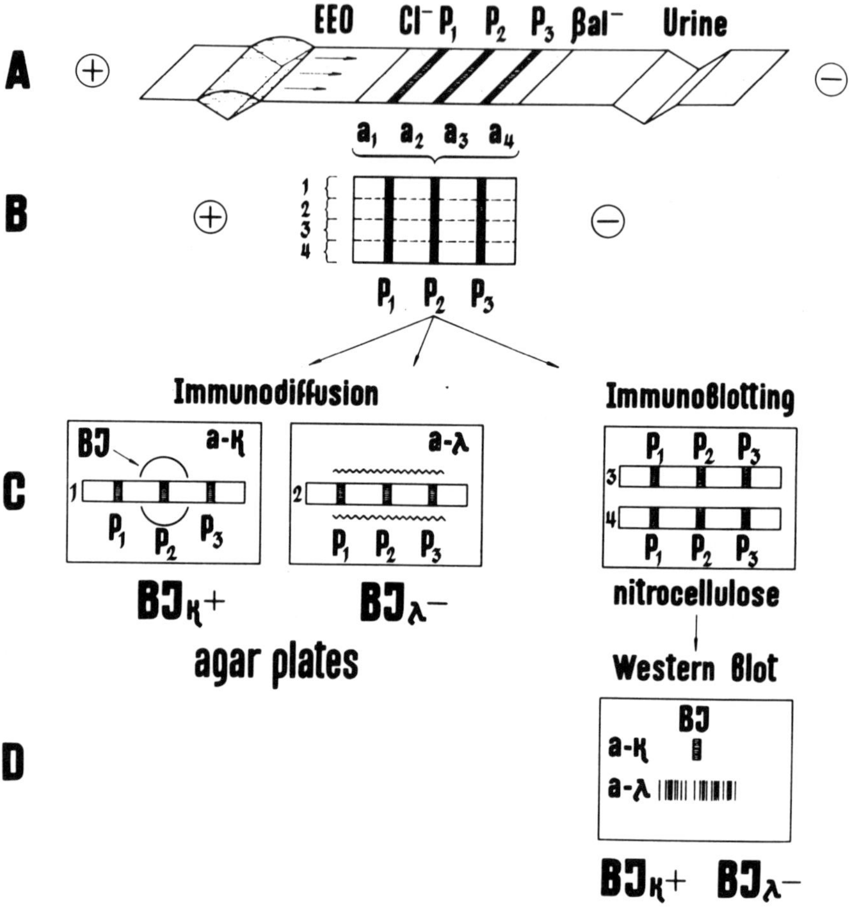

Fig. 4. Schematic representation of the detection of Bence Jones protein (BJP). **A:** Isotachophoretic separations of urinary proteins on cellulose acetate membrane. P_1, P_2, P_3: protein bands; a_1, a_2, a_3, a_4: ampholytic spacers; EEO: electroosmotic flow. "Cathodic" (right) and "anodic" (left) folds are shown. **B:** Area of membrane with separated proteins. 1–4: sections of the membrane. **C:** Immunodetection: a-κ and a-λ, plates covered by agar gel, mixed with anti-κ and anti-λ, respectively. BJκ and BJλ, Bence Jones protein of κ and λ chains, respectively. **D:** Immunoblotting: Western blot developed by anti-κ and anti-λ, respectively. (From Abelev et al., 1990, with permission).

The area with separated proteins was dissected on four strips alongside the electrophoresis axis (Fig. 4B). Two strips were overlaid on agar or agarose gel plates mixed with anti-κ or anti-λ Ig-light chain immune sera, respectively. After overnight diffusion the precipitate was formed, the shape of which demonstrated the presence or absence of electrophoretically homogeneous band of light chain (Fig. 4C). The presence of a homogeneous band of one light chain type against the background of a heterogeneous chain of the alternative type served as the evidence of monoclonal light chain, or BJP, in the patients' urine. The precipitin line was finely inspected after drying and staining the gel plate. If the amount of light chain was below the limit of sensitivity of the method, that is, less than ~1 μg/mL, then another variant of immunodevelopment was applied: immunoblotting. For this the CAM area with separated proteins was pressed by vacuum to the NCM. The protein bands were transferred by diffusion to NCM and fixed on it. Then NCM was treated by milk proteins to block all the protein-binding sites on the NCM. Then the strip of NCM was used for ITP, and the protein bands were consequently treated with monoclonal antibodies (MAb) to Ig κ, λ, or γ chains, followed by goat polyclonal serum to mouse IgG, MAb to horseradish peroxidase, and the peroxidase itself. After development in peroxidase substrate (a mixture of diaminobenzidine [DAB] and chloronaphtol) the black staining of the immune complexes was developed (Fig. 4D), which revealed light chains to the level of approx 10 ng/mL.

4. Results

4.1. Bence Jones Protein (BJP) Produced by Neoplastic B-Cells In Vitro and In Vivo

It is well known that neoplastic plasma cells produce monoclonal Ig (MIg) accompanied by a large amount of monoclonal L-chains (ML). The latter, being present in the blood, were rapidly excreted into urine, wherein they were concentrated and could be easily detected as BJP. However, until the last decade it was commonly accepted that BJP is very rare in other B-cell malignancies, such as chronic lymphocytic leukemia (CLL) and non-Hodgkin's lymphoma (NHL) (*see* Bergsagel and Pruzanski, 1979).

The first work demonstrating a quite different situation was that of Pierson et al. (1980), who extracted L chains from urine of CLL patients by anti-L-chain immunosorbent, eluted them with subsequent concentration, and analyzed them by zonal electrophoresis. Pierson et al. demonstrated a homogeneous band of L chain of one type (κ or λ) against a background of electrophoretically heterogeneous alternative L chain in 8 of 14 cases. Although this work was very convincing and demonstrative, their way of revealing BJP was rather complicated, not quantitative, and doubtless not applicable as a routine clinical procedure.

Just at that time we were looking for an application of ITP-CAM, which was very suitable to reveal electrophoretically homogeneous protein present in trace amounts in solution. Indeed, ITP-CAM combined with immunodiffusion permitted BJP to be revealed easily in about 60% of patients with CLL and related diseases (Abelev et al., 1983).

Similar results were independently obtained by Stevenson et al. (1983), who used isoelectric focusing for preliminary concentration and separation of urine proteins, and immunofixation for identification of BJP. Then Pascali and Pezzoli, using 200- to 500-fold urine concentration, were able to detect BJP in more than half of the cases of CLL and NHL (Pascali and Pezzoli, 1986; Pezzoli and Pascali, 1986). We have continued to look for BJP in B-cell neoplasia and have published observations of two nonoverlapping groups of CLL–NHL patients with comparable results (Sinitsina et al., 1988; Abelev et al., 1990). Moreover, we were able to demonstrate that BJP is a very adequate marker for monitoring chemotherapy of these patients and even for the detection of residual malignant clone during complete clinical remission (Abelev et al., 1990). In our opinion, ITP-CAM is the most appropriate technique for BJP detection in both laboratory and clinical conditions. Below is described in more detail our approach and results concerned with BJP in CLL and NHL.

First we would like to describe the detection of BJP in B-cell lines of Burkitt's lymphoma or Epstein-Barr immortalized B-cell lines of the same patients. These cell lines were produced by Lenoir (IARC, Lyon) and maintained in different laboratories. We used the cultural media from cell lines of S. Torgsteinsdottir (Institute of Tumor Biology, Karolinska Institute, Stockholm) (Aliva-Carino et al., 1987). There were investigated eight Burkitt's lymphoma (BL) cell lines and five lymphoblastoid cell lines (LBL). Six BL lines revealed BJP in the media, whereas all LBL lines demonstrated mono- or oligoclonal L chains when investigated by ITP-CAM in combination with ITP-immunoblotting (Fig. 5). These data illustrate the regular production of free light chains by most proliferating B-cells—neoplastic or immortalized. They show also that ITP-CAM is an absolutely adequate technique for detection of small amounts of free light chains in cultural media containing a large excess of calf serum.

Now we turn to BJP detection in the patient's urine. We shall describe this procedure in more technical detail. The small aliquot (~5 mL) of daily urine was centrifuged, filtered through a 0.45-μm Millipore filter, dialyzed against leading buffer solution 0.06*M* Tris-HCl, pH 6.7) overnight, and stored at –20°C until use.

Before ITP-CAM, each urine was titrated in double-diffusion gel against eight test systems, consisting of anti-κ, anti-λ, anti-μ, anti-γ, anti-α, anti-$\beta_2 m$, anti human serum albumin, and anti human transferrin paired with the corresponding antigens, taken in optimal dilutions. A large excess of κ or λ suggested the BJP of the respective type. Anyway, it was useful to know the titer of L chains for choosing the optimal urine sample for ITP. Usually the sample volume for the pilot ITP was 50 μL with 30 μL of 2.5% ampholine, pH 3.5–10, diluted in leading buffer solution. After 3.5–4 h of ITP at 300 V, the final separation of urinary proteins took place in the area between two folds (Fig. 4A). The gel was dissected into three strips: one stained by BPB and then restained with Coomassie brilliant blue, and the others overlaid onto two agarose plates, containing 7% of anti-κ or anti-λ respectively. After overnight diffusion the plates were washed, pressed, and stained according to Axelsen

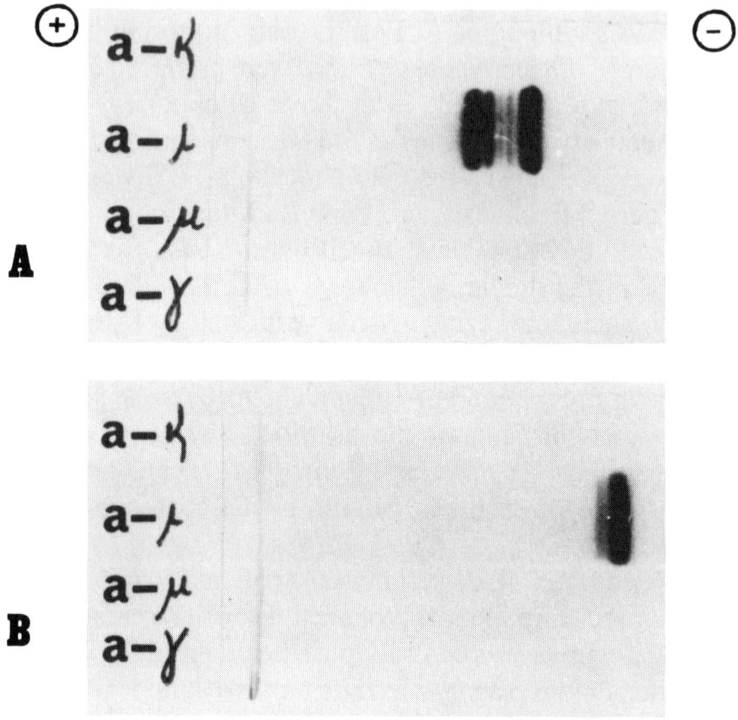

Fig. 5. Western blots of cultural media of lymphoblastoid (LCL) and Burkitt's lymphoma (BL) cell lines. **A:** Cultural media of WW-I-LCL developed by the following MAbs: anti-κ (α–κ), anti-λ (α–λ), anti-μ (α-μ), and anti-γ (α–γ) chains, goat antimouse IgG, and MAbs to horseradish peroxidase and peroxidase. (Oligoclonal free λ chains, no κ chains). **B:** Cultural media of BL cell line, WW-I-BL, developed as above (monoclonal λ chain).

et al. (1973) to reveal precipitin lines. The presence of a clear homogeneous protein band on the stained strip coinciding with precipitin band on one of the plates served as evidence in favor of the presence of BJP (Fig. 6). The titer of the corresponding chain and the area under its band were proportional to the amount of BJP in the sample and could be used for rough calculation of the antigen level. Several separate samples could be taken in one analysis.

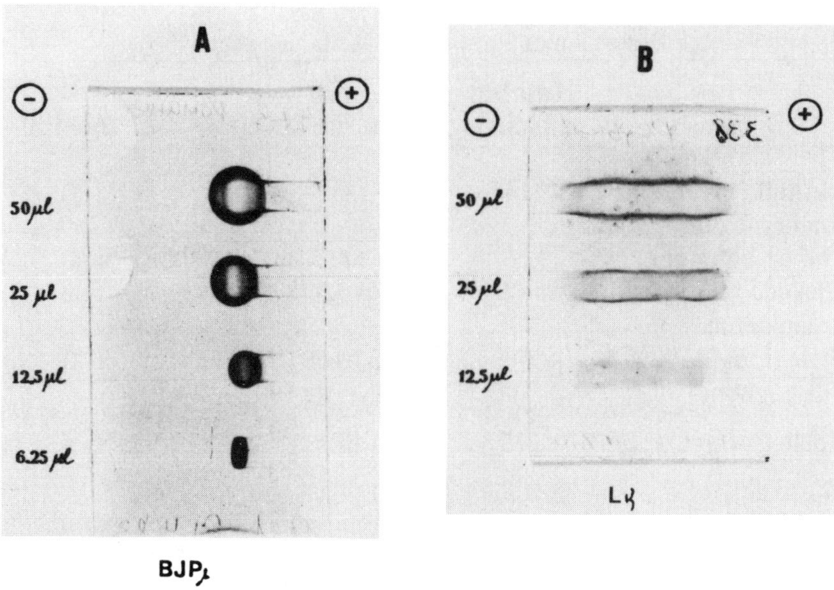

Fig. 6. Bence Jones protein (**A**) and heterogeneous L chains (**B**) revealed by ITP-CAM in combination with immunodiffusion. Urine doses are shown. (From Abelev et al., 1990, with permission).

Tables 1 and 2 contain the results of two nonoverlapping groups of B-cell malignancies analyzed by ITP-CAM combined with immunodiffusion. It is clear that in about half the cases BJP could be used as a marker for CLL and NHL, whereas all the cases of Waldenström macroglobulinemia were accompanied by this tumor marker. The presence of BJP did not correlate to clinical peculiarities of these diseases.

However, the changes of BJP level in the urine were positively correlated to clinical response to chemotherapy. In 19 of 23 cases of patients shown in Table 1, a full coincidence with the response to chemotherapy was obtained. In several cases it was possible to follow during several months patients with changing remissions and relapses. Two such cases are shown in Figs. 7 and 8. Two features should be stressed here: first, the very close coincidence between the changes in BJP level and the clinical picture,

Table 1
Bence Jones Protein in B-Cell Neoplasia[a]

Diagnosis	Number of patients	BJP-positive (BJP+/total)	κ	λ	Biclonal
Multiple myeoloma	14	11 (0.8) (+2?)	6 :	5 :	0
Waldenström macroglobulinemia	3	3 (1)	3 :	0 :	0
Chronic lymphocytic leukemia	42	24 (0.57)	20 :	2 :	2
Non-Hodgkin's lymphoma	56	33 (0.59)	29 :	2 :	2
Total	115	71 (0.62)	58 :	9 :	4
Normal	11	–	–	–	–
Other diseases	28	–	–	–	–

[a]After Abelev et al., 1990.

Table 2
Monoclonal Ig in Patients with Chronic Lymphocytic Leukemia and Non-Hodgkin's Lymphoma[a]

Diagnosis	Number of patients	With monoclonal Ig: Only in serum	Only in urine	In serum and urine	Positive/ total
Chronic lymphocytic leukemia:					
Benign type	6	–	–	1	1/6 (0.16)
Malignant type	35	–	25	3	28/35 (0.8)
Tumoral	28	–	17	–	17/28 (0.6)
Bone marrow	5	–	1	–	1/5 (0.2)
Splenomegalic	3	–	2	–	2/3 (0.66)
Hairy cell	8	–	–	–	0/8 (0.0)
Non-Hodgkin's lymphoma	30	–	7	1	8/30 (0.27)

[a]After Sinitsina et al., 1988.

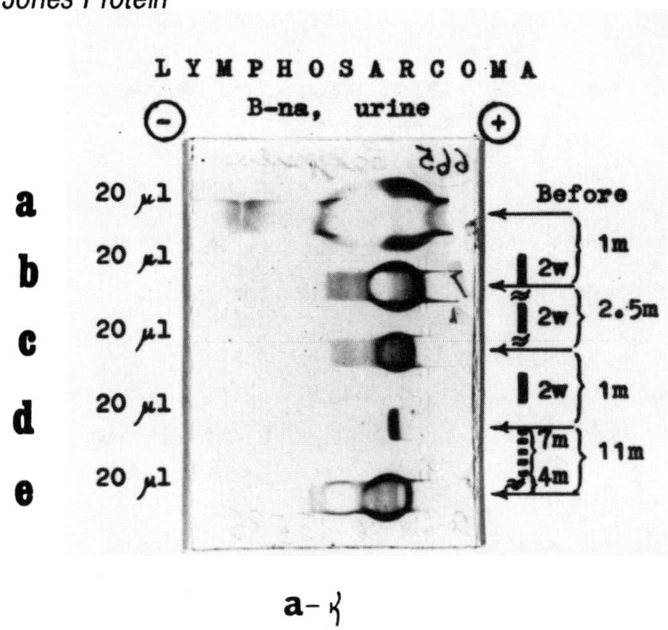

Fig. 7. Dynamics of urinary Bence Jones protein during chemotherapy of patient B-na. ITP-CAM combined with immunodiffusion. The same volume (20 μL) of urine was used in the analyses. Black column (right): periods of chemotherapy: w, weeks; m, months; d, days.

and second, that BJP did not disappear completely during the course of the disease. The marker of malignant clone persisted in all stages of the disease. One case is especially demonstrative in this respect (Fig. 9A). The patient with acute lymphoblastic leukemia responded to treatment by decrease in BJP, and after several courses he entered full clinical remission with disappearance of spleen and lymph-node enlargement and with a normal blood count. ITP-CAM combined with immunodiffusion could not reveal BJP in his urine. However, ITP-CAM in combination with immunoblotting detected the trace amounts of BJP in his urine in this period (Fig. 9B) with the later rise in its level and severe relapse (Abelev et al., 1990).

The further study of residual disease and the possibilities to predict relapse is most important in this field. It must be noted also that MAbs to idiotype of Ig or BJP, which are ideal antigenic markers for a malignant clone, can be used for treatment of CLL and NHL,

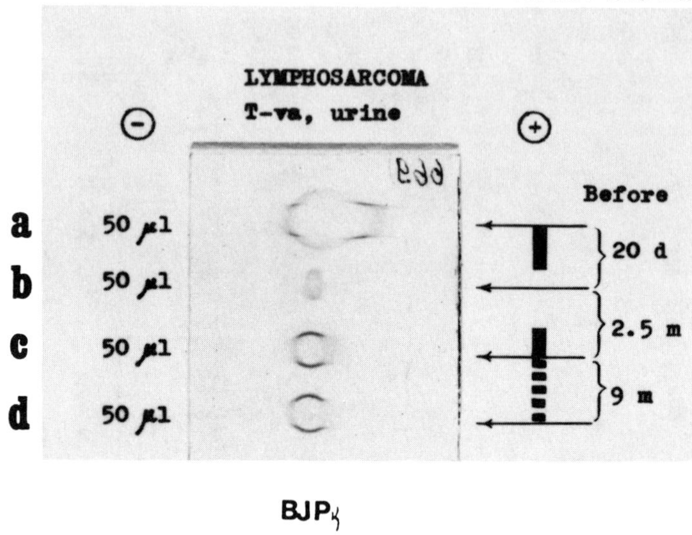

Fig. 8. Dynamics of urinary Bence Jones protein during chemotherapy of Patient T-va. ITP-CAM combined with immunodiffusion. Designations as in Fig. 7.

and this possibility is being actively investigated at present (Wrightham et al., 1987; Bankert et al., 1989; Brown et al., 1989). It is logical to propose that a residual clone during remission might serve as the best target for such treatment.

5. Perspectives: Quantitative Multiantigen Assay

ITP on nitrocellulose membranes has created very broad and flexible possibilities for semiautomatic performance of multistep immmochemical reactions, for instance, immunoblotting (Abelev and Karamova, 1989) and epitope comparison of different MAbs Abelev et al., 1989).

If one has MAbs to several antigens and other polyclonal antibodies to different epitopes of these antigens, then it will be possible to fix these MAbs one after another on the strip so that they will be situated in the area of the counterflow. Then the mixture of the antigens followed by polyclonal antibodies (e.g., of rabbit origin) to other epitopes should be included into the counterflow and

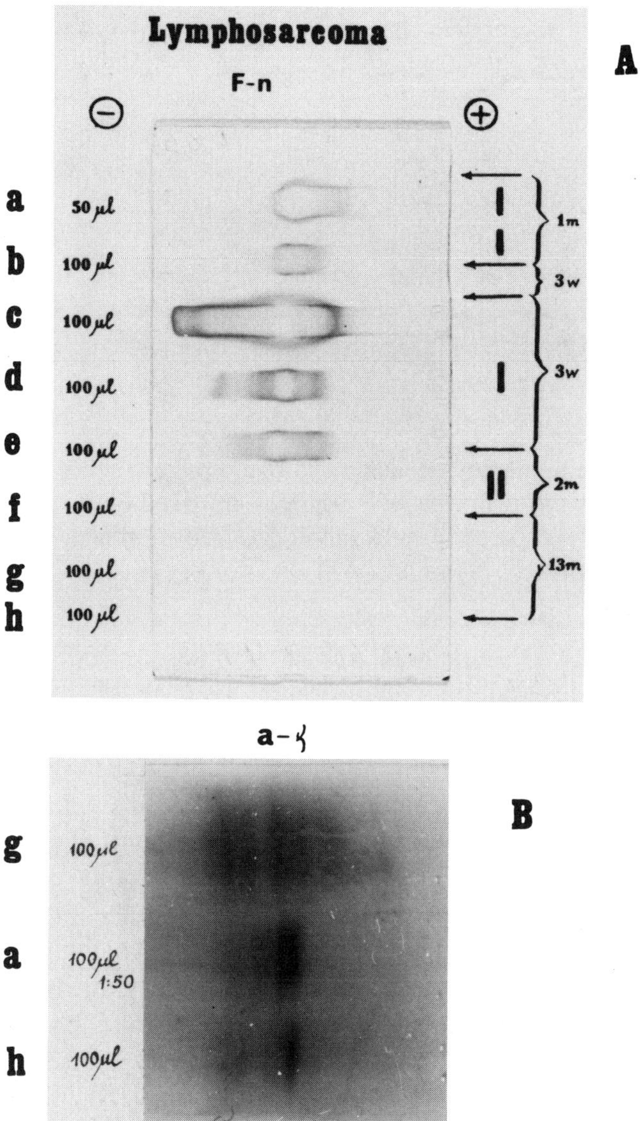

Fig. 9. Dynamics of urinary Bence Jones protein during chemotherapy of patient F-n. **A:** ITP-CAM combined with immunodiffusion. Designations as in Fig. 7. **B:** ITP-CAM combined with Western blotting. Development by monoclonal anti-κ, and then as in Fig. 5.

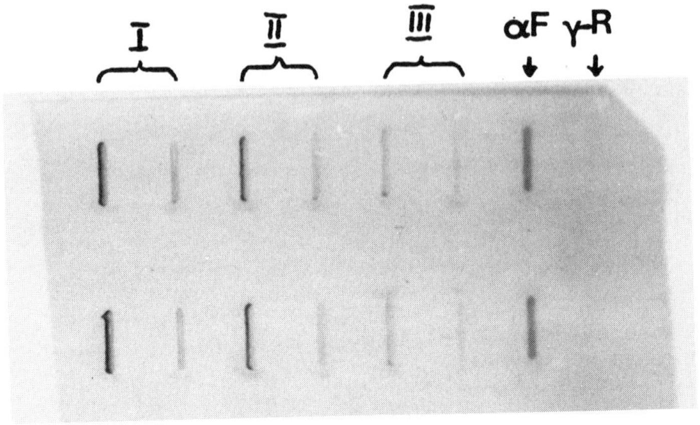

Fig. 10. Simultaneous detection of α-fetoprotein subfractions. Three pairs of MAbs to different AFP epitopes are fixed on the NCM (I–III). αF, total AFP preparation; γ-R, rabbit IgG. Development by successive treatment with AFP, rabbit anti-AFP and donkey peroxidase-conjugated antirabbit IgG.

next-peroxidase-conjugated antirabbit IgG. In this case, the antigens will be fixed on the corresponding antibodies, and they will bind to rabbit polyclonal antibodies, which will be visualized by enzyme-conjugated antirabbit IgG. If the dose of enzyme-conjugated antibody is chosen to detect a certain amount of rabbit IgG and the latter is fixed on NCM as a closing band, then the total amount of conjugate will be distributed among the zones of different antigens and the rest will be bound by the closing band. Densitometry of the distributed dye will give the quantitative data of antibody bound of different MAbs. It is clear that rabbit polyclonal antibodies might be replaced by mouse enzyme-conjugated MAbs to epitopes other than those used for the antigen fixation.

We illustrate the above proposals by an example of the detection of human AFP subfractions distinguished by the presence or absence of certain epitopes, which are recognized by three different MAbs (Fig. 10). This system is essentially a three-antigen mixture.

Obviously this principle could be used for quantitative decomposition of complex antigenic mixtures. The possibility of using relatively large volumes of the sample to be analyzed (about, and more than, 200 μL/cm) and immunoenzyme development makes this method highly sensitive in addition to its semiautomatic performance.

References

Abelev, G. I. and E. R. Karamova (1982), *Zh. Vses. Khim. O-va (USSR)* **27,** 429–475.

Abelev, G. I. and E. R. Karamova (1984), *Anal. Biochem.* **142,** 437–444.

Abelev, G. I. and E. R. Karamova (1987), *Sov. Med. Rev. F. Oncol.* **1,** 85–118.

Abelev, G. I. and E. R. Karamova (1989), *Mol. Immunol.* **26,** 41–47.

Abelev, G. I., E. R. Karamova, E. G. Bragina, N. E. Andreeva, and H. V. Kruglova (1990), *Int. J. Cancer* **46,** 351–355.

Abelev, G. I., E. R. Karamova, N. E. Andreeva, A. A. Ushakov, E. V. Chernokhvostova, and G. P. German (1983), *Immunologiya (USSR)* **6,** 33–37.

Abelev, G. I., E. R. Karamova, A. K. Yazova, and A. I. Gussev (1989), *Mol. Immunol.* **26,** 49–52.

Avila-Carino, J., S. Torsteindottir, B. Ehlin-Henriksson, G. Lenoir, G. Klein, E. Klein, and M. Musucci (1987), *Int. J. Cancer* **40,** 691–697.

Axelsen, N. H., J. Krøll, and B. Weeke, eds. (1973), in *Manual of Quantitative Immunoelectrophoresis,* Universitetsforlaget, Oslo, pp. 30–35.

Bankert, R., S. Yokota, S. Ghosh, E. Mayhew, and Y.-H. Jou (1989), *Cancer Res.* **49,** 301–308.

Bergsagel, D. E. and W. Pruzanski (1979), in *Immunodiagnosis of Cancer* (Herberman, R., and K. McIntire, eds.), Marcel Dekker, New York, pp. 450–472.

Brown, Sh., R. Miller, S. Horning, D. Cherwinski, S. Hart, R. McElderry, T. Basham, R. Warnke, Th. Merigan, and R. Levy (1989), *Blood* **73,** 651–661.

Chrambach, A. (1980), *Mol. Cell. Biochem.* **29,** 23–26.

Haglund, H. (1970), *Sci. Tools* **17,** 2–13.

Pascali, E. and A. Pezzoli (1986), *Acta Haematol.* **75,** 193–198.

Pezzoli, A. and E. Pascali (1986), *Scand. J. Haematol.* **36,** 18–24.

Pierson, J., T. Darley, G. Stevenson, and M. Virji (1980), *Br. J. Cancer* **41,** 681–688.

Sinitsina, T. V., N. E. Andreeva, and G. I. Abelev (1988), *Ther. Arch. (Russ.)* **5,** 50–53.

Stevenson, F. K., M. Spellerberg, and J. L. Smith (1983), *Br. J. Cancer* **47,** 607–612.

Wrightham, M., A. Tutt, M. Glennie, T. Hamblin, G. T. Stevenson, and F. K. Stevenson (1987), *Blood* **69,** 919–923.

Chapter 23

Multiple Testing with Cancer Markers

Adolf L. Pohl

1. Introduction

The exponentially growing interest in cancer markers (Sell, 1990) requires an organized approach to establish their true practical usefulness for the entire society. This includes medical, social, economical, and humanitarian aspects. Unless powerful statistical methods can be applied for converting cancer marker laboratory data into clinically meaningful answers, the measurements generated may raise more interpretational problems than they solve.

Diagnosis and monitoring of cancer by tumor-associated antigens present two major problems. First, there are so many malignant diseases with concomitant signs, symptoms, and laboratory data that the clinician sometimes fails to recall all of the diagnostic information that he or she needs. On the one hand, too many tests are requested from the laboratory, but on the other hand, certain tests are missed although they could contribute essential information. Errors in differential diagnosis might, therefore, result fre-

From: *Serological Cancer Markers* Edited by Stewart Sell ©1992 The Humana Press, Totowa, NJ

quently from errors of omission. Second, we are still quite ignorant of the multitude of benign diseases and physiological conditions that produce confusing elevations of cancer marker serum levels.

The great importance of an early recognition of a possible carcinoma and the severe medical problems in differentiating between disease categories require new and functional approaches in data evaluation. The lack of individual cancer marker tests with satisfactory sensitivity and specificity leads to investigating the combined discriminatory power of several cancer markers. The basis for multiple testing with cancer markers are the quite reasonable assumptions that (1) earlier diagnosis of cancer or recurrence will result in a more favorable disease course and outcome, (2) a whole battery of cancer markers, when compared to a single test, will detect cancer or recurrence much earlier and thereby improve survival, and (3) multiple testing can provide additional information not contained in single tests, thus allowing the identification of several groups of patients, each with a different probability of therapy response. However, emphasis should be placed on which cancer marker tests are cost-effective and which should be performed only in specific situations.

Over the past decade, an enormous impetus to the implementation of multivariate statistical analysis has resulted from the availability of computer-based systems for data processing. Software that provides a detailed statistical analysis of results from multiple measurements and cumulative reports is of enormous use to the clinical chemist and clinician who wishes to extract the maximum information from his data.

This review summarizes the state of the art of multiple cancer marker testing and evaluation. However, the art is not easily codified.

1.1. Scope and Requirements

Only a minor part of cancer marker tests is evaluated critically with the aid of proper statistical techniques and viewed simultaneously with the clinically relevant information. Currently, experienced physicians are integrating laboratory test results and other items of information about the patient mostly by intuition into a coherent pattern. Optimal interpretation would require that all relevant parameters be taken into account, properly weighted, relative to each other.

This task can be achieved by application of multivariate statistical techniques using all statistical methods that simultaneously analyze more than two variables on a sample of observations. Multivariate statistical analysis can perform evaluations in which all relevant variables are processed simultaneously, and it has proven to provide clear objective quantitative judgments (Albert and Harris, 1987; Goldschmidt, 1987). Moreover, multivariate statistical analysis helps in making objective choices between redundant tests and can speed up the abolition of outdated tests.

However, the size and complexity of the software programs available for multivariate evaluation of clinical laboratory data (e.g., BMDP, SAS, SPSS, SYSTAT/SYGRAPH) demands the help of practicing statisticians and the use of a large, efficient central computer facility with workstations in the laboratory. Comprehensive computer-based cumulative reporting systems are essential, as is the possibility to develop selected data bases from past laboratory records so that results appropriate to different kinds of patients can be obtained.

It is time to establish standard criteria for the evaluation of multiple testing programs to compare and select the most useful cancer markers for the differential diagnosis, prognosis, and follow-up of various malignancies. Objectively selecting the most useful tests from among the large number of available cancer markers could contribute significantly to the economics of cancer patient care.

1.2. Problems and Pitfalls

Cancer marker testing has its intrinsic pitfalls. The rational interpretation of cancer marker values not only requires clearly defined medical goals, but depends on the validity of the measurements, i.e., the analytical accuracy and the application of the proper statistical procedures.

Even a single cancer marker, when tested serially, produces multiple results and creates its own kind of multivariate problem with respect to the time dimension. Consequently, dealing with several cancer markers on repeated occasions leads to a complicated statistical problem. Therefore, the twin rule for the use of multiple cancer markers should be observed: minimize and optimize them. In other words, keep them economical but make them functional. In general, the clinical effectiveness of cancer markers should have been demonstrated individually prior to their combination in a multiple set.

1.2.1. Conflicting Results from Multiple Testing

The simultaneous assay of multiple markers is based on the premise that tumors, because of their inherent heterogeneity, may synthesize a broad spectrum of tumor-associated antigens. Though today's technology can provide virtually limitless amounts of data, only unreasoned medical thinking demands the measurement of as many laboratory parameters as attainable with little thought to the contribution of each of those measurements to the final diagnosis. The intuitive reasoning that "the more one measures the more one knows" leads not only to an arbitrary selection of cancer markers, but is simply and fundamentally wrong. A multitude of cancer marker tests may result in a poor understanding of the physiological condition of a patient. If the patient is suffering from a disease for which only one or two cancer markers are truly diagnostic, the other tests are only adding "noise," diverting attention, or, by use of a multivariate reference region based on all the tests, actually obscuring the diagnostic signal. Thus, the clinical chemist or clinician should never ignore valid individual test results.

One of the basic problems in the interpretation of multiple cancer marker data is finding structure in large sets of empirically gathered information. To avoid superfluous information from multiple assays, a selection must be made. The ever increasing use of new tumor-associated antigens demands the implementation of objective and standardized statistical methods (e.g., multivariate regression or discriminant analysis) for selecting those cancer marker panels that are most cost-effective and meaningful in clinical practice. Hence, establishing the optimal combination of cancer markers for oncological decision making takes considerable time and effort, starting with defining precisely the medical needs and selecting the proper cancer markers that provide medically useful information in that particular clinical setting.

Assuming that cancer marker tests have been properly evaluated, selected, and combined to provide medically useful information, then analytical quality becomes the paramount requirement to be met if test results are to be useful in caring for patients. Errors must be kept so small that they do not cause any misinterpretations. Too many users of cancer marker test kits have been under the misapprehension that marker values are precise and accurate. But every measurement procedure is subject to a certain amount of imprecision and inaccuracy. Imprecision is described by the standard deviation or coefficient of variation that is at least in the range of 5–30% for common cancer markers. Cancer marker tests are used in recognition of their imperfection. There is surprisingly little interest in the "true" values when performing measurements of cancer markers. Two replicate measurements are usually done in cancer marker testing, which is often insufficient to determine whether the value in a patient's sample is correct and equivalent to the "true" value. Thus, the analytical performance of cancer marker tests must be evaluated to assure that they can provide medically useful test results. The damage of poor experimental performance is irreparable. No amount of fancy statistical computer analysis can extract much information from a set of false data.

1.2.2. Falsely Abnormal Results

The major disadvantage of uncritically using multiple markers is related to the nonspecific nature of all cancer markers currently known. Including several such markers in a panel tends to magnify this specificity problem. Applying a separate univariate reference range to each cancer marker in a multiple set will often, by chance alone, indicate apparent abnormalities. As the number of tests increases, so too does the probability of at least one false positive result. Simply counting the number of positive cancer marker results gives to all tests equal weight. It does not account for the higher sensitivities of the better tests.

Since no cancer marker in current use is truly cancer-specific, conflicting results are always arising when more than one test is performed. Setting the specificity for each cancer marker, at 95%, e.g., leads to a statistical and clinical dilemma, since the likelihood that a patient without cancer will be correctly identified as "non-diseased" exponentially decreases with the number of cancer marker tests performed (Pohl et al., 1988). The implication of this relationship is shown in the following examples:

No. of tests performed (n)	Combined specificity (0.95^n)
1	0.95
4	0.81
7	0.70
10	0.60
13	0.51

Consequently, a person who undergoes 13 independent laboratory determinations has, by chance alone, a probability of only 51% of being classified as "normal" even if he or she is perfectly healthy!

In order to alleviate this problem inherent in multiple cancer marker testing, I recommend in the present review the application of multivariate statistical analysis. This statistical tool provides a basis for testing the performance of multiple cancer markers over multiple clinical states. It allows the combining and weighting of cancer marker tests in panels for an improved differential diagnosis of various types of cancer. But many more studies are required to collect the necessary data needed to properly evaluate the clinical value of cancer marker panels.

1.3. Reference Regions

Reference regions for laboratory parameters are generally based on data from apparently healthy persons. Even when correctly indicating the presence of disease, they are of little value for a specific diagnosis. The task of differential diagnosis, for example, requires comparable data from age-matched patients with the diseases one wants to distinguish. The Working Group on Tumor Marker Criteria has recently drafted minimal demands to be met for the establishment of such reference values and indicated the conditions for correct interpretation of cancer marker alterations (Bonfrer, 1990). For laboratory tests with specific applications (e.g., diagnosis and/or monitoring of tumors; assessment of prognosis), the conventional normal ranges derived from healthy volunteers or blood donors or laboratory personnel are not appropriate. Instead of the traditional "upper level of normal," decision levels are required that account for the specific clinical situation, e.g., the need for surgical or other aggressive intervention.

Especially in cancer patients, the marker value at which the risks of nonintervention exceed the risks of intervention is exceedingly more important than the value at which results become "abnormal" by the arbitrary standard of the 97.5th percentile of values from healthy volunteers. This dilemma has led in oncological practice to very individual "action levels" of experienced clinicians, which do not correspond to the traditional "normal range."

1.3.1. Univariate Reference Ranges

Establishing the univariate reference range between two disease categories usually starts with plotting the histogram of the cancer marker values vs their frequency in the population sample investigated. Since cancer marker values are rarely normally distributed, the calculation of reference ranges has to be preceded by a transformation procedure (e.g., logarithmic, quadratic, and so on). Finding the underlying Gaussian distribution in a mixed population is not simple.

The combination of such univariate reference ranges results in an increasing number of irrelevant outliers (*see* 1.2.2.). Using multiple univariate reference ranges may produce more than the expected number of false positives even if the tests are uncorrelated. Hence, cancer markers cannot be viewed in isolation.

1.3.2. Multivariate Reference Regions

To avoid fruitless verification procedures of sporadic univariate false positive results, multivariate reference regions have been recommended (Boyd and Lacher, 1982), allowing relatively straightforward models to be formulated for the analysis of multiple data. Multivariate reference regions can be applied for every given combination of clinical, chemical, and hematological variables. A multivariate normal density distribution of p variables has the form of an ellipsoid in the p-dimensional space.

Mutual dependencies of laboratory parameters can result in striking differences between multiple univariate reference ranges and multivariate reference regions. In case the parameters are uncorrelated, this difference is less marked (Albert and Harris, 1987).

However, both approaches, multiple univariate reference ranges as well as multivariate reference regions, suffer from the fact that they are dependent of the set of laboratory parameters that is under evaluation. Moreover, the interpretation of observed test results by means of the reference region, whether univariate or multivariate, is not entirely satisfying because it allows only a dichotomous ("yes" or "no") decision. No account is made for the degree of abnormality. Yet a person's state of health is a continuous variable, which could be very different between two sets of test values just inside the reference region.

1.3.3. Marker Frequency Distribution and Normalization

Cancer marker values seldom follow the ideal Gaussian normal frequency distribution. Their most common departure from normality is a positive skewness and leptokurtotic (peaked) shape of the distribution curve.

However, for the application of multivariate statistical analysis, multivariate normality of the cancer marker data is required. To test whether the independent variables (e.g., cancer marker values) to be used in multivariate analysis can be reasonably thought to be normally distributed, the nonparametric Kolmogorov-

Smirnov one-sample test or the Chi-square goodness-of-fit test should be applied.

Normalization can be achieved in a one- or two-stage transformation by applying a mathematical function (logarithmic, quadratic, and so on) to compress the scale for the higher values (Linnet, 1987). Because the same transformation has to be applied to all control- and patient-sample values, a good approximation for all groups is difficult to find. Alternatively, nonparametric tests may be used.

1.4. Sample Size for a Study

Large cancer marker data banks are an essential condition for the proper and effective application of multivariate statistical techniques. Only if the data bank is sufficiently large can it be split up into a test set and a training set. The results are depending heavily on the accuracy and completeness of the data sets and on the reliability of the diagnoses. When multiple tests are being compared in a study, all tests should be performed on all subjects.

In multivariate techniques, the minimal ratio of patients vs features (e.g., cancer markers or other independent variables) per group should be at least three patients per feature; i.e., the maximum permissible number of independent variables to be investigated should be less than 30% of the number of patients in the smallest disease class. Statistically speaking, too many features (independent variables) will result in unstable estimates of the differences between the class centroids.

1.4.1. Sampling Patient Populations

No two sets of human subjects are identical. Even unbiased, truly random patient samples differ from sample to sample because of statistical variations. Thus, if tests being evaluated are not applied to the same group of subjects, observed differences in test performance may reflect differences in the subjects rather than differences in actual test efficacy.

Sensitivity ("positivity in disease") and specificity ("negativity in health") of a cancer marker test in a specific clinical situation both heavily depend not only on the decision (cutoff) level, but also on the study population chosen. If, for example, the reference group consists only of young, healthy blood donors, the test will appear to have a much better specificity than when applied to an age-matched control group with the diagnostically confusing benign disease. Conversely, the sensitivity strikingly increases when the test is applied to patients who have advanced or metastatic cancer than when applied to patients who have stable or limited disease.

2. Differential Diagnosis by Multiple Cancer Markers

In order to assess how well a cancer marker test performs in discriminating between different disease groups, it is mandatory to use another, independent, method to classify the groups. This independent diagnostic standard may be the findings of surgery, the result of a biopsy or autopsy, or the clinical outcome of patients after follow-up. After such independent classification of disease status, a decision (cutoff) level usually is selected for the diagnostic test that separates the patients from the reference population. Some misclassifications inevitably occur because of the overlap between the groups. Moreover, by selecting and using a decision level for a cancer marker, this originally continuous variable changes into a dichotomous one (like X-ray) that can be merely interpreted in terms of "yes" or "no." If the study is not a multiparametric one, it becomes difficult to compare different diagnostic tests, except when their cutoff levels have been chosen at the same predefined specificity (e.g., 95%).

2.1. Development of Diagnostic Criteria

The true performance of cancer markers can be established provided they are compared to "hard" clinical data, i.e., the classification of patients into groups must be based on reliable data. This demand was put forward by A. Malkin at the First International

Conference on Human Tumor Markers (Munich, 1982).* Therefore, diagnostic criteria, like cancer markers, must be permanently examined and checked and reexamined, in order to select those that can aid optimally to decide on treatment or prognosis. For many conditions, the biopsy is the gold standard, but even this procedure may be subject to failure. For example, the presence of metastatic cancer in the liver can never be excluded with certainty even at autopsy.

To ensure that the clinical diagnosis is truly independent and not influenced by the cancer marker tests under evaluation, it should be done "blindly," i.e., without knowledge of the laboratory test results. The criteria for the clinical diagnosis should be as objective as feasible. When the diagnosis must rest on subjective evaluation of clinical or morphological patterns, such as radionuclide scans or immunocytochemical cell smears, the diagnosis for each patient should reflect the consensus of at least two experts who each diagnosed blindly and independently.

In such a multiparametric study, a cancer marker vs disease group matrix has to be constructed. The influence of other cancer-related variables has to be taken into account as well, e.g., the prior probabilities for the disease groups in question may be calculated from the laboratory records. The respective conditional probabilities may be the incidence ratios based on the records of the hospital.

If a study of this kind demonstrates inconsistencies in the diagnostic criteria for some malignancies, such disagreement among different researchers should lead to revision of diagnostic criteria until consensus is reached. In the end, there should be an essential agreement among physicians and clinical chemists about the optimum set of cancer markers for that specific clinical question.

2.2. Strategy for Diagnostic Workup

The optimal utilization of laboratory data can be attained not by isolated consideration of individual cancer marker results, but

---

*Discussion remark: 'If good laboratory results are compared with soft clinical data — one gets garbage."

by an integrated view of the entire information contained in a patient's data set. If signs, symptoms, laboratory data, and diseases are grouped in a logical way, then diagnosis can be considered to be a taxonomic process resulting from pattern recognition. Hence, medical diagnosis could be viewed as a pattern recognition procedure (Uhr, 1963).

Diagnostic decision trees (Fineberg, 1980; Weinstein and Fineberg, 1980) can be helpful classification schemes to formulate tentative diagnoses.

2.3. Diagnostic Categories

Performance of a laboratory test (cancer marker) is commonly assessed by its ability to correctly classify patients into two subgroups, one having malignant disease or recurrence and thus needing treatment, and the other being unaffected. Usually, there is overlap in the test results and the cancer marker cannot distinguish well between the groups. Cancer marker tests are far from being perfect yet.

2.3.1. Sensitivity, Specificity, Predictive Value, and Diagnostic Efficiency

Sensitivity is the proportion of the diseased population that is correctly identified at the chosen cutoff level. Specificity is the proportion of the nondiseased control group that is correctly identified as nondiseased by the test at the selected cutoff level. Sensitivity and specificity both depend on the choice of the cutoff (decision) level and vary inversely. Moving the decision level from higher toward lower test values increases sensitivity and negative predictive value, but at the same time decreases specificity and positive predictive value. The decision level should, therefore, be selected exclusively with respect to the specific clinical purpose.

The positive predictive value is the fraction of positive test results that are true positives. This is often rather low in cancer markers, when the false positive rate of a test is high compared to the prevalence, resulting in many more false positive results than true positive results.

Diagnostic efficiency is defined as the fraction of results that are correct, that is, true positives and true negatives divided by all results. It is a combination of the predictive value of a positive result and the predictive value of a negative result.

Sensitivity and specificity vary as the decision level varies. Predictive values and diagnostic efficiency vary with both decision level and prevalence of the disease in the study population.

Sensitivity and specificity are concepts related to a laboratory test whose originally continuous values have been dichotomized by use of an arbitrary decision (cutoff) level. Naive cancer marker users sometimes implicitly assume that one sensitivity–specificity pair characterizes a test because they accept a conventional, often arbitrarily chosen "reference" (cutoff) value as the "correct" one for the test. This, however, is only one of multiple possible decision levels for a given cancer marker test in one specific clinical situation. This test will have one set of sensitivity–specificity pairs in one clinical situation, but may have a different set of pairs when applied to another clinical situation in which the patient group tested is different.

For continuous laboratory variables, like cancer markers, with clinical interpretation depending on the actual value of the test result, this dichotomization process entails a substantial loss of information.

2.3.2. Likelihood Ratio, ROC Curve

To retain the full information of continuous quantitative laboratory results, it was suggested to transfer the results to the probability of whether the disease (cancer) is present or absent. The likelihood ratio is defined for a certain result obtained on the patient as the probability of the disease being present (sensitivity) divided by the probability of the disease being absent (1-specificity) (Van der Helm, 1979; Albert, 1982).

Contrarily to the very limited concept of sensitivity and specificity, the likelihood ratio is applicable to both discrete and continuous variables, either separate or combined in a multivariate profile. The calculation of the likelihood ratio does not depend on the assumption that symptoms or laboratory results occur independently. Recently, however, the application of the likelihood ratio has been questioned as being unnecessarily complicated (Gerhardt and Keller, 1986).

The complete clinical performance of a cancer marker test is represented best by displaying its paired true and false positive rates for all possible decision levels in a given clinical setting. The classical graphical way of displaying this diagnostic ability of a test at various decision levels is obtained by plotting its true positive rate (sensitivity) vs the false positive rate (1-specificity) in a so-called receiver operating characteristic (ROC) curve (Swets, 1979). Each point on the ROC curve represents a pair of sensitivity–specificity rates corresponding to some decision level.

A cancer marker test is clinically efficient at a decision (cutoff) level where both sensitivity and specificity are high, i.e., where the ROC curve is closest to the upper left corner of the diagram, where sensitivity and specificity both reach 100%. Conversely, a clinically useless test has a ROC curve running diagonally from lower left to upper right corner of the diagram, i.e., the true and false positive rates are more or less identical for any given decision level; therefore, its discriminatory value is not better than tossing a coin.

The ROC curve can also be constructed as a plot of the true positive rate (sensitivity) vs true negative rate (specificity), thus moving the curve to the right side with the perfect point (100% sensitivity, 100% specificity) being the upper right corner instead of the upper left one.

2.4. Clinical Decision Analysis

Clinical decision analysis and cost-effectiveness analysis offer tools to evaluate cancer marker tests for their clinical efficacy and economic feasibility (Beck, 1982, 1986). Pauker and Kassirer (1980) presented a formal model of three options involving clinical decisions and laboratory tests: (1) treating without testing, (2) withholding treatment without testing, and (3) performing a diagnostic test and treating if the result is "positive." Data on tumor marker test performance can be used in simple decision tree models for selecting appropriate cutoff levels and to evaluate decision rules for specific clinical problems. Since any diagnostic test result should prompt a course of action, the multiple cancer marker testing strategy should lead to the medical paradigm: treat, test, or observe. Such decision models can be constructed as flowcharts, not to give a single answer, but to provide insights into a complex problem. They can be explored with computer support under a variety of assumptions. Decision analysis could assist the clinical chemist in the task of assessing the clinical efficacy of multiple cancer markers and devising economical strategies for their proper use. For each diagnostic strategy, the average costs per patient and the average gain in health benefit, expressed as quality-adjusted life years, should be evaluated (Weinstein, 1981).

2.5. Discriminant Analysis and Regression Analysis

Linear discriminant analysis based on normality assumptions (i.e., multinormal) provides a handy method for interpreting multiple cancer markers for differential diagnosis. Unfortunately, it can be quite difficult to find a single transformation function that can normalize the distributions of the same test in each of several diseased populations.

The logistic discrimination analysis is based on parametric assumptions about the likelihood ratios rather than the individual probability distribution of a cancer marker in each diseased group, as in the multinormal approach. Its applicability, therefore, is much wider. The continuous variables (cancer marker values) need not necessarily be normally distributed, but can be skewed in one group and fairly symmetric in another. Logistic discriminant analysis is thus recognized as a satisfactory approximation to most differential diagnostic situations encountered in clinical and laboratory practice (Albert and Harris, 1987).

2.5.1. Stepwise Cancer Marker Selection

Cancer marker selection is required for (1) medical, (2) economical, and (3) statistical reasons.

1. A multitude of laboratory tests may present so much distraction that the really important information can become obscure or hidden.
2. By proper test selection, a cutdown of costs can be achieved in the clinical laboratory without loss of important information.
3. In a diagnostic setting, a ratio of one variable (e.g., cancer marker) to minimal three objects (patients) is required for multivariate statistical analysis.

The task of selecting only those cancer markers that jointly provide a satisfactory solution to a given, e.g., differential diagnostic, problem in clinical oncology can be performed by multivariate

- regression analysis,
- principal component analysis with cluster analysis, or
- stepwise discriminant analysis.

The most familiar multivariate technique is discriminant function analysis, first proposed by Fisher (1936). This technique seeks to find linear functions of the independent variables (cancer markers) that best discriminate between different groups of patients, these groups having been defined *a priori* by independent clinical diagnosis (*see* 2.1.). The reliability of the clinical diagnosis should exceed 90% correctness in every patient group! The discriminant function obtained has the following structure: $D = ax_1 + bx_2 + cx_3 + \text{const.}$, x being cancer markers. A questionable case is assigned to the group in which its cancer marker measurements yield the largest numerical value of the classification function.

2.5.2. Minimizing the Number of Tests

In realistic clinical situations, in which there are many cancer marker tests and several possible diseases or stages of the same disease, the aid of an experienced statistician equipped with a good computer facility and powerful statistical software (e.g., BMDP, SAS, SPSS, SYSTAT/SYGRAPH) becomes essential to select the best subset of cancer markers that works well in that specific situation. The selection of too few cancer markers may result in a biased and inconsistent group allocation of questionable cases, whereas too many variables may yield reliable results but create redundant information and unnecessary high costs.

2.5.3. Selection of the Best Marker Combination

The choice of the optimal cancer marker combination depends on the clinical problem. If an important therapeutic decision rests on the test result, then maximal specificity is required. On the other hand, if, e.g., all individuals possibly affected by a certain malignancy are to be identified to undergo invasive diagnosis, then the marker combination should have maximal sensitivity.

There are, of course, other clinical situations for which similar minimization techniques can be applied. Instead of choosing the minimum number of tests to discriminate between different cancer stages, it could be valuable to choose optimum sequence rules to decide what sequence of examinations (cancer marker tests, sonography, X-ray, CT scan) would be optimal for a cancer patient or to minimize the costs associated with such tests without any loss of relevant information.

3. Prognostic Categories

Medical prognosis, i.e., predicting the future medical condition of a cancer patient based on information about the patient's present condition is an important area in which multiple cancer marker determinations could help the physician's daily decisions. The outcome (dependent) variable may be binary: remission or recurrence, favorable or unfavorable. Sometimes, more than just two possibilities are defined: for example, complete remission, partial remission, stable disease, and progressive disease. Cancer marker measurements available may be at one time only or from cumulative reports.

To check and improve the prognostic efficacy of multiple cancer markers, multivariate statistical techniques should be applied to study their correlation with disease activity and outcome parameters.

3.1. Outcome Prediction

To estimate an individual patient's chances for each of the above-mentioned outcome categories, the application of logistic probability functions and the calculation of a risk index is suggested by Albert and Harris (1987). To allocate this patient into one of three disease groups, for example, we need to know two discriminant functions. To predict the probability for one of three possible outcomes, for the same patient, only one risk index and the two cutoffs between the three outcome groups are required.

It has been recommended (Anderson and Philips, 1981) that prediction be based on the ratios of posterior to prior probabilities to calculate the individual risk index of a patient.

The application of multivariate statistical techniques to multiple measurements of cancer markers at a given time can be used not only to allocating a patient to one of several disease categories or to predict the individual prognosis, but also to make decisions for the best therapy.

3.2. Response Curves

If serial cancer marker measurements are available, this accumulated information can be used to assess the patient's risk. Serial measurements of a single marker may be thought of as forming a response curve to the disease process. Both the shape and size of such a response curve can give valuable information for outcome prediction. If the cumulative report consists of repeated measurements of several cancer markers then a "multivariate response curve" can be defined. The concepts of discriminant analysis may be extended to the study of multivariate response curves (Albert, 1983) that can be used to classify a given patient's response curve to the prognostic group it resembles most.

Thus, multivariate statistical techniques can be used to derive risk indices and predict outcomes of cancer patients from a set of cancer marker data. Cancer markers bringing none or repetitious information can be discarded and those related to outcome and providing jointly the best predictive efficiency can be selected on a statistically sound basis. However, many more studies are required for various markers and in a variety of tumors to establish any advantage of cancer markers in predicting recurrence over conventional diagnostic procedures and clinical examination.

4. Cancer Patient Monitoring

Cancer marker serial results represent a multivariate situation even when only one analyte is involved. The patient is building up a data base of results over time. Each new result will be interpreted by the physician in terms of its agreement or lack of agreement with the pattern of preceding results. Considering the time dimension in follow-up creates a problem to be solved by multivariate analysis. Consequently, dealing with several analytes on repeated occasions can lead to a complicated statistical problem.

4.1. Trend Analysis of Cancer Marker Data

The task of cancer patient management is still a difficult one, though particularly important for a successful outcome. Many cancer patients present a confusing picture for the physician who directs their follow-up care. Consequently, the physician is pressed hard to recall all of the diagnostically relevant information that is available from the laboratory.

To avoid offhand interpretations, predictions of tumor recurrence should be based on a statistically sound evaluation of the individual patient's own record of past cancer marker measurements, provided this record contains at least the minimum number of observations required to make such a prediction (Ladenson, 1975). For example, when the record consists of only one earlier cancer marker measurement, we shall have to utilize within-person variances obtained from a reference set of individuals in order to develop a statistical guideline for evaluating the second measurement.

Cancer marker estimates are derived from the initial values and applied to forecast future values by using autoregressive, moving average, random walk, or trend statistics (Albert and Harris,

1987). As more and more observations are made over time, each tested against its forecast range, the probability of finding a result outside its range by chance alone increases. Before concluding that the patient's state has been significantly altered, at least two successive test results should have the same trend. Winkel et al. (1982) have suggested in a pioneering study the use of two threshold upper limits at each sampling time. One is set relatively high so that a single outlier would not be falsely taken as an indication of cancer recurrence, the other is set much lower to trap series in which an actual recurrence had generated at least two consecutive or three nonconsecutive high values. The two threshold levels were calculated from simultaneous binomial probability equations.

4.2. Multivariate Time Series

The simultaneous assay of several cancer markers in monitoring therapy and in the detection of recurrent disease may offer the opportunity to find a significant change in one or more markers, thus overcoming their nonspecificity and insensitivity, and giving clinically useful lead times. When analyzing multiple serial data, there are four state probabilities at any given sampling time: (1) steady state, (2) change in level, (3) change in slope, and (4) outlier. These state probabilities, computed sequentially, are the primary output for clinical attention. Their computed values depend in part on arbitrary, but experience-based, numerical settings for the relative magnitudes of the variance terms under different possible states (Harris et al., 1980).

The detection of medically significant changes in a patient's condition by computerized monitoring of multiple laboratory parameters could be performed, e.g., by the multivariate first-order autoregressive time-series statistics (Harris et al., 1980; Harris and Yasaka, 1983). This multiparametric time-series analysis could be useful for an objective, computerized extraction of the clinically relevant information from serial laboratory data containing much more, but not relevant, information ("separation of signal and noise") in a number of applications:

1. Forecast of prognosis;
2. Estimation of remission or disease recurrence; and
3. Optimum therapy control in cancer patients.

However, multivariate time-series analysis with serial correlation among successive cancer marker measurements (the general autoregressive model or the nonstationary random walk model) is not only complicated mathematically but, in sequential mode, makes heavy demands on computer time. Therefore, it seems not yet practical for the clinical laboratory.

4.3. Missing Observations

The absence of data usually raises problems. As clinical data are collected, some patients will have incomplete records; sometimes data are missing or unusable, creating problems of computation, evaluation, and interpretation. Many statistical programs require complete sets of data in equal subclass sizes and eliminate any series with a missing value on any variable. In such cases, the data matrix may be updated by imputing single missing values by the methods decribed in some detail by Anderson (1946), Sokal and Rohlf (1981), Steel and Torrie (1981), and Yates (1933), respectively. Such an estimate of missing values obviously does not supply any additional information, but can only facilitate the analysis of the remaining data. However, this is a risky procedure, especially if a hypothesis is to be tested.

References

Albert, A. (1982), *Clin. Chem.* **28,** 1113–1119.
Albert, A. (1983), *Stat. Med.* **2,** 95–106.
Albert A. and E. K. Harris (1987), *Multivariate Interpretation of Clinical Laboratory Data,* Marcel Dekker, New York.
Anderson, J. A. and P. R. Philips (1981), *Appl. Statist.* **30,** 22–31.
Anderson, R. L. (1946), *Biomed. Bull.* **2,** 41–47.
Beck, J. R. (1982), *Clin. Lab. Med.* **2,** 751–777.
Beck, J. R. (1986), *Clin. Chem.* **32,** 1707–1713.
Bonfrer, J. M. G. (1990), *Tumor Biol.* **11,** 287–288.
Boyd, J. C. and D. A. Lacher (1982), *Clin. Chem.* **28,** 259–265.

Fineberg, H. V. (1980), *Bull. Cancer* **67,** 395–404.
Fisher, R. A. (1936), *Annals of Eugenics* **7,** 179–188.
Gerhardt, W. and H. Keller (1986), *Scand. J. Clin. Lab. Invest.* **46 (Suppl. 181),** 1–74.
Goldschmidt, H. M. J. (1987), *The Application of Multivariate Statistical Analysis in Clinical Chemistry and Haematology,* RBGG, Tilburg.
Harris, E. K., B. K. Cooil, G. Shakarji, and G. Z. Williams (1980), *Clin. Chem.* **26,** 383–391.
Harris, E. K. and T. Yasaka (1983), *Clin. Chem.* **29,** 25–30.
Ladenson, J. (1975), *Clin. Chem.* **21,** 1648–1653.
Malkin, A. (1982), First International Conference on Humor Tumor Markers, Munich.
Pauker, S. G. and J. P. Kassirer (1980), *N. Engl. J. Med.* **302,** 1109–1117.
Pohl, A. L., B. Worofka, R. Dudczak, and M. Schemper (1988), *J. Tumor Marker Oncology* **3,** 387–397.
Sell, S. (1990), *Clin. Lab. Med.* **10,** 1–37.
Sokal, R. R. and F. J. Rohlf (1981), *Biometry,* Freeman, New York.
Steel, R. G. D. and J. H. Torrie (1981), *Principles and Procedures of Statistics,* McGraw-Hill, Singapore.
Swets, J. A. (1979), *Invest. Radiol.* **14,** 109–121.
Uhr, L. (1963), *Psychol. Bull.* **60,** 40–73.
Van der Helm, H. J. and E. A. H. Hische (1979), *Clin. Chem.* **25,** 985–988.
Weinstein, M. C. (1981), *Med. Decision Making* **1,** 309–330.
Weinstein, M. C. and H. V. Fineberg (1980), *Clinical Decision Analysis,* Saunders, Philadelphia, pp. 12–36.
Winkel, P., M. W. Bentzon, B. E. Statland, H. Mouridsen, and O. Sheike (1982), *Clin. Chem.* **28,** 2057–2067.
Yates, F. (1933), *Empir. J. Exper. Agr.* **1,** 129–142.

Chapter 24

New Cancer Products

Predicting Market Success

N. Coleman Owen

1. Introduction

Worldwide markets for research-use and clinical immunodiagnostics (in vitro) utilized for cancer-patient testing will be approx $200 million (US dollars) in 1991 and are projected to exceed $500 million in 1996 (*see* Table 1). Today's commercial products for cancer testing consist, for the most part, of monoclonal-antibody-based reagents. Commercial DNA-probe products for cancer testing are just beginning to emerge. In vitro diagnostic cancer markets are growing at 20–25% annually and can be expected to continue to grow at this rate for at least the next five years. Even when the in vitro diagnostic product market for monoclonal-antibody-based cancer reagents exceeds $500 million in 1996, the emergence of an array of DNA-probe methods for cancer-patient testing will be just at the beginning of establishing a major clinical-laboratory market for DNA-probe cancer tests. In the years between 1995 and 2000, and beyond, these emerging DNA-probe products for testing of cancer patients will fuel the same dramatic percentage

From: *Serological Cancer Markers* Edited by Stewart Sell ©1992 The Humana Press, Totowa, NJ

Table 1
Immunodiagnostic Cancer Test Markets,
Estimated US Dollars in Millions[a]

Region	Market Size 1991	Market Size 1996
North America	$100	$220
Europe	80	220
Japan	40	100
Rest of world	10	30
Total	$230	$570

[a]Source: Fritzsche Pambianchi and Associates.

increases in annual growth of the commercial "in vitro diagnostic" cancer market that has been observed in recent years as a result of the emergence of monoclonal-antibody (MAb) reagents.

Cancer detection, diagnosis, patient staging, and monitoring are accomplished by the physician using a multiplicity of tools. The increasing value of in vitro diagnostic tests for use by the physician with cancer patients is attributable in large part to the availability of improved tests that use "biotechnology" reagents (i.e., monoclonal antibodies and DNA-probes) as components of the "cancer tests."

The ideal cancer test is one that would provide presymptomatic diagnosis for an otherwise undetectable cancer. The most critical element of improved survival for cancer patients is early diagnosis. The desire for early detection leads one immediately to the concept of a "universal" marker for cancers that can be detected in the blood or urine. Unfortunately, no such marker is known at this time. Many investigators now suspect that the growing knowledge of carcinogenesis, resulting in large part from our improving biotechnology laboratory reagents, suggests that the ideal cancer product may never be discovered, because no such single, universal cancer-screening marker may exist. If this is true, the medical community and the laboratory marketplace can expect to continue to see an array of discretely different new "cancer diagnostics" for use with specific cancers, introduced initially for research use only, with a very small percentage of tests eventually appearing as products for the clinical laboratory.

The number of new MAb reagents and DNA-probe reagents developed annually in universities, private research foundations, and commercial research and development programs has gone beyond realistic tracking or counting. Thousands of new antibodies and DNA-probes are developed annually as research tools, during investigations into the processes of carcinogenesis. Several hundred of these research tools show sufficient promise to the respective investigator that the antibody or probe is used to some extent in new or ongoing investigations in cancer research. Dozens and dozens of these research tools are exchanged among investigators and are used and cited in research publications. A smaller number of the more thoroughly developed research tools begin to show promise as potential clinical-laboratory reagents. At this point the research tool begins to be shared more widely among academic investigators and/or becomes available commercially as a "research use only" reagent. Later the reagent may become a true clinical-laboratory product, approved by the US Food and Drug Administration (and similar agencies in other countries) for the reporting of patient data to make clinical decisions.

Most entries into the in vitro diagnostic "cancer products" market will not achieve significant commercial success. An even larger number will not achieve the level of commercial success envisioned at the time of their respective introductions. How can one evaluate emerging cancer products, particularly MAb and DNA-probe reagents, with respect to their probable market acceptance? Are there some fundamental indicators (and comparators) to permit a knowledgeable estimate of the extent of potential commercial success for a new cancer test? Yes, we suggest that there are such indicators. Many different "market-success indicators" could be considered for an emerging, commercially sponsored laboratory product, not the least of which is the resource base of the commercial house introducing the product. Obviously, large, well-funded, and well-staffed companies are predictably better equipped for success than are small, emerging firms with no established sales organization or market position.

A primary objective of this chapter is not only to provide a perspective on the current size and projected growth rate for cancer-testing markets (Table 1), but, more important, to provide for the reader who is not in a commercial setting an approach to evaluating new and proposed market entries for both the probability of success and the extent and rate of the probable success.

The scientists who develop new cancer tests, and the business teams who commercialize the tests, often become so convinced of the new test's attributes that they may lack objectivity when predicting the extent and timing of the product's market success. Many cancer-test developers truly believe that their new test is, in reality, the broadly applicable, singularly available "cancer-screening test" that is sought as the ideal cancer-testing product. In the midst of typical, enthusiastic predictions by the developers of the new cancer test, how can one sort through the background noise to determine if, in fact, it may be a superior product? Basically, think like a cancer physician.

Cancer tests have several potential uses for the physician. Among these uses are the following: to screen asymptomatic patients; to screen a high-risk population; to confirm a clinical diagnosis; to "stage" a known cancer patient; and/or to monitor a cancer patient's response to therapy. Table 2 provides examples of in vitro diagnostic products used for these applications. MAb technology has provided significant new tools for the development of tests for certain of these applications, although the hope that this technology would deliver one or more "cancer-screening tests" for asymptomatic patients has not been realized. It is now thought by many investigators that developing a screening test was too optimistic a goal, at least for those antigen sources used in the 1980s. DNA-probes offer a similar promise for new cancer tests and for many people now represent what is thought to be the basis for tomorrow's ideal cancer test.

Table 2
Objective of an In Vitro Diagnostic Cancer Test[a]

Objective	Examples of laboratory tests
Screen asymptomatic patients	Fecal occult blood
Screen high-risk patients	Complete blood count (CBC)
	Pap smear
Confirm a suspected clinical diagnosis	CEA; PSA
	T- and B-cell testing
"Stage" a known cancer patient	Histology
	Immunohistochemistry
	Estrogen receptors
Monitor response to therapy	CEA; PSA
	CA 125
	T- and B-cell testing

[a]Source: Fritzsche Pambianchi and Associates.

1.1. World Market Opportunities

The total potential market size available for a new cancer test is determined by several factors. The patient pool available for a laboratory cancer test is related to the number of patients who develop a specific cancer each year (the incidence), the number of patients in a high-risk category (e.g., age, sex, known risk factors) who will be tested, and/or the number of patients with clinical symptoms of pathologies that are sufficiently similar to those of a particular cancer to require a differential diagnosis (e.g., benign vs malignant tumors). The patient pool for a cancer-patient-monitoring test is determined by the number of people who survive the cancer (prevalence) and who have undergone or are still undergoing treatment.

Figures 1 and 2 show the top eight cancers in terms of incidence or cancer deaths to emphasize that there are sometimes different opportunities for tests used for diagnosis than there are for tests used for monitoring cancer patients who are still alive. Uter-

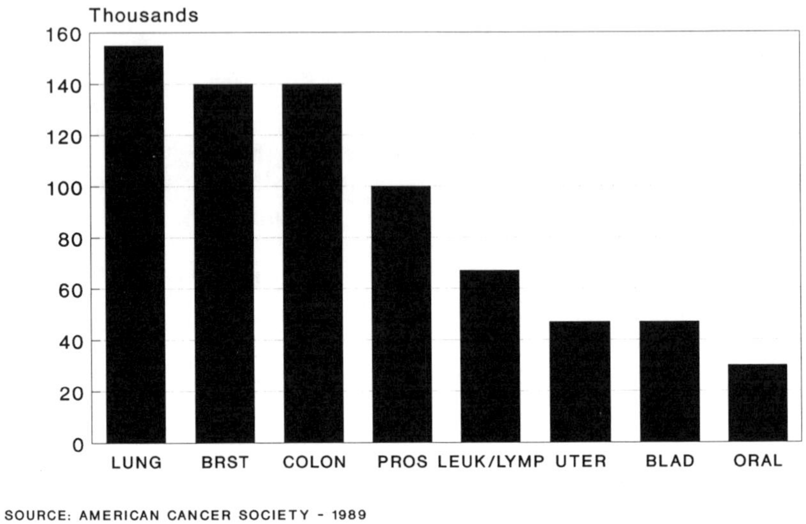

Fig. 1. Incidence of the top eight cancers (US only).

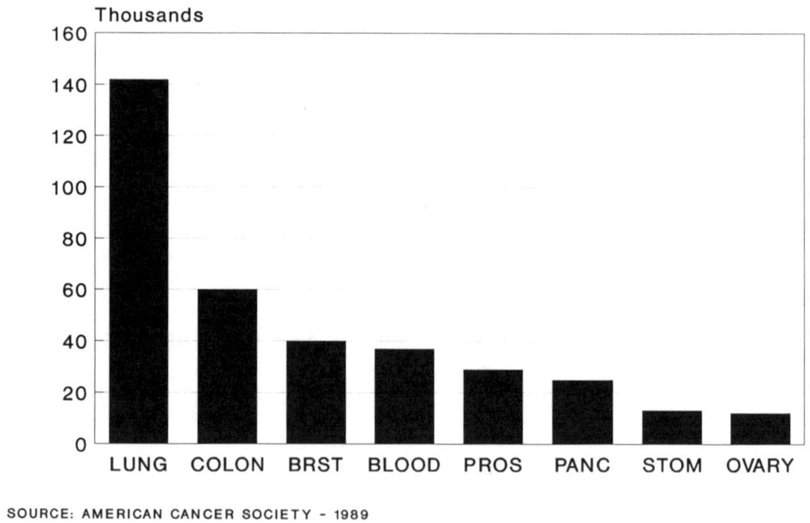

Fig. 2. Cancer deaths from the top eight cancers (US only).

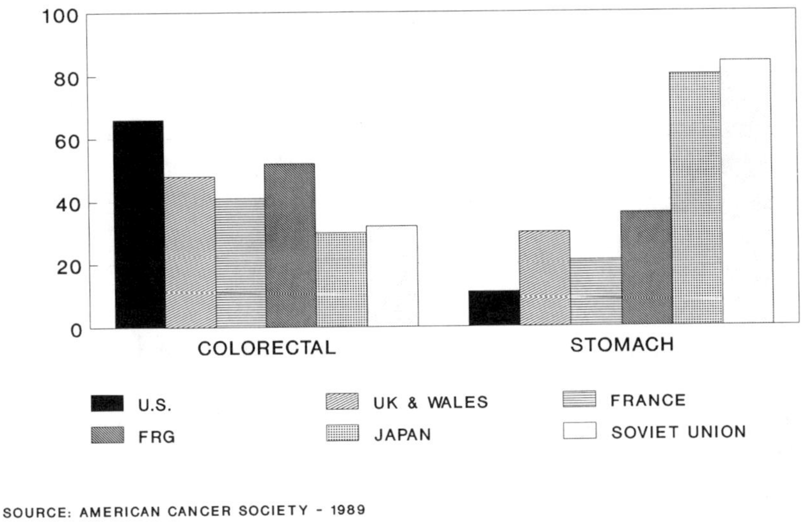

Fig. 3. Death rates for selected cancers (per 100,000 by country).

ine, bladder, and oral cancers show up in the "top eight" category based on cancer incidence, but pancreatic, stomach, and ovarian cancers are included in the "top eight" based on cancer deaths. There are also different market opportunities based on sex differences, with lung cancer the number-one killer in males, but breast cancer the number-one killer in females. Prostate cancer ranks number three in mortality for males (vs number five overall) and ovarian cancer is number five in females (vs number 13 overall). One needs to recall these basic facts regarding characteristics of incidence, prevalence, and high-risk categories as one reviews descriptions of the potential market opportunity for a new cancer test.

Analogous differences can be cited when incidence and mortality is tracked among the different races of the world. The opportunities for a new cancer test will differ among the US, Japan, and Europe because of differences in the types of cancers that predominate in each area (Fig. 3). Deaths (per capita) from certain cancers (i.e., colorectal) do not vary widely among the different countries.

Thus, the market opportunities for products for colorectal cancer are essentially consistent worldwide, based on population distribution and socioeconomic factors for the respective countries. In contrast, stomach cancer is a dominant cancer in Japan and the Soviet Union, but not in the US or Western Europe. Therefore, simple "rule-of-thumb" market-opportunity projections based solely on population data may be largely irrelevant for a particular cancer test. The adoption of Centocor's CA 19-9 as a frequently used test for stomach cancer in Japan, for instance, is best understood in context of these worldwide statistics. In the US CA 19-9 is used primarily as a marker for pancreatic cancer. One product may not enjoy equal success in the US, Japan, and Europe, or it may enjoy success in several countries, but for totally different reasons and with widely different market opportunities compared to total population statistics.

Lung cancer statistics emphasize interesting market differences. There are differences in incidence between the sexes, with deaths consistently higher among males than among females (Fig. 4). Differences such as these may also have an impact on the physician specialty initially seeing the high-risk patient category. Determining high-risk groups may determine which physician specialties are the most important to target for product introductions, for instance. Strength of distribution channels among general practitioners may be critical in the US, but access to gastroenterologists may be important in Japan for the same "cancer product" (e.g., CA 19-9).

Opportunity in the world market is now routinely considered by marketers of new laboratory diagnostic tests, just as they consider the world market for new pharmaceuticals. The costs of developing and obtaining regulatory approval for a new cancer-associated laboratory product are too great to think only in terms of the local market. However, as cancer products truly become more and more "specific" to a particular cancer, the impact of different worldwide rates of cancer incidence and prevalence must be considered as markets are projected. The rule of thumb for laboratory diagnostic reagents has, for several years, been that the US and Western Europe markets were essentially equal in size. Japan's laboratory-

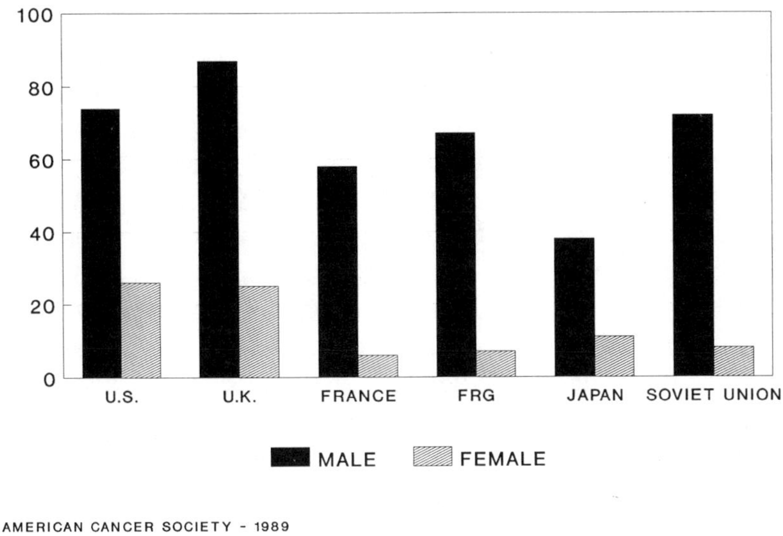

Fig. 4. Lung cancer (male vs female).

reagents market has been considered to be approx 50% of the size of either of the two other major world markets. The "rest-of-world" market has been considered to be about 10% of that of the more developed countries. This rule of thumb is no longer true, either generally speaking or particularly for cancer tests. Europe now frequently represents a larger market for a laboratory diagnostic reagent than does the US. This will more and more frequently be the case with the integration of Eastern Bloc countries into the new European Common Market. Based on the incidence of the subject cancer for a new cancer test of interest, Japan may be dramatically more important in considering total opportunities for the cancer test than its population statistics suggest. What has been acceptable in calculating glucose markets and typical "wet chemistry" markets is less and less reliable and certainly will not hold for specific cancer tests.

Despite the failure to date to deliver cancer screening tests, MAbs have had a significant impact in the past 10 years on the cancer-testing market because of the delivery of new (and improved) immunoassays for testing tumor-associated markers. The original tumor-associated-antigen immunoassay, a test for carcinoembryonic antigen (CEA), is now a "monoclonal" rather than a "polyclonal" reagent, at least as provided by most commercial suppliers. The tumor-associated markers introduced by Centocor Inc. (Malvern, PA), such as CA 19-9, CA 125, CA 15-3, and the company's array of other cancer-marker products, have been based on monoclonal reagents from the time the markers were defined. Approaches to the identification of intracellular markers that correlate to cancer, such as the approach of Matritech Inc. (Cambridge, MA), which is developing tests to detect components of the architectural framework of cells, such as the intermediate filaments of cell nuclei, may require the specificity of MAb technology to identify the target marker.

The MAb version of the first commercially significant test for prostate-specific antigen (PSA) was introduced by Hybritech Inc. (San Diego, CA). In less than two years it became number two in dollar volume among immunoassay cancer tests, measured in market sales. CEA remains the largest-selling single immunoassay product for cancer-patient testing.

Why has the PSA cancer test met with resounding commercial success, as have certain of the Centocor products, when so many new products have been unsuccessful? The remainder of this chapter describes some of the underlying causes of the observed differences in market acceptance and success, and is intended to assist the reader in identifying certain key aspects describing a new test that can be considered when estimating the probability of a test's commercial success and also when predicting the order of magnitude of the product's success.

1.2. Four Market-Success Indicators

As a preliminary assessment of the market potential for a new cancer test one can consider four parameters as key indicators. These indicators (*see* Table 3) are

1. The claims made for the product;
2. The regulatory strategy to be followed for product approval;

Table 3
Test Parameters and Their Impact on Evaluation[a]

Parameter	Impact
Claims for intended use	Determines market segment to be served; more important, is a "reality test" of the specified objectives for the test.
Regulatory classification	Defines the time-line to market availability and the extent of probable widespread use.
Format of test	Defines where the test can be used; the equipment required for use, e.g., gamma counters, luminometer, or NMR instrument; and the skill level of technicians required; defines the total number of immediately available market users.
Specimen required	Defines patient access and skill, expense, and trauma involved in acquiring the test specimen; e.g., urine specimen or tissue biopsy.

[a]Source: Fritzsche Pambianchi and Associates.

3. The test format to be offered; and
4. The test specimen required for the product.

This is a simplified description of the many parameters that might be evaluated to assess the market opportunities and probable success of a new product. Such issues as if the product is unique (i.e., patent-protected); the total number and relative strength of competitors; the channel of market distribution chosen; the pricing strategy; the differential utility of the new test compared to alternative, emerging, or existing in vitro diagnostic tests; and finally the resource base and extent of commitment of the commercial firm introducing the product will each affect both the rate of market penetration and the total market share achieved. Those qualifications noted, the objective of this chapter is to provide a perspective on four "common denominators" that will always be crucial to the potential initial market success of a new cancer product intended for the clinical laboratory.

1.2.1. Claims for Intended Use

As one considers the potential market response to a new in vitro test, the first criterion to investigate very critically is the claim for the intended use of the test. Table 2 lists potential claims and the intended use for a new cancer test. The potential claims cited are not comprehensive, but are only examples. The objective of the list is to remind the reader that no single immunodiagnostic test that is in routine use is intended for screening patients for cancer. Those laboratory tests that are used to "screen" asymptomatic patients for cancer (in the broadest sense of the term "screen"), such as the fecal occult blood test and Pap smear, are not based on either MAbs or DNA-probes. Further, at least in the opinion of the author, the US Food and Drug Administration or similar government agencies in other countries are not likely to approve, in the next five years, any immunodiagnostic tests (or DNA-probe tests) as "cancer-screening tests" for use with asymptomatic patients.

Every marker that, to date, has been approved by the FDA for clinical use is approved as a monitoring test or a confirmation test, not as a primary diagnostic test for symptomatic patients. That is, the tumor markers are used to predict the prognosis of a patient who has already been diagnosed with cancer, to confirm an already-suspected cancer, to monitor patients for the recurrence of metastatic disease, or to monitor the effects of therapy.

It is not likely that any of the currently available MAb or DNA-probe tests will be used as a primary diagnostic test, that is, to determine if an asymptomatic patient has a cancer. The available tests have finite, limited applications because the tests detect late-stage disease and are also not usually specific to only one tumor type. Until a marker can discriminate early-stage disease and until the marker is specific to one tumor type, it is unlikely that these markers will be useful as a primary clinical diagnostic tool.

With respect to claims for the intended use of a product, one can often predict the probable market success and physician acceptance of a new cancer test, based on consideration of the initial claims made in a company's early product literature and announcements. The more grandiose the claims and the broader and less distinct these claims are with respect to serving a particular subset of cancer patients, the more immediately suspect one should be about the probability of significant commercial success. Conversely, the more finite and limited the claims for the initial intended use of a product, regarding both its intended use (e.g., monitoring post-surgical metastatic colon cancer patients) and the specific patients to be served (e.g., differentiation between chronic myelogenous leukemia [CML] and acute lymphocytic leukemia [ALL]), the more immediately credible the test will be to the medical community. Ironically, not only do more finite claims often improve the product's immediate (though limited) market success, they also suggest greater potential for expanded future uses that are broader than the initial claims. The cancer test with very specific supporting data and claims actually stands a superior chance for serious investigation and adoption by the medical community for additional "off-label" applications (i.e., claims not made in the package insert or "directions for use") than does the cancer product that promises at the outset to be the ultimate cancer-screening test. The "off-label" applications are often for use with patients who, although not included in the original data, represent a logical extrapolation of these data to other patients (or cancers) by the respective patient-treating physician.

The reason for a greater probability of market success for the product with more limited claims is straightforward. A basic marketing fact that our firm continually emphasizes to our health-care-industry clients is that clinicians understand all too well that cancer is not a single disease. No single test is likely to be broadly applicable as a "screen" for an array of different cancers. The marketing emphasis to our industry clients is that with a new product they should always strive "to be something to somebody."

A product has a much better chance for commercial success if the developers have the courage to ignore the always-available, ever-expanding total world population of "potential cancer-test users," as counted by cancer incidence and prevalence data, and instead target very specifically a finite population of patients. The recommendation is to be of value to a finite patient group (i.e., differentiating CML from ALL), rather than to try to be everything to everyone (i.e., a "cancer-screening test"). Too often, however, "cancer" is discussed in reference to new commercial test opportunities just as it is in the lay press, that is, as if cancer were a single disease; this frequently results in an overstatement of commercial opportunities for a new cancer test, especially by entrepreneurs raising money for a new venture. The cancer statistics, usually taken from a credible source, such as the American Cancer Society (ACS) or the World Health Organization (WHO), are too often multiplied by a projected market penetration rate per year and by a proposed value (price) per test or per procedure, with the objective of yielding a projected total world-market opportunity in the next five or 10 years. Such grossly simplified descriptions of product opportunities and "cancer-market opportunities" are usually as misrepresentative of the realistic commercial potential for the particular proposed product as is a description of "cancer" as if it were a single disease.

A more complete description of the marketing recommendation made to our clients is always to strive "to be something to somebody; because if you try to be everything to everybody, you will end up being nothing to nobody" (pardon the grammar). In other words, the market will often ignore the product for which the broadest claims are made specifically because the claims are too broad or nebulous to establish interest for use with a *particular* patient category. Clinicians have learned that broad claims are often a clue to a paucity of hard data on specific cancer patients who will benefit from a new cancer test. A lack of data is, of course, a much more critical flaw to immediate market success than violating a marketing recommendation like the one mentioned.

As an example of the recommendation "to always be something to somebody," consider the opportunity for new leukemia tests.

Manufacturers often refer to the total "leukemia"-incidence figures from the American Cancer Society as the basis for projections of commercial opportunity for new leukemia tests. In fact, oncologists have become so skilled at differentiating among the multiple manifestations of "leukemia" that many oncology clinical services now have physicians on staff who specialize in patients with a particular *form* of T-cell leukemia, and the B-cell leukemias or the lymphomas are routinely segregated (clinically) from other leukemias. Yet all of these different forms of the blood-cell cancers may be grouped together in gross incidence/prevalence "leukemia" statistics and used to forecast "the market." A brief consideration of the clinical information known about a given cancer, such as differential diagnosis and management of the subject cancer in the context of the claims made for the new product, will provide the inquirer with significant perspective on how real the predicted market opportunity is with respect to what is estimated by the test's commercial backers.

1.2.2. Regulatory Strategy

Market opportunities for commercial in vitro cancer products should be considered with respect to the regulatory classification of a new product. Products may be introduced "for research use only," essentially with minimal supporting data and with no product "claims," or they may be introduced after acquisition of appropriate regulatory agency approvals for "in vitro diagnostic use." This is a very specific term indicating US FDA approval for use of the product to test patients and for clinicians to use the test results in decision making for the specific indications that are cited in the product's package insert or directions for use.

"Research use" products are not intended (or permitted) by a regulatory agency, such as the US FDA, to be used in making a clinical diagnosis. Third-party reimbursement from Medicare, Blue Cross, and private insurance firms is not usually provided for "research use only" products. This lack of reimbursement authorization limits the extent of commercial adoption by clinical laboratories.

Tests intended for use with cancer patients must undergo a relatively comprehensive regulatory review. In the US the process is referred to as a "pre-market-approval" (PMA) application to the FDA. The process of obtaining approval for a new cancer-patient test is significantly more comprehensive, time-consuming, and expensive than the simpler "510k" regulatory path by which a US manufacturer proves to the FDA that the proposed product is "substantially equivalent" in results to an existing, previously approved clinical laboratory test. The "510k" procedure requires 30 to 90 days after submission to obtain market clearance, and no formal clinical trials are required. The PMA requires at least six months (and two years is not unheard of) to obtain approval, and the PMA often includes the requirement for true prospective clinical trials. Even with submission of data from formal clinical trials there is no guarantee that regulatory approval for marketing for the proposed product claims will be granted.

Thus, the regulatory strategy for a new cancer test becomes another important element to consider with respect to a product's total market potential. Commercial tests for PSA offer a recent example of the impact that regulatory classification has on sales and market penetration. PSA immunoassay tests have been available for several years as "research use only" products. In 1987 they were generating less than $5 million annually in worldwide revenues. Upon achieving "in vitro diagnostic use" approval in the US (via the PMA process), the total annual revenues approached $20 million in 1989, the second year following receipt of such approval. Note that products measuring the same PSA marker had been available for approximately five years and had generated a sales volume cumulatively lower than the revenues achieved during the second year of "PMA approved" sales of a PSA product. Importantly, almost the complete increase in PSA sales revenues has been captured by the manufacturer of the single approved product (Hybritech Inc.). There has been no "carry-along effect" in the marketplace for the "research use only" PSA products that continue to be available, even though the research-use-only tests are available at a substantially lower price per test than the approved product.

The phenomenon to note is that a particular immunoassay (or DNA-probe) for cancer testing will be limited to relatively small worldwide revenues unless formal regulatory-agency approval is obtained. A few hundred research-use-only cancer-marker products are commercially available worldwide. The total annual sales for all such products probably do not exceed the annual revenues for the "approved" commercial cancer-marker products, CEA, PSA, and α-fetoprotein (AFP). (Note that certain immunoassay products, such as PAP and hCG, are also used for cancer-patient testing. However, these products originally received regulatory clearance based on the respective product's ability to measure the PAP or hCG molecules in the specimen, but were not approved for an intended use as a clinical indication of cancer. These markers are not discussed in detail because the focus of this chapter is on products that would enter the market as new indicators for cancer.)

Without a credible regulatory strategy and the necessary resources to obtain approval for clinical use, the emerging product, even if it offers value when used with cancer patients, will be subject to a fairly low limit on the potential market available. Most "research use only" reagents generate total annual revenues to the manufacturer of less than $10,000 (US dollars). A research-use-only product that achieves $100,000 in annual sales is extremely unusual. The total number of research-use-only commercial products that have achieved sustained annual sales of $1,000,000 is probably less than five or ten worldwide.

Contrast the dozens and dozens of research-use monoclonals and DNA-probes, each with annual sales of a few thousand dollars, and the tens of millions of dollars of annual sales for CEA, or the $20 million in sales achieved by PSA in its second full year after receiving regulatory approval. The importance of regulatory approval and its relationship to significant market penetration becomes evident.

1.2.3. Format of Test

Cancer tests are most often performed by skilled medical technologists in sophisticated clinical laboratories. As a result, a simple, rapid, convenient test is not a requirement for successful market penetration. If the clinical result has value and an innovator has the only test available, the medical community will adopt and utilize the test, obtain the required specimen, and deliver it to those few locations with the technical skill and capital equipment to deliver the test result.

When the second commercial test for the same marker becomes available, however (assuming that the second test demonstrates similar accuracy and other performance characteristics), the features of the test format, such as radioactive or nonradioactive label, time to result, instrumentation required, number of pipeting steps, calibration requirements, and other ease-of-use and economic issues (e.g., price of test, including technician time), become important factors of the market success.

The format determines in large part the location at which a test can be performed. Does it require the latest and most sophisticated model luminometer, for instance? Does the laboratory have to acquire new, specialized, proprietary instrumentation before the test can be added to its menu of offerings? Are special technician skills required, or must new licenses or administrative approvals be obtained by the laboratory in order to handle radioactive materials or other toxic substances in order to perform the test? To the extent that the inherent design of the test format bypasses these issues for the intended end users, the larger will be the base of immediate potential customers. If any laboratory that has an enzyme-linked immunosorbent assay (ELISA) plate reader can perform the new cancer test, for instance, then the number of immediate potential users is limited only by the current availability of such instruments and the total patient need.

Contrast a new cancer test offered in a conventional ELISA format and a new cancer test that requires a new, relatively expensive luminometer to obtain results. The rate of potential penetration for the latter test is limited not only by the requirement to educate the potential customer to the advantages of the new cancer marker, which may be a significant requirement in itself, but also by the time required to obtain agreement to acquire the new instru-

Table 4
Tumor-Marker Assays

Reagent	Assay	Advantage	Disadvantage
Antibody	RIA	High sensitivity	Short half-life Special handling Special disposal
Antibody	EIA (ELISA, EMIT, FIA)	High sensitivity Not a safety hazard	
Antibody	*In situ*	Permit direct correlation with histology	Frozen sections Tissue biopsy
Antibody	Flow cytometry	Rapid testing of large-volume blood cells	Specialized instrumentation
Antibody	Western blot	Specific and sensitive	Labor-intensive Difficult protocol
DNA probe	Southern blot	Specific	Labor-intensive Difficult protocol
DNA probe	*In situ*	Permits direct correlation with histology	Frozen sections Tissue biopsy
Hormone receptor	RIA; ELISA; *In situ*	High sensitivity Histology correlation (*in situ*)	Tissue biopsy

ment that is a precondition for using the new test. With the delivery of new, valuable clinical information, and with no competition from simpler methods to measure the same cancer marker, the format requiring the new instrument will be adopted. However, the format will not be successful at the same rate of immediate market penetration as a typical ELISA-format test, if other performance parameters are equal.

Table 4 lists formats of tests that are commonly used for tumor markers. Initially the radioimmunoassay (RIA) was the format used exclusively to test for CEA. The radioimmunoassay technique crossed over from use in the research laboratory to the clinical lab-oratory, and came into widespread use in clinical laboratories in the 1970s. Currently RIA has been replaced for many applications by a variety of enzyme immunoassays. The original innovator with a radioisotopic assay for CEA, Roche Diagnostics, has seen dramatic erosion of its former 100% share of the CEA market. In large part the erosion was the result of the introduction of a competitive CEA format, a nonradioisotopic ELISA introduced by Abbott Laboratories. Using enzymes as the signal molecule to detect the antibody marker offers considerable advantages for many laboratories when compared to the radioisotopically labeled product format. The radioactive products are considered an unnecessary health hazard by some laboratories, and the isotope requires administrative tracking and expensive disposal methods that are not required for enzyme-labeled assays.

Many of today's DNA-probe tests are carried out using the Southern blot technique, which is a labor-intensive molecular biology method that does not transfer easily to the clinical laboratory. Since molecular techniques have not been routinely used by the pathologist or clinical-laboratory specialist, manufacturers of commercial DNA-probes must educate these practitioners in techniques of molecular biology, along with providing new reagents to assure that accurate results are obtained. Several manufacturers have simplified the method to make it more adaptable to a clinical laboratory, but the first-generation Southern blot test format includes difficulties inherent in the format itself. An easier, more "fail-safe" format that delivers the same patient information would be of significant market interest.

An FDA-approved DNA-probe that is used as a clinical reagent is the human papilloma virus (HPV) probe, which is available in a Southern blot format and an *in situ* format. Two strains (of approx 60 known strains) of human papilloma virus (HPV 16 and HPV 18) are associated with genital warts in patients who develop cervical cancer. Two other strains of the virus (HPV 6 and HPV 11) are present in genital warts, but are not correlated to the development of cervical cancer. The correlation between HPV 16/18 and cervical cancer resulted in the introduction of this viral probe as a proposed adjunctive diagnostic test (with the Pap smear) for cervical cancer in asymptomatic women.

Although many university-based teaching and research hospitals have adopted the use of HPV testing, the general population of physicians remains on the sidelines, waiting for more correlative data to accumulate before they adopt or recommend HPV testing. To some extent the difficulty of initiating a routine clinical-laboratory method utilizing the current Southern blot format impedes adoption by community hospitals and smaller laboratories.

HPV testing with DNA-probes is also available as an *in situ* assay. The long-term objective of commercial suppliers for the product is for the test to be used along with each of the more than 30 million (US only) Pap smears done each year. Since the *in situ* test is currently restricted to use with fresh tissue sections, HPV testing is still fairly limited in scope. Manufacturers of the test are working on adapting the test format to permit its use with formalin-fixed specimens stored in paraffin blocks, so that archival material can be used to further validate the test accuracy retrospectively by correlating HPV data to cancer-patient data.

In situ testing for tumor markers is emerging as especially useful for diagnosing heterogeneous tumors. Abbott Diagnostics offers an ELISA kit as well as an *in situ* kit for estrogen-receptor (ER) testing of breast cancer patients. Since a breast cancer is a tumor that is made up of several cell types, such as connective tissue stroma and blood vessels as well as epithelial tumor cells, it is important to many physicians to know which cancer cells in the tissue sample correlate to the ER data. Using an ER result obtained from a homogeneous ELISA test specimen, it is possible that a negative result is a false negative if the tissue that was sampled did not contain many tumor cells, but a majority of stroma and blood-vessel cells, which would be expected to test negative for ER. A false negative result in cancer testing can be a life-threatening mistake. With an *in situ* analysis it is possible to identify the cell type that is ER-positive, so that an accurate diagnosis can be made. Here we have an example of a more procedurally cumbersome format (*in situ* vs ELISA) that offers important additional value to the clinician and is used in spite of the inconvenience.

The use of T- and B-cell antibody markers (which are approved as "research use only" products) to "diagnose" blood-cell cancers is almost routine at many large hospital centers, in spite of the requirement for expensive equipment to run the assays. This is an example of the only test available requiring a major commitment of capital for purchase of an instrument. The use of flow cytometry to assay for these markers has grown considerably since its introduction in the 1970s, and the use of the technique will continue to grow for the next several years. Eventually more-specific DNA-probes may displace antibody markers for leukemias and lymphomas. Already on the horizon and in research testing are DNA-probes for T- and B-cell receptors. These receptor probes potentially detect an earlier stage of the disease than can MAb cell-surface markers and therefore may differentiate between those T- and B-cells that are now perceived as "null" cells by the antibody markers. It is likely that, when reliable probes are available or an alternative test format to flow cytometry is designed, such competition will affect the flow-cytometry market.

Test format is, then, another parameter that should be considered and compared among potential new product offerings. Generally, for a new cancer test the format will be straightforward. A quantitative immunoassay using an ELISA format or fluorescent format will be most common in the next several years. Visual-end-point assays that do not require an instrument; "dipstick" assays and rapid-filtration-format immunoassays, such as those pioneered by Hybritech in its "ICON"™ products; and other new rapid, simple formats not yet commercially obtainable will eventually be available and will become important formats for cancer testing.

Test format becomes a very important determinant of the market-share performance of one test brand vs another when the same cancer marker is available from several suppliers. Format should always be carefully considered as an indication of market performance when multiple product offerings exist. If an initial format is somewhat different procedurally or technically demanding it may be acceptable. For future years, however, it is important to future market share that the manufacturer recognizes (with the initial product offered) the format problems and has a second-generation product format already in development.

1.2.4. Specimen Required

Integral to being able to access the market immediately with a new test is the test specimen required. Specimens required for cancer products may vary from truly noninvasive test samples, such as saliva or urine, which can be collected by the patient or a nonskilled technician, to commonly acquired specimens that employ invasive procedures, such as peripheral blood, tissue biopsy, bone-marrow aspirate, or cerebrospinal-fluid sampling. These later specimens may require a physician, surgeon, or uniquely skilled nurse or paramedical technician to obtain the specimen.

The willingness of a physician to use a test that provides additional information for cancer management will depend on the physician's consideration of not only the financial cost to the patient, but also the inconvenience and pain associated with obtaining the test specimen. Obviously, the greater the inconvenience and pain for the patient, the greater the probable diagnostic or prognostic benefit must be before the physician will order the test. Tests that can be carried out on a peripheral-blood specimen, urine, or other readily available body fluid will be adopted most rapidly and utilized most frequently in those situations in which the physician is not certain of the extent of the incremental value provided by the new test.

Future cancer tests, in the opinion of the author, will more and more frequently be based on specimens that are more difficult to obtain. Obtaining difficult specimens will not be a negative market factor as long as new, valuable information is provided that is not otherwise available. Tissue-biopsy specimens and bone-marrow aspirates will become the required specimen for many of tomorrow's most valuable cancer tests, particularly for MAb and DNA-probe *in situ* assays, when tests using these specimens can provide valuable staging and prognostic information along with and complementary to the data already obtained using traditional histology. The reader should be aware, however, of the differential value that is required from a test result requiring such specimens, before physicians will readily adopt such tests.

Data from emerging cancer products that propose to use a specimen obtained invasively should be compared with other clinical information that can be obtained using peripheral blood or other body fluids. The value of the new cancer test may very well justify the use of an invasive procedure (or the specimen may already be obtained invasively as a routine element of cancer management), but the product developer must not ignore the logistics of specimen access in the enthusiasm of defining the new marker at the molecular level.

1.3. Trends in Cancer-Testing-Product Technologies

Solution-phase specimens as the test specimen for cancer-marker immunoassays, such as CEA, PAP, AFP and hCG, have been dominant in market share ever since the immunoassay principle was widely applied to cancer-patient testing. Classic histological studies and recognition that many (indeed, most) solid tumors are heterogeneous in their tissue type are factors stimulating increased interest in the *in situ* assay as an important adjunct to the histological sample. The tumor-marker antibody or DNA-probe that is linked to a signal molecule, such as a radiolabel, or to an enzyme, such as horseradish peroxidase, represents a refinement in histological staining and adds another dimension of specificity not available with traditional stains, such as hematoxylin and eosin or Wright's stain. The added information represents added value to the physician in terms of diagnosing and treating the patient. Major market opportunities will be generated in cancer testing using both antibody and DNA-probe *in situ* methods in coming years.

In an effort to increase the specificity of cancer markers there will be an eventual displacement of many MAbs by DNA-probes for certain clinical-laboratory applications in cancer testing, since

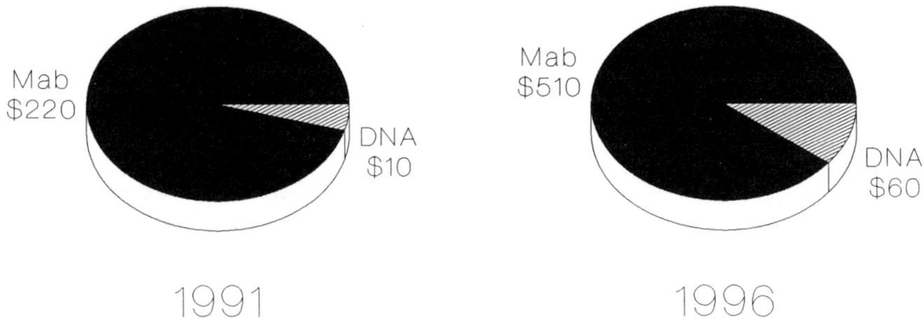
Mab
$220
DNA
$10
1991
Mab
$510
DNA
$60
1996

Fig. 5. Cancer markets by method (dollar amounts in millions).

these genetically based probes are capable of detecting the early and causal events of carcinogenesis. This displacement is not, however, anticipated to have any significant impact on the clinical-laboratory market within the next five years. The use of DNA-probes in research-use applications, in contrast, is already well established. The study of oncogenes with DNA-probes has provided a dramatic new method for studying the causal basis of carcinogenesis.

Figure 5 shows the current (1990) and projected (1995) markets for both MAbs and DNA-probes. MAb diagnostic products for cancers total about $200 million and should exceed $500 million in five years. The clinical-laboratory market for DNA-probes for cancer testing is less than $10 million and growth for clinical tests is not expected to achieve more than $50–75 million by 1995. New cancer tests based on DNA-probes can be expected, however, to develop into major new markets by the year 2000 and beyond.

In some cases new and emerging MAbs to oncoproteins will be even more specific and more useful than DNA-probes as diagnostic laboratory tools for specific cancers. For example, the *bcr/abl* probe detects both ALL and CML, but the MAbs to the gene products, which are fusion proteins expressed by the *bcr* and the *abl* genes, can be used to distinguish between ALL and CML. Since the two fusion proteins differ in molecular weight, these proteins potentially permit a differential diagnosis between the two diseases. The *bcr* DNA-probe will identify 98% of CML patients, but only

50% of ALL patients. The *bcr/abl* fusion protein in ALL patients has a mol wt of 190; the same gene's fusion protein in CML patients has a mol wt of 210, thereby making it possible to distinguish ALL from CML by using MAbs to the two fusion proteins.

Many comments are made that DNA-probes will eventually displace MAb reagents as the reagents of choice for cancer-patient testing. The reader should note, however, that the prior example, differentiating ALL and CML patients, suggests a situation for cancer-patient testing that may apply to other cancers. DNA-probes may be used to show that a gene is present in a particular cancer, to indicate that a gene is absent (anti-oncogenes), or to indicate that a gene is amplified. In some cases, however, when there are no differences detected at the gene level, a MAb to the oncogene protein product(s) may become the basis of a useful test. An oncogene product may be easier to detect, and it may be of as great (or greater) clinical value as is information on the gene itself. Be cautious about early reports of the demise of MAbs for cancer testing because of the emergence of DNA-probes. DNA-probes may, in the process of generating huge new markets for DNA-probes for cancer testing, also define significant new market opportunities for MAb reagents that detect oncoproteins.

Monoclonal antibodies as reagents used with solution-phase specimens for immunoassays and for *in situ* tests for immunohistochemistry have become routine as adjunctive tools in determining the prognosis of cancer patients. ER (and progesterone[PgR]) assays, for instance, are now used routinely for patients who have undergone a mastectomy for breast cancer. In addition to a histological examination of a lymph-node biopsy to determine if a patient's tumor is metastatic, the breast tumor itself is examined for the presence of ERs. If the tissue is ER-positive, the first choice of therapy is hormonal. If endocrine hormone therapy fails, chemotherapy is necessary.

An emerging DNA-probe that has been studied in early clinical trials is the DNA-probe to the oncogene *Her-2-neu*. *Her-2-neu* is the name given by Genentech Inc. (South San Francisco, CA) to the probe that identifies the oncogene initially named by different investigators as *erb-B*, *neu*, and *Her-1*, each of which represent the same gene. Dennis Slamon (UCLA) used the *Her-2-neu* probe to confirm that this oncogene was present in the breast tumors of lymph-node-negative breast cancer patients. The presence of *Her-2-neu* correlated to a poor patient prognosis. In terms of therapy, when the *Her-2-neu* oncogene is detected, Slamon's results suggest that aggressive chemotherapy should be administered. Based on data to date, breast cancer patients that are *Her-2-neu*-negative do not need to undergo the aggressive, debilitating, and often life-threatening side effects of chemotherapy. Although still a research-use-only tool, some clinical laboratories are already offering the *Her-2-neu* test to their clients. If regulatory approval is sought (and obtained) for use of this DNA probe as an in vitro diagnostic product, the market for this probe can be predicted to expand manyfold.

This potential *Her-2-neu* product provides an example of a product that provides additional value to a finite patient group. The innovator that introduces the test with proper regulatory approval can anticipate rapid adoption and market development, even with the requirement for a biopsy specimen and an *in situ* method that may be procedurally difficult. New data of clinical value would offset these problems. The innovator would need to be aware, however, of the need to simplify the method and make as "user-friendly" as possible, especially as the second supplier aproached market entry.

In the future DNA-probes will have a significant impact as laboratory tools for cancer diagnosis and management. The probes will be used for both identification and determination of the tumor's genetic makeup, and will also test for the presence of viral pathogens associated with a particular cancer type. For example, a cancer-associated DNA-probe that is already commercially available is used to test for the presence of the human papilloma virus (HPV).

The long-term trend in clinical diagnosis and monitoring is toward more-specific markers. Enzymes and hormones as markers for cancer-patient use have been displaced in large part by immuno-assays for the respective enzymes or hormones and by MAbs to new markers. Eventually many of the monoclonal cancer markers will be displaced by DNA-probes that are even more specific. To the extent that existing MAb cancer tests are to be displaced, the impact of DNA-probes on the monoclonal-reagent market is not expected to be seen for at least five years. Very few DNA-probes have been studied to date in the formal clinical trials that are required for an assay to become an accepted, FDA-approved clinical assay.

2. Summary

The research tools that are the basis for new commercial clinical-laboratory cancer products are primarily MAbs, with DNA-probes just beginning to emerge. Thousands of new potential product reagents are discovered annually in various university, private research foundation, and commercial laboratories. A small percentage of the discoveries, totaling about 100 annually, become visible as research-use-only commercial products for further investigation. Only a handful of these new research products introduced annually will be pursued to the point of development of a product for the clinical laboratory for use in patient diagnosis and/or disease management.

Many factors can be considered with respect to predicting the probable market success of a late-stage research-use-only product or soon-to-be-introduced clinical-laboratory product. Four "common denominator" parameters that provide perspective on both the probable rate of acceptance of a new cancer product and the extent of total market penetration are important among the many parameters that can be analyzed. These parameters are the initial claims proposed for use of the product; the regulatory status and strategy for the product; the format chosen for the test method; and the test specimen required. These parameters, when considered both independently and with respect to other cancer tests, provide a very functional way to preliminarily analyze and assess market opportunities and projections for an emerging cancer test.

These parameters should be considered with respect to a commercial product in the broader context of awareness that cancer is not a single disease. A close look at product claims that intuitively imply that cancer is a single disease entity, test formats that ignore the existing infrastructure of laboratory resources, and test specimens that are inconsistent with current cancer-management practices can be very illuminating with respect to estimating the realistic market opportunity. Finally, review and critical assessment of regulatory strategy and planning can provide significant insight into the total market opportunity.

Consideration of these four parameters, long before one has to sort out the arguments about the merits of one MAb vs another, can predict more clearly the opportunity for a particular product.

Chapter 25

Comments

J. V. Klavins

The term "tumor markers" emerged recently to define substances that are produced by tumor cells in larger quantities than, or uniquely when compared with, nontransformed cells. This definition serves practical clinical application, as is evident in this book. The term "tumor markers" can be defined still more narrowly as substances that can be measured in body fluids to monitor the course of the disease. Although interest in such markers is recent, more than 150 years ago there was already a marker: Bence Jones protein for multiple myeloma.

To some extent such tumor markers can be used in the prognosis, and only occasionally, for the diagnosis. For example, α-fetoprotein and human chorionic grandrotropin in a patient with suspected germ-cell neoplasm would indicate tumor-containing yolk sac and trophoblast-like cells.

The exceptions to this narrower definition are the chromosome studies, and cytoskeletal and, more recently, oncogenic investigations. The nature of these markers, which are not circulating in body fluids, but are present in the cells, is still the most important indicator of a neoplasm.

From: *Serological Cancer Markers* Edited by Stewart Sell ©1992 The Humana Press, Totowa, NJ

For more than a century, efforts have been exerted to find markers that are specific or unique for malignant neoplasms. So far, the only identified specific marker of clinical interest is the idiotype of the B-cell lymphoma. Antiidiotype antibodies have been tested in the treatment of patients with this disease.

The search continues for specific markers. They would be applied in diagnosis and screening for malignant neoplasms. Presence or absence of a specific marker would indicate the effect of therapy. Furthermore, various chemotherapeutic agents and radiation could be specifically targeted to tumor cells without affecting normal tissues.

The other kinds of markers are oncofetal and tumor-associated. The oncofetal markers are gene products expressed during embryonic development and by malignant neoplasms. Examples of this kind of marker are α-fetoprotein and carcinoembryonic antigen.

Historically, the relationship of embryonic tissues to malignant neoplasms was observed and reported for the first time by Durante, more than 100 years ago. Thus Durante, a few years before Cohnheim, was the proponent of the embryonic theory of cancer; not Cohnheim, as frequently has been mentioned in medical history. Durante postulated his theory on the basis of morphological similarities, but now we find that there is also a biochemical similarity among embryonic and tumor cells.

The tumor-associated markers are substances produced by differentiated cells. They are produced in much larger quantities by tumor cells than by differentiated normal cells. An example of a tumor-associated marker is serum calcitonin. In the serum of patients with medullary carcinoma of thyroid, calcitonin is significantly elevated compared with normal levels.

All such presently available markers are useful in following up patients with the disease to evaluate the effect of the therapy and imminent recurrence. Because of their nonspecific nature, these markers cannot be utilized in diagnosis, with just a few exceptions. They cannot be used for screening purposes. It could be possible to set up a screening system with multiple markers. However, there would still be some neoplasms that would escape this system by not producing sufficently high levels of a marker. In addition, such a system—use of a panel of different markers—would be economically prohibitive. The cost of tumor-marker analysis is considerably higher than that of other clinical biochemistry tests.

All tumor markers can be classified as universal and limited-distribution. The universal markers are those like carcinoembryonic antigen, produced by different kinds of malignant neoplasms. A marker with limited distribution is produced by only a certain type or a related group of neoplasms, e.g., calcitonin produced by medullary carcinoma of thyroid.

An ideal tumor marker would be a universal specific marker. Such a marker may not exist. Even circulating specific markers with limited distribution (except antiidiotype antibody to B-cell lymphoma) have not been detected.

Yet there is ample opportunity to investigate the existence of undetected oncofetal markers. There may exist oncofetal gene products in the earliest stages of embryonic development, which may be related more to transformed cells than to normal undifferentiated cells. The efforts in diagnosis, for example, determining the localization of metastases and treatment with labeled chemotherapeutic agents or radionuclides, could be greatly facilitated by such markers.

It is conceivable that methodologies using radionuclide-labeled monoclonal antibodies to such markers could be developed to discriminate between small foci of the tumor and nonspecific or specific binding in small quantities to otherwise normal cells. It may also be possible, by the use of monoclonal antibodies, to direct the chemotherapeutic agents more selectively to tumors with oncofetal markers than is being done now by subjecting all cells equally to these substances.

The disadvantage of using presently available oncofetal markers in diagnosis and therapy is their presence in appreciable amount in normal, basal, undifferentiated cells in many tissues, e.g., basal cells of mucosa, bone marrow, and lymphatic tissues.

It can be expected that more markers will be detected that are expressed in most of the earliest stages of embryonic development and by tumors, but to a lesser extent or not in detectable amounts by normal, undifferentiated cells. Such oncofetal markers would exhibit greater specificity than those that are available at the present time.

In my view this volume is a very important, stimulating factor for future research as well as clinical application of tumor markers.

References

Bence Jones, H. (1847), *Lancet* **2,** 88–92.
Durante, F. (1874), *Arch di Mem de Osservaz. di Chirurg. Pract.* **11,** 217–226.

Index